AF575246

Infections in Hematology

Georg Maschmeyer • Kenneth V.I. Rolston
Editors

Infections in Hematology

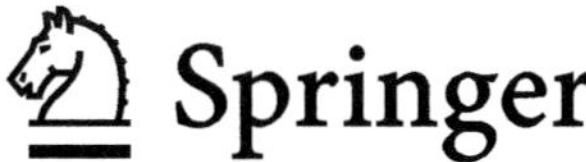

Editors
Georg Maschmeyer
Department of Hematology
Oncology and Palliative Care
Klinikum Ernst von Bergmann
Potsdam
Germany

Kenneth V.I. Rolston
Department of Infectious Diseases
Infection Control and Employee Health
The University of Texas
M.D. Anderson Cancer Center
Houston, TX
USA

ISBN 978-3-662-43999-9 ISBN 978-3-662-44000-1 (eBook)
DOI 10.1007/978-3-662-44000-1
Springer Heidelberg New York Dordrecht London

Library of Congress Control Number: 2014956548

Printed on acid-free paper

Springer is part of Springer Science+Business Media (www.springer.com)

Introduction

Despite substantial advances in supportive care, infections remain the leading cause of morbidity and mortality in patients with hematologic malignancies and in hematopoietic stem cell transplant(HSCT) recipients. The etiology of infection in this patient population continues to evolve, especially with the development of new immunomodulatory therapies, which produce profound and prolonged immunosuppression and are associated with a wide array of pathogens. The widespread use of antimicrobial therapy for various indications (prophylaxis, empiric and/or preemptive therapy, specific or targeted therapy, and suppressive therapy) has to some extent led to the emergence of multidrug-resistant pathogens producing newer diagnostic and therapeutic challenges. These challenges are compounded by the relative paucity of novel antimicrobial agents being developed to combat resistant pathogens and have led to the revival of some older antimicrobial agents. Our objective for this textbook was to provide updated information regarding all aspects of the management of infections in this high-risk patient population. This information is presented in five distinct sections of the textbook, each section dealing with a specific and unique aspect.

Part I describes the current epidemiology of infections, with particular focus on infections associated with relatively newer therapeutic modalities (e.g., monoclonal antibodies, nucleoside analogues) and on infections seen in various patient subgroups (e.g. acute leukemias, malignant lymphomas, HSCT recipients). Part II features discussions about risk stratification in febrile neutropenic patients and the diagnostic approaches currently employed in such patients in order to arrive at a specific diagnosis as promptly as possible. Part III covers the various therapeutic strategies in febrile neutropenic patients including those with fever of unknown origin and specific sites of infection (e.g., pulmonary, central venous catheter associated, gastrointestinal, and central nervous system infections). Antimicrobial therapy including important pitfalls, toxicities, and interactions is covered in Part IV. Part V provides information on various aspects of infection prevention, an area which is of increasing importance in the current era of multidrug-resistant pathogens.

It is our sincere hope that this textbook will be of use to all those who take care of patients with hematologic malignancies and HSCT recipients. We wish to thank all the authors who have so generously given their time and expertise toward the completion of this volume, and we dedicate it to our patients, who continue to provide us with the incentive and inspiration to seek new knowledge on a daily basis.

Potsdam, Germany — Georg Maschmeyer
Houston, TX, USA — Kenneth V.I. Rolston

Contents

Part I

Epidemiology: Infections in Patients with Hematologic Malignancies

Infections in Patients with Acute Leukemia

1

Kenneth V.I. Rolston

Contents

1.1 Introduction

Patients with acute leukemia are at increased risk of developing infections both as a result of the leukemia and its treatment [1]. Neutropenia is the primary risk factor associated with the development of infection, with the severity and frequency of infection increasing as the absolute neutrophil count drops below 500 cells/mm^3, as initially described by Bodey and colleagues [2]. Other risk factors may be present including impaired cellular or humoral immunity, breakdown of normal barriers such as the skin and mucosal surfaces, and vascular access catheters and other

K.V.I. Rolston
Department of Infectious Diseases, Infection Control and Employee Health, The University of Texas, M.D. Anderson Cancer Center, Houston, TX, USA
e-mail: krolston@mdanderson.org

G. Maschmeyer, K.V.I. Rolston (eds.), *Infections in Hematology*,
DOI 10.1007/978-3-662-44000-1_1

foreign medical devices. Multiple risk factors are often present in the same patient. Additionally, the frequent use of antimicrobial agents for various indications (prophylaxis, empiric therapy, pre-emptive administration, specific or targeted therapy, and occasionally maintenance or suppressive therapy) has an impact on the nature and spectrum of infections, with the emergence/selection of multidrug-resistant (MDR) organisms being of particular concern [3–7]. Bacterial infections tend to occur early on in a neutropenic episode, with fungal infections being uncommon at this stage. If neutropenia persists, the risk for fungal infections increases. There are periodic changes in the epidemiology/spectrum of infection in patients with leukemia. It is important to conduct periodic epidemiologic and susceptibility/resistance surveys, especially at institutions dealing with large numbers of such patients, in order to detect these shifts and changes in susceptibility/resistance patterns, since empiric therapy is largely based on this information [8, 9]. Such surveys are conducted every 3–5 years at our institution.

Fever (defined by the Infectious Diseases Society of America as a single oral temperature of 38.3 °C (101 °F) or a temperature of >38.0 °C (100.4 °F) sustained over a 1 h period) is the most consistent sign of infection and occurs with or without focal signs or symptoms [10]. Greater than 90 % of episodes of fever in neutropenic patients with acute leukemia are likely to be caused by an infection. Noninfectious causes include drug fever, fever related to the underlying malignancy, transfusion reactions, or allergic reactions. This chapter will focus on the current epidemiology of infections in patients with acute leukemias. Infections that occur in patients with malignant lymphomas and those that occur as a consequence of treatment with specific modalities (e.g., monoclonal antibodies and nucleoside analogs) will be dealt with separately.

1.2 Nature of Febrile Episodes

Febrile episodes in neutropenic patients have been classified into three distinct categories:

- Clinically documented infections (presence of clinical or radiographic features of infection such as cellulitis or pneumonia, without microbiologic confirmation)
- Microbiologically documented infections (positive cultures from any significant site)
- Unexplained fever – formerly fever of unexplained origin (FUO) – (fever, but no positive cultures or clinical/radiographic features of infection)

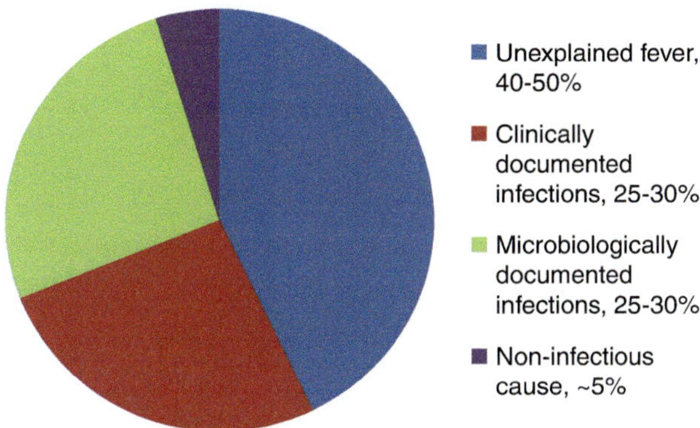

Fig. 1.1 Nature of febrile episodes in neutropenic patients

1.3 Clinically Documented Infections

Clinically documented infections account for 25–30 % of febrile episodes in neutropenic patients (Fig. 1.1). They are defined by the presence of a site suggestive of an infection such as cellulitis, pneumonia, esophagitis, or enterocolitis, without microbiological documentation of the causative pathogen for the infection. This may be due to various reasons including the use of antimicrobial prophylaxis, which can render microbiologic cultures negative and/or a blunted inflammatory response resulting in lack of specimens (e.g., sputum) to culture. The vast majority of these episodes respond to empiric antimicrobial therapy, providing indirect evidence that they are due to an infectious process.

1.4 Microbiologically Documented Infections

Microbiologically documented infections also account for 25–30 % of febrile episodes in neutropenic patients (Fig. 1.1). The majority of these are monomicrobial (i.e., caused by a single pathogen), but polymicrobial infections are being documented with increasing frequency. Recent data show that ~15–25 % of bacteremias in neutropenic patients, including catheter-related infections, are polymicrobial [11–13]. Infections involving deep tissue sites are predominantly polymicrobial [14]. These include neutropenic enterocolitis, perirectal infections, complicated skin/skin structure infections, and pneumonia. The majority of polymicrobial infections are caused by multiple bacterial pathogens (gram-positive, gram-negative, and occasionally anaerobic organisms) although bacterial and fungal or bacterial and viral infections can also co-exist.

Table 1.1 Common sites of infection in patients with acute leukemia

Site of infection[a]	Frequency (%)
Respiratory tract[b]	30–40
Bloodstream[c]	15–20
Urinary tract	10–15
Skin and skin structure	8–10
Intestinal tract[d]	5–8
Other sites[e]	10–15

[a]Approximately 15–20 % of patients will have multiple sites of infection (data from survey conducted at MD Anderson Cancer Center – 2012)
[b]Includes paranasal sinuses, upper respiratory tract, lungs, and infections such as empyema
[c]Includes primary and catheter-related bacteremia
[d]Includes neutropenic enterocolitis, perianal infections, cholangitis
[e]Includes meningitis, brain abscess, septic arthritis, and other uncommon sites

1.5 Sites of Infection

The most common and important sites of infection in patients with acute leukemia are listed in Table 1.1. Overall, the respiratory tract is the most common site of infection. Approximately 25 % of patients with acute leukemia will develop a pulmonary infiltrate during an episode of neutropenia lasting 10 days or longer. Other parts of the respiratory tract including the oropharynx, upper airways, and the paranasal sinuses are also frequent sites of infection. Most pulmonary infiltrates are secondary to an infectious process (bacterial and fungal organisms predominate) although it is often quite difficult to establish a specific microbiologic diagnosis. Noninfectious causes of pulmonary infiltrates such as alveolar hemorrhage and drug toxicity are much less common. Consequently, empiric therapy directed against anticipated pathogens is generally administered in such patients and can be modified if confirmatory microbiologic data become available. The management of patients with pulmonary infections/complications is discussed in detail else where. Approximately 15–20 % of patients with acute leukemia and neutropenia will develop a bloodstream infection. These include primary bacteremias and central line-associated infections. Gram-positive bacteria are isolated most often (~75–80 % of the time) with organisms colonizing the skin (e.g., *Staphylococcus* species, *Bacillus* species, *Corynebacterium* species) being predominant [13–16]. In patients with oral or intestinal mucositis, viridans group streptococci (VGS), enterococci (including VRE), and enteric gram-negative organisms are common pathogens [17, 18]. The frequency of gram-negative bacteremia is lower in patients receiving antibacterial prophylaxis with agents such as the fluoroquinolones, than in patients not receiving prophylaxis [19, 20]. Fungemias occur ~4–6 % of the time, are caused most often by *Candida* species, and are often associated with indwelling central venous catheters [21–24]. With the exception of *Fusarium* species, invasive mold infections seldom cause fungemia [25, 26]. A small proportion of bacteremic infections are caused by nontuberculous mycobacteria [27].

Urinary tract infections are documented in 10–15 % of patients with acute leukemia, especially in patients requiring the placement of short-term or long-term urinary drainage catheters. Gram-negative bacterial pathogens such as *Escherichia coli* predominate although *Candida* species are not uncommon in patients with urinary catheters, stents, or other devices and in those that have received multiple courses of broad-spectrum antibacterial therapy for previous episode of neutropenic fever.

Common skin and skin structure infections include cellulitis, infections at phlebotomy or other puncture wounds, and surgical site infections in patients who have undergone recent surgery. Uncommon, but more serious infections include pyomyositis (occasionally caused by *E. coli*) and necrotizing fasciitis [28]. These conditions usually require surgical intervention in addition to antimicrobial therapy. Even less common are primary cutaneous mold infections [29, 30].

Infections along the gastrointestinal tract are not uncommon. Prior to the frequent use of antifungal prophylaxis, thrush and esophagitis caused mainly by *Candida* species (occasionally by herpes viruses) were commonplace. Azole and echinocandin prophylaxis has rendered these infections largely of historical interest. Neutropenic enterocolitis (typhlitis) occurs primarily in patients with acute leukemia who receive therapy with agents (e.g., cytosine arabinoside, in combination with idarubicin or another anthracycline) that cause high-grade intestinal mucositis although it is being described with increasing frequency in patients receiving other mucotoxic antineoplastic agents such as the taxanes and vinorelbine [31–33]. Perirectal infections occur more often in patients with preexisting local lesions such as fissures and hemorrhoids [34]. True abscess formation is uncommon in patients with severe and prolonged neutropenia, but surgical drainage is almost always beneficial [35, 36].

1.6 Spectrum of Bacterial Infection

Recent epidemiologic data document a predominance of gram-positive pathogens from microbiologically documented infections [13–16]. Unfortunately, these data focus on monomicrobial bacteremic infections, and do not provide details from most other sites of infection, or from polymicrobial infections. This gives an incomplete and skewed view about the microbiology of these infections since bacteremias are caused most often by gram-positive organisms that colonize the skin, whereas infections at most other sites (lung, intestinal tract, urinary tract) have a predominance of gram-negative pathogens [14]. Additionally ~80 % of polymicrobial infections have a gram-negative component, and ~33 % are caused by multiple gram-negative species [11]. When all sites of infection and polymicrobial infections are taken into consideration, a substantially different picture emerges, with gram-negative pathogens being almost as frequent as gram-positive pathogens [14]. Indeed, some institutions are now reporting a predominance of gram-negative

Table 1.2 Microorganisms isolated most often from neutropenic patients

Gram positive
Coagulase-negative staphylococci
Staphylococcus aureus (including MRSA)
Viridans group streptococci
Enterococcus species (including VRE)
Corynebacterium species
Beta-hemolytic streptococci (groups A, B, G, and F)
Stomatococcus mucilaginosus
Gram negative
Escherichia coli
Klebsiella species
Pseudomonas aeruginosa
Enterobacter species
Stenotrophomonas maltophilia
Other Enterobacteriaceae
Other non-fermentative gram-negative bacteria
Fungal
Candida species
Aspergillus species
Zygomycetes
Fusarium species
Viral
Herpes simplex virus and varicella zoster virus (reactivation)
Community respiratory viruses

pathogens [37]. Knowledge of local epidemiologic patterns is critical as empiric regimens need to be designed with this information in mind.

1.6.1 Gram-Positive Organisms

The microorganisms isolated most often from neutropenic patients are listed in Table 1.2. The most commonly isolated organisms isolated overall are the coagulase-negative staphylococci (CoNS) [38]. These organisms are generally of low virulence and seldom cause serious or life-threatening infections. Catheter-related bacteremias are the most common infections caused by CoNS. These can often be treated with antimicrobial agents without removal of the offending catheter, although some infections may recur if the catheter is retained [39]. The one exception is *Staphylococcus lugdunensis*, which resembles *S. aureus* in virulence, and infections caused by this species need to be managed like those caused by *S. aureus* [40–42]. Other gram-positive organisms that frequently colonize human skin and often cause infections in patients with leukemia include *Bacillus* species, *Corynebacterium* species, and *Micrococcus* species [43–49]. Like CoNS, the most common infection caused by these organisms is catheter-related bacteremia. Occasionally more serious infections such as pneumonia, endocarditis, endophthalmitis, and meningitis develop. The organisms are uniformly susceptible to vancomycin, linezolid, and daptomycin, whereas susceptibility to other agents is variable. Most patients respond to appropriate antimicrobial therapy, and infection-related mortality is low. It is not clear whether removal of the infected catheter is always necessary for response; however, recurrent infections seem to be more frequent if the catheter is retained [45, 48, 50]. As mentioned earlier, infections caused by *S. aureus* are more virulent and are associated with substantial morbidity and mortality [51]. In some cancer treatment centers, ~40–60 % of these organisms may be methicillin resistant, although institutional and regional differences do occur, with resistance rates <10 % in the Netherlands or Scandinavian countries. Some of these isolates have also developed tolerance or reduced susceptibility to vancomycin (the so-called MIC creep), and slow response to, or overt failure of vancomycin therapy has been reported especially in infections caused by organisms with vancomycin MICs of >1.0/ml [51–56]. In a recent study of MRSA bacteremia in cancer patients from a comprehensive cancer center, a high treatment failure rate for vancomycin (52 %) was demonstrated, and a vancomycin MIC of >2/ml was found to be an independent factor for vancomycin failure [57]. Based on this and similar reports, the current recommendation is to consider therapy with alternative agents such as linezolid or daptomycin for infections caused by organisms with reduced susceptibility to vancomycin [58–60].

Alpha-hemolytic or viridans group streptococci are major components of human oral microflora. For many years, they were considered contaminants or organisms of low virulence, even in neutropenic patients. However, subsequent clinical experience has shown that they are responsible for serious, life-threatening infections in this patient population [61, 62]. The most consistent predisposing factor for infection by these organisms appears to be high-dose chemotherapy with agents such as cytosine arabinoside that induce severe mucosal damage, thereby facilitating entry of these organisms into the bloodstream [63]. Other probable predisposing factors include antimicrobial prophylaxis with fluoroquinolones that might encourage selection and overgrowth of these organisms and treatment of chemotherapy-induced gastritis with antacids or histamine type 2 (H2) antagonists [64–66]. *Streptococcus mitis*, *S. sanguis*, and *S. salivarius* are the predominant species [18, 67]. Bacteremia is the most common manifestation. In some patients, a rapidly progressive and disseminated infection (sometimes referred to as the streptococcal toxic shock syndrome) occurs involving the bloodstream, lungs, central nervous system, and skin [68]. Despite prompt and aggressive antimicrobial therapy, the mortality associated with this syndrome is 25–35 %. Of increasing concern are reports that 20–60 % of VGS are nonsusceptible or overtly resistant to penicillin [18, 68]. This has limited the utility of penicillin G and other penicillins for the prevention and treatment of these infections. All isolates are currently susceptible to vancomycin, although tolerance has been described [18, 69–72]. The use of antibiotic combinations may be necessary, especially against tolerant organisms. These organisms are also susceptible to the newer-generation quinolones (e.g., moxifloxacin), daptomycin, and linezolid, but clinical experience with these agents is limited.

The enterococci reside primarily in the intestinal tract and cause a variety of infections such as bacteremia, urinary tract infection, endocarditis, intra-abdominal/pelvic infections, biliary tract infections, and occasionally pneumonia and meningitis. They are seldom primary pathogens but are seen most often following prolonged therapy with broad-spectrum cephalosporins or carbapenems to which they are intrinsically resistant. Increased use of vancomycin especially in neutropenic cancer patients was at least in part responsible for the emergence of vancomycin-resistant enterococci (VRE) globally, and these organisms now account for 15–30 % of all enterococcal isolates [4]. Fecal colonization with VRE is not uncommon in patients with acute leukemia and recipients of stem cell transplantation [73, 74]. Approximately 30 % of patients with VRE fecal colonization will go on to develop bacteremia or other significant infections with these organisms following chemotherapy, and some experts recommend the empiric use of agents with activity against VRE when such patients develop fever during an episode of neutropenia [10, 75]. Attempts at eradicating fecal colonization with VRE have been singularly unsuccessful. Consequently, infection control measures to reduce transmission of VRE are of overriding importance.

1.6.2 Gram-Negative Bacilli

The gastrointestinal tract serves as an important source of infection in neutropenic patients, with the predominant pathogens being enteric gram-negative bacilli. The use of antibacterial prophylaxis in high-risk patients including those with acute leukemia has led to a reduction in the frequency of documented gram-negative infections, although some centers are reporting a reversal of this trend [19, 20]. Nevertheless, gram-negative infections, when they do occur, are generally associated with greater morbidity and mortality than infections caused by their gram-positive counterparts. Multiple surveillance studies have shown that *E. coli, Klebsiella* spp., and *P. aeruginosa* remain the three most commonly isolated gram-negative organisms from neutropenic patients and collectively cause 65–75 % of microbiologically documented gram-negative infections [76–79]. Other Enterobacteriaceae such as *Enterobacter* spp., *Citrobacter* spp., *Serratia* spp., and *Proteus* spp. are less common, although institutional differences do exist. Despite the overall decline in the frequency of gram-negative infections in neutropenic patients, there has been an increase in the proportion of such infections caused by non-fermentative gram-negative bacilli (NFGNB) such as *Acinetobacter* spp., non-aeruginosa *Pseudomonas* spp., and *Stenotrophomonas maltophilia* [80]. Collectively, NFGNB now cause ~38 % of documented gram-negative infections, a proportion that has gradually increased over the years. The overall spectrum of infections caused by gram-negative bacilli is wide, with pneumonia, primary and catheter-related bacteremia, and urinary tract infection being common – Table 1.3.

P. aeruginosa is the most frequently isolated and the most important pathogenic NFGNB in this setting and causes between 15 and 20 % of all gram-negative infections [13–16]. Additionally, it is the most common gram-negative organism isolated

Table 1.3 The spectrum of infections caused by *Pseudomonas aeruginosa* and other gram-negative bacilli

Bacteremia – primary and catheter related
Pneumonia, empyema, lung abscess[a]
Urinary tract infection – primary and catheter related
Neutropenic enterocolitis (typhlitis)
Perirectal infection/abscess[a]
Skin and skin structure infection (ecthyma)
Cholangitis/biliary tract infection
Abdominal/pelvic/hepatic abscess[a]
Otitis externa/mastoiditis
Keratitis/endophthalmitis
Osteomyelitis/septic arthritis
Prostatitis

Data from infectious diseases consultation records at MD Anderson Cancer Center

[a]Abscess formation is uncommon in patients with severe and prolonged neutropenia

from polymicrobial infections [11, 12]. These organisms have the propensity for developing resistance to antimicrobial agents by multiple mechanisms [81, 82]. A recent study demonstrated that the risk factors associated with multidrug-resistant *P. aeruginosa* infections were the use of a carbapenem as monotherapy for >7 days, a history of *P. aeruginosa* infection in the preceding year, and a history of chronic obstructive pulmonary disease [83]. Consequently, the antimicrobial stewardship program at our institution has targeted the prolonged use of carbapenem monotherapy, with a resultant decrease in the frequency of infections with MDR *P. aeruginosa* [84]. *Stenotrophomonas maltophilia* colonization/infection rates in neutropenic patients, especially those with acute leukemia and recipients of HSC transplantation, have increased considerably over the past two to three decades. Surveillance studies conducted at the University of Texas MD Anderson Cancer Center have documented an increase in the proportion of *S. maltophilia* from 2 % of all gram-negative bacilli isolated in 1986 to 7 % in 2012. Patients with prolonged neutropenia, those exposed to broad-spectrum antibiotics, especially the carbapenems, and those requiring mechanical ventilation have a higher risk of infection, although these infections are also seen in patients without traditional risk factors [85, 86]. The shift from trimethoprim/sulfamethoxazole (TMP/SMX) which has potent activity against *S. maltophilia*) to the fluoroquinolones (which are much less active against *S. maltophilia*) as the preferred agents for antimicrobial prophylaxis in high-risk neutropenic patients may also have contributed to the increase in infections caused by these organisms. TMP/SMX has been and remains the agent of choice for the treatment of infections caused by *S. maltophilia*, but in vitro resistance to it appears to be increasing [85, 87]. Ticarcillin/clavulanate also has reliable activity, whereas other beta-lactams such as ceftazidime, cefepime, and piperacillin/tazobactam have variable activity against these organisms. The newer quinolones such as moxifloxacin are more active than older agents such as ciprofloxacin and levofloxacin [80]. Minocycline and the novel glycylcycline – tigecycline, are also active against many *S. maltophilia* isolates [88]. Clinical experience with agents other than TMP/SMX and ticarcillin/clavulanate is limited. Combination regimens based on the susceptibility of individual isolates are often employed [89].

Other less common but important NFGNB include *Acinetobacter* spp., *Achromobacter* and *Alcaligenes* spp., *Burkholderia* spp., *Chryseobacterium* spp., and non-aeruginosa *Pseudomonas* species such as *P. putida* and *P. fluorescens* [90–96]. The clinical importance of these organisms has increased in recent years as they frequently cause outbreaks and MDR infections. Many outbreaks can be traced to sources such as contaminated dialysis fluid, chlorhexidine solution, deionized water, and mechanical ventilators.

1.7 Fungal Infections

Whereas bacterial infections predominate during the first 7–10 days of severe neutropenia, invasive fungal infections start to develop as neutropenia persists. Prior to the availability of agents like fluconazole, invasive candidiasis with or without hematogenous dissemination was common, with *Candida albicans* being the predominant species isolated. The frequency of invasive candidiasis has been substantially reduced with the routine usage of antifungal prophylaxis (azoles, echinocandins) in high-risk patients, with manifestations like *Candida* esophagitis, and chronic disseminated (hepatosplenic) candidiasis becoming increasingly of historical interest [97]. The use of some of these agents also led to the emergence of *Candida* spp. other than *Candida albicans* as frequent pathogens in this setting, although *C. albicans* continues to be the single most common species isolated [98, 99]. Regional differences have been documented with a preponderance of different *Candida* species at different centers [21, 22, 100–102]. These differences may represent divergent use of antifungal prophylaxis and/or geographic diversity. Consequently, local epidemiologic and susceptibility data should be used to guide empiric and targeted therapy. Other yeasts that are encountered in this setting include *Trichosporon beigelii*, *Malassezia furfur*, *Saccharomyces cerevisiae*, and occasionally *Hansenula anomala* [103, 104].

The risk of hematogenous dissemination with various yeasts is greater in patients who have indwelling vascular catheters and chemotherapy-induced mucositis or graft versus host disease [99, 105]. Currently, catheter removal in addition to appropriate antifungal therapy is recommended, although this strategy is by no means universally accepted [106–108]. Most *C. albicans* isolates maintain susceptibility to fluconazole and itraconazole. The newer triazole agents such as voriconazole also have potent activity against most pathogenic yeasts. The echinocandins appear to be effective for the treatment of candidiasis caused by most *Candida* species [106]. Treatment of candidiasis with polyenes is seldom necessary. Despite appropriate therapy, the overall mortality in cancer patients with candidemia (which is mainly due to the severity of the underlying disease) approaches 40 % [98]. Disseminated *T. beigelii* infections respond less frequently than disseminated candidiasis [104].

Invasive mold infections, due primarily to *Aspergillus* species, are the most frequent cause of serious, often life-threatening infections in patients with neutropenia that persists for more than 2 weeks [109]. Other risk factors include impaired cellular immunity, prolonged corticosteroid administration, allogeneic stem cell transplantation, and advanced age [103]. *A. fumigatus* is the predominant species isolated but non-fumigatus species of *Aspergillus* are emerging as significant pathogens [110–113]. The most common site of involvement is the lungs leading to invasive pulmonary aspergillosis (IPA). Other common sites of involvement include the paranasal sinuses, the central nervous system, the heart and pericardium, the liver, the kidneys, and occasionally, bones and joints. Cough, dyspnea, and hemoptysis are the classic manifestations of IPA but may be absent or muted in many patients due to severe immunosuppression leading to a blunted inflammatory response. Persistent fever in patients with prolonged neutropenia, despite appropriate antibiotic therapy, should raise the suspicion of invasive fungal infection including IPA. Most infections are diagnosed by computerized tomography (CT) imaging. Classic findings include nodular or wedge-shaped densities, the halo sign, and cavitary lesions [114, 115]. These findings change and evolve over time, and in response to therapy, consequently the performance of serial CT imaging has been found to be useful in monitoring patients with IPA. *Aspergillus hyphae* are angioinvasive in nature and result in release of fungal antigens into the bloodstream. Serologic testing to detect galactomannan or beta-D-glucan has been evaluated for the early diagnosis of invasive aspergillosis. The former appears to be more useful than the latter and may also be a predictor of outcome [116–120]. The use of these tests in conjunction with CT imaging has been discussed in various guidelines for the diagnosis and management of invasive fungal infections in neutropenic patients and HSCT recipients [121–123].

Several mold-active agents are now available for the prevention and treatment of invasive aspergillosis. These include amphotericin B and its lipid formulations, itraconazole, voriconazole, posaconazole, and the echinocandins. A detailed discussion of antifungal prophylaxis and therapy is beyond the scope of this chapter, but recent guidelines addressing these issues are available [121–125]. Although still uncommon, zygomycosis (mucormycosis) has emerged as an increasingly important infection in the past 15–20 years especially in patients with hematologic malignancies and HSCT recipients [99, 126, 127]. The increasing frequency of zygomycosis has at least in part been attributed to the use of voriconazole for various indications such as antifungal prophylaxis and empiric, pre-emptive or targeted therapy of invasive fungal infection [128–132]. The most common organisms isolated include *Rhizopus* species, *Mucor* species, and *Cunninghamella* species. Common sites of infection include the paranasal sinuses and orbit, the lungs, skin, and the central nervous system, with pulmonary manifestations being predominant in neutropenic cancer patients. Generalized dissemination occurs in up to 5 % of patients. Clinical features are often indistinguishable from other common mold infections. Early diagnosis of zygomycosis is important for timely therapeutic intervention, and ultimately, reduced mortality and improved survival. Conventional methods for laboratory assessment for zygomycosis include direct examination, cytopathologic examination, and histopathologic examination of respiratory and other relevant specimens. The use of immunohistochemical stains, fluorescent and in situ hybridization, or in situ polymerase chain reaction (PCR) may also be useful. Cultures from various specimens are often negative. There is increased reliance on diagnostic imaging such as CT of the paranasal sinuses and chest, which may reveal early findings even before the development of localizing symptoms [133, 134]. Unlike invasive aspergillosis where recent diagnostic and therapeutic advances have improved overall survival, the outcome of patients with hematologic malignancies who develop zygomycosis has not improved significantly [126, 127, 135]. Only two systemic antifungals have reliable activity against these organisms – amphotericin B and its lipid formulations and the new triazole, posaconazole. Recent guidelines advocate the lipid preparations of amphotericin B as first-line therapy, with posaconazole and combinations of caspofungin with lipid preparations of amphotericin B as second-line therapy [136, 137]. Surgery is recommended for rhinocerebral and soft tissue infections. Reversal of underlying risk factors is important. The duration of therapy remains unclear and should be guided by resolution of all associated symptoms and findings. Maintenance therapy and/or secondary prophylaxis should be considered in patients who remain severely immunosuppressed. Other uncommon but important molds that cause invasive infections in patients with hematologic malignancies include *Fusarium* species and *Scedosporium* species [138]. Unlike most other molds, fungemia is common in patients with fusariosis and may occur in ~40 % of patients [139]. Involvement of the paranasal sinuses, lungs, skin, and disseminated infection is also relatively common. Optimum therapy remains to be defined, and the overall outcome is poor. The incidence of Scedosporium infection appears to be increasing, with cases of *S. prolificans* generally occurring after 2000 [140]. As with fusariosis, optimum therapy remains to be defined, and the overall prognosis is poor.

1.7.1 Viral Infections

Viral infections per se are uncommon in patients with hematologic malignancies who do not receive HSCT. Most HSV and VZV infections in this setting result from reactivation of the latent viruses from previous exposure, and primary infections are rare [141, 142]. Most US adults are HSV-1 or HSV-2 seropositive, and reactivation can occur in up to 60 % of patients undergoing intensive chemotherapy for hematologic malignancies. Reactivation usually occurs soon after chemotherapy, while patients are still severely neutropenic, and much of the morbidity caused by oral mucositis has been attributed to HSV reactivation in this setting. Consequently, several guidelines recommend HSV prophylaxis in patients undergoing HSCT or remission induction therapy for leukemia [10, 143]. Reactivation of latent VZV also occurs but to a lesser extent, and the risk is considered insufficient to warrant routine prophylaxis.

Over the past two decades, the importance of community respiratory viruses as significant causes of morbidity and mortality in HSCT recipients and patients with hematologic malignancies has been recognized [144–150]. These include human influenza viruses (A and B), respiratory syncytial virus (RSV), human parainfluenzae viruses, human metapneumovirus, human coronaviruses, and human rhinoviruses. Many of these (e.g., the influenza viruses and RSV) have a seasonal preponderance, although some are encountered year round. Upper respiratory tract infections (URTI) predominate, with rhinorrhea being the most common manifestation. Progression to lower respiratory tract infection (LRTI) can lead to respiratory failure and a fatal outcome depending on host factors and the intrinsic virulence of specific viruses. Testing for respiratory viruses is recommended in high-risk patients. Specimens for diagnostic testing include nasopharyngeal swabs, washes, or aspirates, tracheal aspirates, and bronchoalveolar lavage specimens. Laboratory tests include nucleic acid amplification testing, direct antigen detection, and isolation of the virus by cell culture. Optimum therapy for most of these infections remains to be determined (except for human influenza viruses). Pooling of published studies from various centers in the absence of sufficiently powered, randomized, controlled trials, suggests that treatment of LRTI with ribavirin and intravenous immunoglobulin may improve outcome in RSV infections [151]. This approach is also used to prevent the development of LRTI in HSCT recipients with URTI.

1.8 Summary

Infections cause a substantial amount of morbidity and mortality in patients with acute leukemia and other hematologic malignancies. Neutropenia is the predominant predisposing factor, although other factors also contribute to the development of infection. Bacterial infections predominate during the initial phases of severe neutropenia. Invasive fungal infections develop in patients with persistent and profound neutropenia. Viral infections appear to be increasing in frequency and severity. Early diagnosis and the administration of pre-emptive therapy, especially when dealing with invasive fungal infections, are important as infection prevention. The development of resistance and the limited availability of therapeutic agents with activity against resistant pathogens are areas of global concern. As a result, programs for antimicrobial stewardship and infection control need to be strictly adhered to.

References

1. Crawford J, Dale DC, Lyman GH. Chemotherapy-induced neutropenia: risks, consequences, and new directions for its management. Cancer. 2004;100:228–37.
2. Bodey GP, Buckley M, Sathe YS, Freireich EJ. Quantitative relationships between circulating leukocytes and infection in patients with acute leukemia. Ann Intern Med. 1966;64:328–40.
3. Edmond MB, Ober JF, Weinbaum DL, Pfaller MA, Hwang T, Sanford MD, et al. Vancomycin-resistant Enterococcus faecium bacteremia: risk factors for infection. Clin Infect Dis. 1995;20:1126–33.
4. Kern WV, Klose K, Jellen-Ritter AS, Oethinger M, Bohnert J, Kern P, et al. Fluoroquinolone resistance of Escherichia coli at a cancer center: epidemiologic evolution and effects of

discontinuing prophylactic fluoroquinolone use in neutropenic patients with leukemia. Eur J Clin Microbiol Infect Dis. 2005;24:111–8.
5. Fihman V, Le Monnier A, Corvec S, Jaureguy F, Tankovic J, Jacquier H, et al. Stenotrophomonas maltophilia–the most worrisome threat among unusual non-fermentative gram-negative bacilli from hospitalized patients: a prospective multicenter study. J Infect. 2012;64:391–8.
6. Lai CC, Wang CY, Chu CC, Tan CK, Lu CL, Lee YC, et al. Correlation between antibiotic consumption and resistance of Gram-negative bacteria causing healthcare-associated infections at a university hospital in Taiwan from 2000 to 2009. J Antimicrob Chemother. 2011;66:1374–82.
7. Sanyal SC, Mokaddas EM. The increase in carbapenem use and emergence of Stenotrophomonas maltophilia as an important nosocomial pathogen. J Chemother. 1999;11:28–33. Rolston.
8. Rolston K. RI, LeBlanc BJ, Streeter HL, Ho DH. Susceptibility surveillance among gram-negative bacilli at a comprehensive cancer center. (A-004). 103 General meeting of American Society of Microbiology, Washington, DC; 2003.
9. Rolston KV. Challenges in the treatment of infections caused by gram-positive and gram-negative bacteria in patients with cancer and neutropenia. Clin Infect Dis. 2005;40 Suppl 4:S246–52.
10. Freifeld AG, Bow EJ, Sepkowitz KA, Boeckh MJ, Ito JI, Mullen CA, et al. Clinical practice guideline for the use of antimicrobial agents in neutropenic patients with cancer: 2010 update by the Infectious Diseases Society of America. Clin Infect Dis. 2011;52:e56–93.
11. Elting LS, Bodey GP, Fainstein V. Polymicrobial septicemia in the cancer patient. Medicine (Baltimore). 1986;65:218–25.
12. Rolston KV, Bodey GP, Safdar A. Polymicrobial infection in patients with cancer: an underappreciated and underreported entity. Clin Infect Dis. 2007;45:228–33.
13. Klastersky J, Ameye L, Maertens J, Georgala A, Muanza F, Aoun M, et al. Bacteraemia in febrile neutropenic cancer patients. Int J Antimicrob Agents. 2007;30 Suppl 1:S51–9.
14. Yadegarynia D, Tarrand J, Raad I, Rolston K. Current spectrum of bacterial infections in patients with cancer. Clin Infect Dis. 2003;37:1144–5.
15. Zinner SH. Changing epidemiology of infections in patients with neutropenia and cancer: emphasis on gram-positive and resistant bacteria. Clin Infect Dis. 1999;29:490–4.
16. Wisplinghoff H, Seifert H, Wenzel RP, Edmond MB. Current trends in the epidemiology of nosocomial bloodstream infections in patients with hematological malignancies and solid neoplasms in hospitals in the United States. Clin Infect Dis. 2003;36:1103–10.
17. Husni R, Hachem R, Hanna H, Raad I. Risk factors for vancomycin-resistant Enterococcus (VRE) infection in colonized patients with cancer. Infect Control Hosp Epidemiol. 2002;23:102–3.
18. Han XY, Kamana M, Rolston KV. Viridans streptococci isolated by culture from blood of cancer patients: clinical and microbiologic analysis of 50 cases. J Clin Microbiol. 2006;44:160–5.
19. Bucaneve G, Micozzi A, Menichetti F, Martino P, Dionisi MS, Martinelli G, et al. Levofloxacin to prevent bacterial infection in patients with cancer and neutropenia. N Engl J Med. 2005;353:977–87.
20. Cullen M, Steven N, Billingham L, Gaunt C, Hastings M, Simmonds P, et al. Antibacterial prophylaxis after chemotherapy for solid tumors and lymphomas. N Engl J Med. 2005;353:988–98.
21. Sipsas NV, Lewis RE, Tarrand J, Hachem R, Rolston KV, Raad II, et al. Candidemia in patients with hematologic malignancies in the era of new antifungal agents (2001–2007): stable incidence but changing epidemiology of a still frequently lethal infection. Cancer. 2009;115:4745–52.
22. Hachem R, Hanna H, Kontoyiannis D, Jiang Y, Raad I. The changing epidemiology of invasive candidiasis: Candida glabrata and Candida krusei as the leading causes of candidemia in hematologic malignancy. Cancer. 2008;112:2493–9.

23. Bodey GP, Mardani M, Hanna HA, Boktour M, Abbas J, Girgawy E, et al. The epidemiology of Candida glabrata and Candida albicans fungemia in immunocompromised patients with cancer. Am J Med. 2002;112:380–5.
24. DiNubile MJ, Hille D, Sable CA, Kartsonis NA. Invasive candidiasis in cancer patients: observations from a randomized clinical trial. J Infect. 2005;50:443–9.
25. Jossi M, Ambrosioni J, Macedo-Vinas M, Garbino J. Invasive fusariosis with prolonged fungemia in a patient with acute lymphoblastic leukemia: case report and review of the literature. Int J Infect Dis. 2010;14:e354–6.
26. Nucci M, Anaissie E. Fusarium infections in immunocompromised patients. Clin Microbiol Rev. 2007;20:695–704.
27. Chen CY, Sheng WH, Lai CC, Liao CH, Huang YT, Tsay W, et al. Mycobacterial infections in adult patients with hematological malignancy. Eur J Clin Microbiol Infect Dis. 2012;31:1059–66.
28. Vigil KJ, Johnson JR, Johnston BD, Kontoyiannis DP, Mulanovich VE, Raad II, et al. Escherichia coli Pyomyositis: an emerging infectious disease among patients with hematologic malignancies. Clin Infect Dis. 2010;50:374–80.
29. van Burik JA, Colven R, Spach DH. Cutaneous aspergillosis. J Clin Microbiol. 1998;36:3115–21.
30. Walsh TJ. Primary cutaneous aspergillosis–an emerging infection among immunocompromised patients. Clin Infect Dis. 1998;27:453–7.
31. Ibrahim NK, Sahin AA, Dubrow RA, Lynch PM, Boehnke-Michaud L, Valero V, et al. Colitis associated with docetaxel-based chemotherapy in patients with metastatic breast cancer. Lancet. 2000;355:281–3.
32. Gomez L, Martino R, Rolston KV. Neutropenic enterocolitis: spectrum of the disease and comparison of definite and possible cases. Clin Infect Dis. 1998;27:695–9. Nesher.
33. Nesher L, Rolston KV. Neutropenic enterocolitis, a growing concern in the era of widespread use of aggressive chemotherapy. Clin Infect Dis. 2013;56:711–7.
34. Schimpff SC, Wiernik PH, Block JB. Rectal abscesses in cancer patients. Lancet. 1972;2:844–7.
35. Barnes SG, Sattler FR, Ballard JO. Perirectal infections in acute leukemia. Improved survival after incision and debridement. Ann Intern Med. 1984;100:515–8.
36. Rolston K, Bodey GP. Diagnosis and management of perianal and perirectal infection in the granulocytopenic patient. In: Jack S, Remington M, editors. Current clinical topics in infectious diseases. Cambridge, MA: Blackwell Scientific Publications; 1989. p. 164–71.
37. Gudiol C, Bodro M, Simonetti A, Tubau F, Gonzalez-Barca E, Cisnal M, et al. Changing aetiology, clinical features, antimicrobial resistance, and outcomes of bloodstream infection in neutropenic cancer patients. Clin Microbiol Infect. 2013;19(5):474–9.
38. Rolston KV, Yadegarynia D, Kontoyiannis DP, Raad II, Ho DH. The spectrum of Gram-positive bloodstream infections in patients with hematologic malignancies, and the in vitro activity of various quinolones against Gram-positive bacteria isolated from cancer patients. Int J Infect Dis. 2006;10:223–30.
39. Raad I, Kassar R, Ghannam D, Chaftari AM, Hachem R, Jiang Y. Management of the catheter in documented catheter-related coagulase-negative staphylococcal bacteremia: remove or retain? Clin Infect Dis. 2009;49:1187–94.
40. Klotchko A, Wallace MR, Licitra C, Sieger B. Staphylococcus lugdunensis: an emerging pathogen. South Med J. 2011;104:509–14.
41. Kleiner E, Monk AB, Archer GL, Forbes BA. Clinical significance of Staphylococcus lugdunensis isolated from routine cultures. Clin Infect Dis. 2010;51:801–3.
42. Fadel HJ, Patel R, Vetter EA, Baddour LM. Clinical significance of a single Staphylococcus lugdunensis-positive blood culture. J Clin Microbiol. 2011;49:1697–9.
43. Banerjee C, Bustamante CI, Wharton R, Talley E, Wade JC. Bacillus infections in patients with cancer. Arch Intern Med. 1988;148:1769–74.
44. Ozkocaman V, Ozcelik T, Ali R, Ozkalemkas F, Ozkan A, Ozakin C, et al. Bacillus spp. among hospitalized patients with haematological malignancies: clinical features, epidemics and outcomes. J Hosp Infect. 2006;64:169–76.

45. Kassar R, Hachem R, Jiang Y, Chaftari AM, Raad I. Management of Bacillus bacteremia: the need for catheter removal. Medicine (Baltimore). 2009;88:279–83.
46. Martins C, Faria L, Souza M, Camello T, Velasco E, Hirata Jr R, et al. Microbiological and host features associated with corynebacteriosis in cancer patients: a five-year study. Mem Inst Oswaldo Cruz. 2009;104:905–13.
47. Adderson EE, Boudreaux JW, Hayden RT. Infections caused by coryneform bacteria in pediatric oncology patients. Pediatr Infect Dis J. 2008;27:136–41.
48. Ghide S, Jiang Y, Hachem R, Chaftari AM, Raad I. Catheter-related Corynebacterium bacteremia: should the catheter be removed and vancomycin administered? Eur J Clin Microbiol Infect Dis. 2010;29:153–6.
49. Ramos ER, Hachem R, Youssef S, Fang X, Jiang Y, Raad I. The crucial role of catheters in micrococcal bloodstream infections in cancer patients. Infect Control Hosp Epidemiol. 2009;30:83–5.
50. Mermel LA, Allon M, Bouza E, Craven DE, Flynn P, O'Grady NP, et al. Clinical practice guidelines for the diagnosis and management of intravascular catheter-related infection: 2009 Update by the Infectious Diseases Society of America. Clin Infect Dis. 2009;49:1–45.
51. Safdar A, Rolston KV. Vancomycin tolerance, a potential mechanism for refractory gram-positive bacteremia observational study in patients with cancer. Cancer. 2006;106:1815–20.
52. Sakoulas G, Moise-Broder PA, Schentag J, Forrest A, Moellering Jr RC, Eliopoulos GM. Relationship of MIC and bactericidal activity to efficacy of vancomycin for treatment of methicillin-resistant Staphylococcus aureus bacteremia. J Clin Microbiol. 2004;42:2398–402.
53. van Hal SJ, Lodise TP, Paterson DL. The clinical significance of vancomycin minimum inhibitory concentration in Staphylococcus aureus infections: a systematic review and meta-analysis. Clin Infect Dis. 2012;54:755–71.
54. Sakoulas G. Daptomycin for soft tissue infection and neutropenia in a myelogenous leukemia patient who failed prior vancomycin therapy. Clin Adv Hematol Oncol. 2008;6:813–5.
55. Rolston KV. Review: daptomycin for the treatment of gram-positive infections in neutropenic cancer patients. Clin Adv Hematol Oncol. 2008;6:815–7.
56. Sakoulas G, Moellering Jr RC. Increasing antibiotic resistance among methicillin-resistant Staphylococcus aureus strains. Clin Infect Dis. 2008;46 Suppl 5:S360–7.
57. Mahajan SN, Shah JN, Hachem R, Tverdek F, Adachi JA, Mulanovich V, et al. Characteristics and outcomes of methicillin-resistant staphylococcus aureus bloodstream infections in patients with cancer treated with vancomycin: 9-year experience at a comprehensive cancer center. Oncologist. 2012;17:1329–36.
58. Liu C, Bayer A, Cosgrove SE, Daum RS, Fridkin SK, Gorwitz RJ, et al. Clinical practice guidelines by the infectious diseases society of america for the treatment of methicillin-resistant Staphylococcus aureus infections in adults and children: executive summary. Clin Infect Dis. 2011;52:285–92.
59. Chaftari AM, Hachem R, Mulanovich V, Chemaly RF, Adachi J, Jacobson K, et al. Efficacy and safety of daptomycin in the treatment of Gram-positive catheter-related bloodstream infections in cancer patients. Int J Antimicrob Agents. 2010;36:182–6.
60. Rolston KV, McConnell SA, Brown J, Lamp KC. Daptomycin use in patients with cancer and neutropenia: data from a retrospective registry. Clin Adv Hematol Oncol. 2010;8:249–56, 90.
61. Bochud PY, Eggiman P, Calandra T, Van Melle G, Saghafi L, Francioli P. Bacteremia due to viridans streptococcus in neutropenic patients with cancer: clinical spectrum and risk factors. Clin Infect Dis. 1994;18:25–31.
62. Tunkel AR, Sepkowitz KA. Infections caused by viridans streptococci in patients with neutropenia. Clin Infect Dis. 2002;34:1524–9.
63. Paganini H, Staffolani V, Zubizarreta P, Casimir L, Lopardo H, Luppino V. Viridans streptococci bacteraemia in children with fever and neutropenia: a case-control study of predisposing factors. Eur J Cancer. 2003;39:1284–9.

64. Elting LS, Bodey GP, Keefe BH. Septicemia and shock syndrome due to viridans streptococci: a case-control study of predisposing factors. Clin Infect Dis. 1992;14:1201–7.
65. Razonable RR, Litzow MR, Khaliq Y, Piper KE, Rouse MS, Patel R. Bacteremia due to viridans group Streptococci with diminished susceptibility to Levofloxacin among neutropenic patients receiving levofloxacin prophylaxis. Clin Infect Dis. 2002;34:1469–74.
66. Prabhu RM, Piper KE, Litzow MR, Steckelberg JM, Patel R. Emergence of quinolone resistance among viridans group streptococci isolated from the oropharynx of neutropenic peripheral blood stem cell transplant patients receiving quinolone antimicrobial prophylaxis. Eur J Clin Microbiol Infect Dis. 2005;24:832–8.
67. Gaudreau C, Delage G, Rousseau D, Cantor ED. Bacteremia caused by viridans streptococci in 71 children. Can Med Assoc J. 1981;125:1246–9.
68. Gassas A, Grant R, Richardson S, Dupuis LL, Doyle J, Allen U, et al. Predictors of viridans streptococcal shock syndrome in bacteremic children with cancer and stem-cell transplant recipients. J Clin Oncol. 2004;22:1222–7.
69. Westling K, Julander I, Ljungman P, Heimdahl A, Thalme A, Nord CE. Reduced susceptibility to penicillin of viridans group streptococci in the oral cavity of patients with haematological disease. Clin Microbiol Infect. 2004;10:899–903.
70. Lyytikainen O, Rautio M, Carlson P, Anttila VJ, Vuento R, Sarkkinen H, et al. Nosocomial bloodstream infections due to viridans streptococci in haematological and non-haematological patients: species distribution and antimicrobial resistance. J Antimicrob Chemother. 2004;53:631–4.
71. Diekema DJ, Coffman SL, Marshall SA, Beach ML, Rolston KV, Jones RN. Comparison of activities of broad-spectrum beta-lactam compounds against 1,128 gram-positive cocci recently isolated in cancer treatment centers. Antimicrob Agents Chemother. 1999;43:940–3.
72. Wisplinghoff H, Reinert RR, Cornely O, Seifert H. Molecular relationships and antimicrobial susceptibilities of viridans group streptococci isolated from blood of neutropenic cancer patients. J Clin Microbiol. 1999;37:1876–80.
73. Matar MJ, Tarrand J, Raad I, Rolston KV. Colonization and infection with vancomycin-resistant Enterococcus among patients with cancer. Am J Infect Control. 2006;34:534–6.
74. Liss BJ, Vehreschild JJ, Cornely OA, et al. Intestinal colonisation and blood stream infections due to vancomycin-resistant enterococci (VRE) and extended-spectrum beta-lactamase-producing Enterobacteriaceae (ESBLE) in patients with haematological and oncological malignancies. Infection. 2012;40(6):613–9.
75. Rolston KV. Letter to the Editor: Regarding: Kraft S, Mackler E, Schlickman P, Welch K, DePestel DD (2011) Outcomes of therapy: vancomycin-resistant enterococcal bacteremia in hematology and bone marrow transplant patients. Supp Care Cancer 19;1969–1974. Support Care Cancer. 2012;20:1117–8.
76. Bodey GP, Ho DH, Elting L. Survey of antibiotic susceptibility among gram-negative bacilli at a cancer hospital. Am J Med. 1988;85:49–51.
77. Rolston KV, Elting L, Waguespack S, Ho DH, LeBlanc B, Bodey GP. Survey of antibiotic susceptibility among gram-negative bacilli at a cancer center. Chemotherapy. 1996;42(5):348–53.
78. Jacobson K, Rolston K, Elting L, et al. Susceptibility surveillance among gram-negative bacilli at a cancer center. Chemotherapy. 1999;45(5):325–34.
79. Rolston KV, Tarrand JJ. Pseudomonas aeruginosa–still a frequent pathogen in patients with cancer: 11-year experience at a comprehensive cancer center. Clin Infect Dis. 1999;29:463–4.
80. Rolston KV, Kontoyiannis DP, Yadegarynia D, Raad II. Nonfermentative gram-negative bacilli in cancer patients: increasing frequency of infection and antimicrobial susceptibility of clinical isolates to fluoroquinolones. Diagn Microbiol Infect Dis. 2005;51:215–8.
81. Aboufaycal H, Sader HS, Rolston K, Deshpande LM, Toleman M, Bodey G, et al. blaVIM-2 and blaVIM-7 carbapenemase-producing Pseudomonas aeruginosa isolates detected in a tertiary care medical center in the United States: report from the MYSTIC program. J Clin Microbiol. 2007;45:614–5.

82. Toleman MA, Rolston K, Jones RN, Walsh TR. blaVIM-7, an evolutionarily distinct metallo-beta-lactamase gene in a Pseudomonas aeruginosa isolate from the United States. Antimicrob Agents Chemother. 2004;48:329–32.
83. Chatzinikolaou I, Abi-Said D, Bodey GP, Rolston KV, Tarrand JJ, Samonis G. Recent experience with Pseudomonas aeruginosa bacteremia in patients with cancer: Retrospective analysis of 245 episodes. Arch Intern Med. 2000;160:501–9.
84. Tverdek FP, Wu C, Mihu C, et al. Antimicrobial stewardship initiative in cancer patients: The MD Anderson Cancer Center Experience. Infectious diseases society of America (IDSA) annual meeting, San Diego. 17–21 Oct Abstract# 37545.
85. Safdar A, Rolston KV. Stenotrophomonas maltophilia: changing spectrum of a serious bacterial pathogen in patients with cancer. Clin Infect Dis. 2007;45:1602–9.
86. Aisenberg G, Rolston KV, Dickey BF, Kontoyiannis DP, Raad II, Safdar A. Stenotrophomonas maltophilia pneumonia in cancer patients without traditional risk factors for infection, 1997–2004. Eur J Clin Microbiol Infect Dis. 2007;26:13–20.
87. Vartivarian S, Anaissie E, Bodey G, Sprigg H, Rolston K. A changing pattern of susceptibility of Xanthomonas maltophilia to antimicrobial agents: implications for therapy. Antimicrob Agents Chemother. 1994;38:624–7.
88. Noskin GA. Tigecycline: a new glycylcycline for treatment of serious infections. Clin Infect Dis. 2005;41 Suppl 5:S303–14.
89. Krueger TS, Clark EA, Nix DE. In vitro susceptibility of Stenotrophomonas maltophilia to various antimicrobial combinations. Diagn Microbiol Infect Dis. 2001;41:71–8.
90. Cayo R, Yanez San Segundo L, Perez del Molino Bernal IC, Garcia de la Fuente C, Bermudez Rodriguez MA, Calvo J, et al. Bloodstream infection caused by Acinetobacter junii in a patient with acute lymphoblastic leukaemia after allogenic haematopoietic cell transplantation. J Med Microbiol. 2011;60:375–7.
91. Turkoglu M, Mirza E, Tunccan OG, Erdem GU, Dizbay M, Yagci M, et al. Acinetobacter baumannii infection in patients with hematologic malignancies in intensive care unit: risk factors and impact on mortality. J Crit Care. 2011;26:460–7.
92. Aisenberg G, Rolston KV, Safdar A. Bacteremia caused by Achromobacter and Alcaligenes species in 46 patients with cancer (1989–2003). Cancer. 2004;101:2134–40.
93. Mann T, Ben-David D, Zlotkin A, Shachar D, Keller N, Toren A, et al. An outbreak of Burkholderia cenocepacia bacteremia in immunocompromised oncology patients. Infection. 2010;38:187–94.
94. Bloch KC, Nadarajah R, Jacobs R. Chryseobacterium meningosepticum: an emerging pathogen among immunocompromised adults. Report of 6 cases and literature review. Medicine (Baltimore). 1997;76:30–41.
95. Simor AE, Ricci J, Lau A, Bannatyne RM, Ford-Jones L. Pseudobacteremia due to Pseudomonas fluorescens. Pediatr Infect Dis. 1985;4:508–12.
96. Anaissie E, Fainstein V, Miller P, et al. Pseudomonas putida. Newly recognized pathogen in patients with cancer. Am J Med. 1987;82:1191–4.
97. Bow EJ, Laverdiere M, Lussier N, Rotstein C, Cheang MS, Ioannou S. Antifungal prophylaxis for severely neutropenic chemotherapy recipients: a meta analysis of randomized-controlled clinical trials. Cancer. 2002;94:3230–46.
98. Pappas PG, Rex JH, Lee J, Hamill RJ, Larsen RA, Powderly W, et al. A prospective observational study of candidemia: epidemiology, therapy, and influences on mortality in hospitalized adult and pediatric patients. Clin Infect Dis. 2003;37:634–43.
99. Maschmeyer G. The changing epidemiology of invasive fungal infections: new threats. Int J Antimicrob Agents. 2006;27 Suppl 1:3–6.
100. Beck-Sague C, Jarvis WR. Secular trends in the epidemiology of nosocomial fungal infections in the United States, 1980-1990. National Nosocomial Infections Surveillance System. J Infect Dis. 1993;167:1247–51.
101. Girmenia C, Martino P, De Bernardis F, Gentile G, Boccanera M, Monaco M, et al. Rising incidence of Candida parapsilosis fungemia in patients with hematologic malignancies: clinical aspects, predisposing factors, and differential pathogenicity of the causative strains. Clin Infect Dis. 1996;23:506–14.

102. Safdar A, Perlin DS, Armstrong D. Hematogenous infections due to Candida parapsilosis: changing trends in fungemic patients at a comprehensive cancer center during the last four decades. Diagn Microbiol Infect Dis. 2002;44:11–6.
103. Safdar A, Armstrong D. Infections in patients with hematologic neoplasms and hematopoietic stem cell transplantation: neutropenia, humoral, and splenic defects. Clin Infect Dis. 2011;53:798–806.
104. Girmenia C, Pagano L, Martino B, D'Antonio D, Fanci R, Specchia G, et al. Invasive infections caused by Trichosporon species and Geotrichum capitatum in patients with hematological malignancies: a retrospective multicenter study from Italy and review of the literature. J Clin Microbiol. 2005;43:1818–28.
105. Koh AY, Kohler JR, Coggshall KT, Van Rooijen N, Pier GB. Mucosal damage and neutropenia are required for Candida albicans dissemination. Plos Pathog. 2008;4:e35.
106. Pappas PG, Kauffman CA, Andes D, Benjamin DK, Calandra TF, Edwards JE, et al. Clinical practice guidelines for the management of Candidiasis: 2009 update by the Infectious Diseases Society of America. Clin Infect Dis. 2009;48:503–35.
107. Nucci M, Anaissie E, Betts RF, Dupont BF, Wu CZ, Buell DN, et al. Early removal of central venous catheter in patients with candidemia does not improve outcome: analysis of 842 patients from 2 randomized clinical trials. Clin Infect Dis. 2010;51:295–303.
108. Brass EP, Edwards JE. Should the guidelines for management of central venous catheters in patients with candidemia be changed Now? Clin Infect Dis. 2010;51:304–6.
109. Steinbach WJ, Marr KA, Anaissie EJ, Azie N, Quan SP, Meier-Kriesche HU, et al. Clinical epidemiology of 960 patients with invasive aspergillosis from the PATH Alliance registry. J Infection. 2012;65:453–64.
110. Denning DW. Invasive aspergillosis. Clin Infect Dis. 1998;26:781–803.
111. Walsh TJ, Groll AH. Overview: non-fumigatus species of Aspergillus: perspectives on emerging pathogens in immunocompromised hosts. Curr Opin Investig Drugs. 2001;2:1366–7.
112. Lass-Florl C, Rath P, Niederwieser D, Kofler G, Wurzner R, Krezy A, et al. Aspergillus terreus infections in haematological malignancies: molecular epidemiology suggests association with in-hospital plants. J Hosp Infect. 2000;46:31–5.
113. Steinbach WJ, Benjamin DK, Kontoyiannis DP, Perfect JR, Lutsar I, Marr KA, et al. Infections due to Aspergillus terreus: a multicenter retrospective analysis of 83 cases. Clin Infect Dis. 2004;39:192–8.
114. Caillot D, Couaillier JF, Bernard A, Casasnovas O, Denning DW, Mannone L, et al. Increasing volume and changing characteristics of invasive pulmonary aspergillosis on sequential thoracic computed tomography scans in patients with neutropenia. J Clin Oncol. 2001;19:253–9.
115. Caillot D, Latrabe V, Thiebaut A, Herbrecht R, De Botton S, Pigneux A, et al. Computer tomography in pulmonary invasive Aspergillosis in hematological patients with neutropenia: an useful tool for diagnosis and assessment of outcome in clinical trials. Eur J Radiol. 2010;74:E173–6.
116. Ostrosky-Zeichner L, Alexander BD, Kett DH, Vazquez J, Pappas PG, Saeki F, et al. Multicenter clinical evaluation of the (1 -> 3) beta-D-glucan assay as an aid to diagnosis of fungal infections in humans. Clin Infect Dis. 2005;41:654–9.
117. Lamoth F, Cruciani M, Mengoli C, Castagnola E, Lortholary O, Richardson M, et al. Beta-glucan antigenemia assay for the diagnosis of invasive fungal infections in patients with hematological malignancies: a systematic review and meta-analysis of cohort studies from the third european conference on infections in leukemia (ECIL-3). Clin Infect Dis. 2012;54:633–43.
118. Wheat LJ, Walsh TJ. Diagnosis of invasive aspergillosis by galactomannan antigenemia detection using an enzyme immunoassay. Eur J Clin Microbiol. 2008;27:245–51.
119. Mennink-Kersten MASH, Donnelly JP, Verweij PE. Detection of circulating galactomannan for the diagnosis and management of invasive aspergillosis. Lancet Infect Dis. 2004;4:349–57.

120. Chai LYA, Kullberg BJ, Johnson EM, Teerenstra S, Khin LW, Vonk AG, et al. Early serum galactomannan trend as a predictor of outcome of invasive Aspergillosis. J Clin Microbiol. 2012;50:2330–6.
121. Maschmeyer G, Beinert T, Buchheidt D, Cornely OA, Einsele H, Heinz W, et al. Diagnosis and antimicrobial therapy of lung infiltrates in febrile neutropenic patients: Guidelines of the infectious diseases working party of the German Society of Haematology and Oncology. Eur J Cancer. 2009;45:2462–72.
122. Maertens J, Marchetti O, Herbrecht R, Cornely OA, Fluckiger U, Frere P, et al. European guidelines for antifungal management in leukemia and hematopoietic stem cell transplant recipients: summary of the ECIL 3-2009 Update. Bone Marrow Transpl. 2011;46:709–18.
123. Walsh TJ, Anaissie EJ, Denning DW, Herbrecht R, Kontoyiannis DP, Marr KA, et al. Treatment of aspergillosis: clinical practice guidelines of the Infectious Diseases Society of America. Clin Infect Dis. 2008;46:327–60.
124. Maschmeyer G. The changing face of febrile neutropenia-from monotherapy to moulds to mucositis. Prevention of mould infections. J Antimicrob Chemother. 2009;63 Suppl 1:i27–30.
125. Cornely OA, Bohme A, Buchheidt D, Einsele H, Heinz WJ, Karthaus M, et al. Primary prophylaxis of invasive fungal infections in patients with hematologic malignancies. Recommendations of the Infectious Diseases Working Party of the German Society for Haematology and Oncology. Haematologica. 2009;94:113–22.
126. Kontoyiannis DP, Wessel VC, Bodey GP, Rolston KVI. Zygomycosis in the 1990s in a tertiary-care cancer center. Clin Infect Dis. 2000;30:851–6.
127. Roden MM, Zaoutis TE, Buchanan WL, Knudsen TA, Sarkisova TA, Schaufele RL, et al. Epidemiology and outcome of zygomycosis: a review of 929 reported cases. Clin Infect Dis. 2005;41:634–53.
128. Marty FM, Cosimi LA, Baden LR. Breakthrough zygomycosis after voriconazole treatment in recipients of hematopoietic stem-cell transplants. N Engl J Med. 2004;350:950–2.
129. Siwek GT, Dodgson KJ, de Magalhaes-Silverman M, Bartelt LA, Kilborn SB, Hoth PL, et al. Invasive zygomycosis in hematopoietic stem cell transplant recipients receiving voriconazole prophylaxis. Clin Infect Dis. 2004;39:584–7.
130. Kontoyiannis DP, Lionakis MS, Lewis RE, Chamilos G, Healy M, Perego C, et al. Zygomycosis in a Tertiary-Care Cancer Center in the era of Aspergillus-active antifungal therapy: a case-control observational study of 27 recent cases. J Infect Dis. 2005;191:1350–60.
131. Pongas GN, Lewis RE, Samonis G, Kontoyiannis DP. Voriconazole-associated zygomycosis: a significant consequence of evolving antifungal prophylaxis and immunosuppression practices? Clin Microbiol Infec. 2009;15:93–7.
132. Trifilio SM, Bennett CL, Yarnold PR, McKoy JM, Parada J, Mehta J, et al. Breakthrough zygomycosis after voriconazole administration among patients with hematologic malignancies who receive hematopoietic stem-cell transplants or intensive chemotherapy. Bone Marrow Transpl. 2007;39:425–9.
133. Georgiadou SP, Sipsas NV, Marom EM, Kontoyiannis DP. The diagnostic value of halo and reversed halo signs for invasive mold infections in compromised hosts. Clin Infect Dis. 2011;52:1144–55.
134. Walsh TJ, Gamaletsou MN, McGinnis MR, Hayden RT, Kontoyiannis DP. Early clinical and laboratory diagnosis of invasive pulmonary, extrapulmonary, and disseminated mucormycosis (zygomycosis). Clin Infect Dis. 2012;54:S55–60.
135. Kontoyiannis DP, Lewis RE. How I treat mucormycosis. Blood. 2011;118:1216–24.
136. Ruping MJGT, Heinz WJ, Kindo AJ, Rickerts V, Lass-Florl C, Beisel C, et al. Forty-one recent cases of invasive zygomycosis from a global clinical registry. J Antimicrob Chemoth. 2010;65:296–302.
137. Skiada A, Lanternier F, Groll AH, Pagano L, Zimmerli S, Herbrecht R, et al. Diagnosis and treatment of mucormycosis in patients with haematological malignancies: guidelines from the 3rd European Conference on Infections in Leukemia (ECIL 3). Haematologica. 2013; 94(4):492–504.

138. Park BJ, Pappas PG, Wannemuehler KA, Alexander BD, Anaissie EJ, Andes DR, et al. Invasive non-Aspergillus mold infections in transplant recipients, United States, 2001–2006. Emerg Infect Dis. 2011;17:1855–64.
139. Campo M, Lewis RE, Kontoyiannis DP. Invasive fusariosis in patients with hematologic malignancies at a cancer center: 1998–2009. J Infect. 2010;60:331–7.
140. Lamaris GA, Chamilos G, Lewis RE, Safdar A, Raad II, Kontoyiannis DP. Scedosporium infection in a tertiary care cancer center: a review of 25 cases from 1989–2006. Clin Infect Dis. 2006;43:1580–4.
141. Wade JC. Viral infections in patients with hematological malignancies. Hematology Am Soc Hematol Educ Program. 2006;1:368–74.
142. Redding SW. Role of herpes simplex virus reactivation in chemotherapy-induced oral mucositis. NCI Monogr. 1990;9:103–5.
143. Flowers CR, Seidenfeld J, Bow EJ, Karten C, Gleason C, Hawley DK, et al. Antimicrobial prophylaxis and outpatient management of fever and neutropenia in adults treated for malignancy: American Society of Clinical Oncology clinical practice guideline. J Clin Oncol. 2013;31(6):794–810.
144. Ohrmalm L, Wong M, Aust C, Ljungman P, Norbeck O, Broliden K, et al. Viral findings in adult hematological patients with neutropenia. PLoS ONE. 2012;7:e36543.
145. Karapinar DY, Ay Y, Karzaoglu Z, Balkan C, Ergin F, Vardar F, et al. Experience of pandemic influenza with H1N1 in children with leukemia. Pediatr Hemat Oncol. 2011;28:31–6.
146. Tavil B, Azik F, Culha V, Kara A, Yarali N, Tezer H, et al. Pandemic H1N1 influenza infection in children with acute leukemia: a single-center experience. J Pediatr Hematol Oncol. 2012;34:48–50.
147. Marcolini JA, Malik S, Suki D, Whimbey E, Bodey GP. Respiratory disease due to parainfluenza virus in adult leukemia patients. Eur J Clin Microbiol. 2003;22:79–84.
148. Chemaly RF, Hanmod SS, Rathod DB, Ghantoji SS, Jiang Y, Doshi A, et al. The characteristics and outcomes of parainfluenza virus infections in 200 patients with leukemia or recipients of hematopoietic stem cell transplantation. Blood. 2012;119:2738–45.
149. Srinivasan A, Wang C, Yang J, Inaba H, Shenep JL, Leung WH, et al. Parainfluenza virus infections in children with hematologic malignancies. Pediatr Infect Dis J. 2011;30:855–9.
150. Torres HA, Aguilera EA, Mattiuzzi GN, Cabanillas ME, Rohatgi N, Sepulveda CA, et al. Characteristics and outcome of respiratory syncytial virus infection in patients with leukemia. Haematologica. 2007;92:1216–23.
151. Hirsch HH, Martino R, Ward KN, Boeckh M, Einsele H, Ljungman P. Fourth european conference on infections in leukaemia (ECIL-4): guidelines for diagnosis and treatment of human respiratory syncytial virus, parainfluenza virus, metapneumovirus, rhinovirus, and coronavirus. Clin Infect Dis. 2013;53:258–66.

Infections in Patients with Malignant Lymphomas

2

Kenneth V.I. Rolston

Contents

2.1 Introduction

The malignant lymphomas represent neoplastic transformation of cells that reside primarily in lymphoid tissues and are the most common hematologic malignancies in man. The American Cancer Society estimates that there will be 9,290 new cases of Hodgkin's lymphoma and 69,740 new cases of non-Hodgkin's lymphoma in the United States in 2013, with over 20,000 estimated deaths [1]. Infections in patients with malignant lymphomas are quite common, and their pathogenesis is multifactorial. Predisposing factors for infection include multiple immunologic deficits caused by the underlying lymphoma (impaired cell-mediated immunity, impaired humoral immunity/hypogammaglobulinemia, impaired neutrophil function, and impaired

K.V.I. Rolston
Department of Infectious Diseases, Infection Control and Employee Health, The University of Texas, M.D. Anderson Cancer Center, Houston, TX, USA
e-mail: krolston@mdanderson.org

G. Maschmeyer, K.V.I. Rolston (eds.), *Infections in Hematology*,
DOI 10.1007/978-3-662-44000-1_2

complement activity) and by various treatment modalities. While neutropenia remains the most common predisposing factor in this subset of cancer patients, it is often superimposed on the other immunologic deficits listed above, each with its unique spectrum of pathogens (although there is some overlap).

2.2 Neutropenia

Neutropenia was recognized almost 50 years ago as a major predisposing factor for infection [2]. The current definition of neutropenia is an absolute neutrophil count of $\leq 500/mm^3$ or $\leq 1{,}000/mm^3$ with an anticipated decline to below 500 cells/mm^3 in the ensuing 48 h [3]. Bacterial infections predominate in the early stages of profound neutropenia, with infections caused by gram-positive pathogens (*Staphylococcus* species, *Streptococcus* species, *Enterococcus* species) being almost twice as common as gram-negative pathogens (*Enterobacteriaceae*, non-fermentative gram-negative bacilli) [4]. Fungal infections (*Candida* species, *Aspergillus* species, and other molds) generally develop in patients with prolonged neutropenia. Infections in neutropenic patients have been dealt with in great detail elsewhere in this volume and will not be discussed further in this chapter.

2.3 Humoral Immunity

Antibodies are produced by B lymphocytes (or B cells) and play a central role in the immune system's response to various infections. They are not directly microbicidal but possess various other mechanisms to help eradicate invading pathogens. For instance, IgM antibodies block pathogens binding to cells and also cause aggregation of infectious agents, which enhances their clearance. Antibody-coated organisms in turn activate monocytes/macrophages and promote the release of the proinflammatory cytokines. IgM antibodies also activate complement proteins which attract phagocytic cells. Responses to polysaccharides are mediated by the IgG class of immunoglobulins and provide protection against encapsulated organisms such as *Streptococcus pneumoniae* and *Haemophilus influenzae*. Impaired opsonization and phagocytosis may lead to fulminant infection with *S. pneumoniae*. Immunoglobulins of the IgA variety defend mucosal surfaces against invading pathogens. Hypogammaglobulinemia is related to deficiencies of both T cells and B cells.

2.4 Cell-Mediated Immunity

Cell-mediated immunity protects the host from a wide spectrum of microbial pathogens. Defects in cell-mediated immunity are common in patients with hematologic malignancies including malignant lymphomas, in recipients of allogeneic hematopoietic stem-cell transplantation (HST), and in patients treated with newer modalities (nucleoside analogs, monoclonal antibodies) and result in an increase in

Table 2.1 Infections in patients with impaired humoral (B-cell-mediated) and cellular (T-cell-mediated) immunity

Bacterial pathogens
Streptococcus pneumoniae
Haemophilus influenzae
Neisseria meningitidis
Nocardia species
Salmonella species
Listeria monocytogenes
Campylobacter species
Legionella species
Capnocytophaga species
Mycobacteria
Fungal pathogens
Aspergillus species
Zygomycetes (*Mucorales*)
Fusarium species
Scedosporium species
Pneumocystis jiroveci
Cryptococcus neoformans
Histoplasma capsulatum (endemic areas)
Candida spp.
Viral pathogens
Cytomegalovirus
Varicella-zoster virus
Herpes simplex virus 1 and 2
Epstein-Barr virus
Human herpes virus 6
Parasites
Toxoplasma gondii
Strongyloides stercoralis
Babesia microti

infections caused by bacterial pathogens such as mycobacteria, *Salmonella* spp., *Nocardia* spp., and *Listeria monocytogenes*; fungal pathogens such as invasive molds, *Candida* spp., *Pneumocystis jiroveci*, and *Cryptococcus neoformans*; a number of viral pathogens such as CMV and other herpes viruses; and *Strongyloides stercoralis* (Table 2.1). The management of infections associated with newer treatment modalities has been discussed in detail elsewhere in this volume. Other infections seen in patients with malignant lymphomas will be discussed below.

2.5 Bacterial Infections

As previously mentioned, infections caused by encapsulated organisms (*Streptococcus pneumoniae, Haemophilus influenzae, Neisseria meningitidis*) have been reported as being more frequent and more virulent in patients with impaired humoral immunity/

hypogammaglobulinemia. However, recent surveys indicate that both *H. influenzae* and *N. meningitidis* are now quite uncommon, even in this setting [5, 6]. This decline is most likely the result of herd immunity due to the availability of effective immunization against these organisms and the practice of administering quinolone prophylaxis in high-risk patients. Infections caused by *S. pneumoniae* are more common but are also on the decline. A recent review of streptococcal bloodstream infections seen at a comprehensive cancer center over a 12-year span documented that the largest number of cases (45.6 %) was caused by *S. pneumoniae*. However, there was a 55 % decline in frequency from the beginning of the review (2000) to the end of it (2011) [5]. These infections were more common in patients with solid organ malignancies than in patients with lymphomas and/or other groups with impaired humoral defense mechanisms. A significant decline in penicillin-resistant *S. pneumoniae* was also documented. Only 4 % of the total pneumococcal bacteremias occurred in an age group in which the 7-valent pneumococcal conjugate vaccine (PCV7) is recommended. The authors hypothesize that the continued vaccination of the pediatric population with PCV7 may be a major method of controlling invasive, antimicrobial-resistant pneumococcal disease in the broad cancer population. Other experts prefer the use of the 13-valent vaccine (PCV-13) for primary vaccination followed by booster vaccination with the 23-valent vaccine (Pneumovax-23) [7].

Nocardiosis is caused by several species of *Nocardia*, the most common of which are *Nocardia asteroides* complex, *N. brasiliensis, and N. otitidiscaviarum* (formerly *N. caviae*). Nocardiosis is uncommon in immunocompetent persons. Approximately half the number of cases occur in individuals with impaired cell-mediated immunity secondary to an underlying malignancy (most often lymphoma) or its treatment. Nocardiosis occurs less often in patients with impaired humoral immunity or with leukocyte abnormalities. T lymphocytes are essential for a host to mount an adequate immune response to *Nocardia* infection. Although T lymphocytes can kill *Nocardia* in vitro, their primary role is to activate macrophages and stimulate a cellular response. Infection usually follows introduction of the organisms into the respiratory tract, although it is also acquired via direct inoculation into the skin.

Data from a relatively large study (43 episodes) of nocardiosis in patients with cancer documented that 64 % of these patients had an underlying hematologic malignancy, with lymphoma being the most common [8]. Lymphocytopenia was present in 54 %, 58 % had received corticosteroids, and 24 % had undergone hematopoietic stem cell transplantation. The most common sites of infection were the lungs (70 %) and soft tissue (16 %). *Nocardia asteroides* complex was the most common species isolated. Central nervous system (CNS) infection and widespread dissemination were uncommon (2 % each). When CNS disease is present, the differential diagnosis is wide and includes other pathogens such as *Cryptococcus neoformans*, *Toxoplasma gondii*, and mycobacteria (predominantly *M. tuberculosis*) which are common in this setting, as well as the underlying malignancy (predominantly lymphoma) itself. Hence, the need for establishing a specific diagnosis is paramount. Trimethoprim/sulfamethoxazole (standard dosage) remains the backbone of therapy. It is often combined with agents such as the carbapenems, tetracyclines, or aminoglycosides [8, 9]. Prolonged treatment (up to 6–12 months) is usually necessary, despite which the mortality rate is around 60 % [10].

Other bacterial infections that occur more frequently in patients with impaired cellular and/or humoral immunity include salmonellosis, legionellosis, listeriosis, and infections caused by *Campylobacter* and *Capnocytophaga* species. Bacteremia is the most common manifestation of salmonellosis, although other manifestations including gastroenteritis, cholangitis, septic arthritis, and meningitis also occur [11–13]. The morbidity and mortality associated with salmonellosis is greater in patients with underlying malignancies than in immunocompetent individuals. Resistance rates to antimicrobial agents commonly used to treat salmonellosis (fluoroquinolones, ceftriaxone) may differ from region to region and appear to be increasing in some parts of the globe, although these organisms generally remain quite susceptible to the carbapenems [12]. Although much less common than salmonellosis, gastroenteritis and bacteremia caused by *Campylobacter* species does occur more frequently in patients with underlying lymphoid and gastrointestinal malignancies. Most cases involve elderly males. In one recent review of *Campylobacter* bacteremia, the rate of resistance to fluoroquinolones was 32 %, but all isolates were susceptible to imipenem, and 99 % were susceptible to amoxicillin/clavulanate [14]. There is a strong association between antecedent infection with *Campylobacter jejuni* and Guillain-Barre syndrome (GBS), with about a quarter of patients who develop GBS giving a history of recent *C. jejuni* infection [15]. This may lead to the generation of antibodies which cause acute axonal damage and result in acute motor axonal neuropathy [16].

Infections caused by *Legionella* species (primarily *Legionella pneumophila*) occur in immunocompromised individuals, including those with malignant lymphomas, as well as in immunocompetent individuals [17]. Often, hospital water systems harbor *Legionella* species, and most cases of hospital-acquired legionellosis can be traced to such sources [18]. Consequently, monitoring of hospital water systems for the presence of *Legionella* (and other potential pathogens) is mandatory, and guidelines for how to do this and how to deal with outbreaks where they do occur have been published [19]. However, patients with malignant lymphomas may also acquire legionellosis from household water or whirlpools that have been inactive for a while. Pneumonia is the most common manifestation, and it cannot be distinguished clinically or radiographically from other forms of pneumonia [20]. The detection of urinary antigens and/or culture on special media is usually required to make a specific diagnosis. The fluoroquinolones and macrolides are used most often for treatment which needs to be longer in duration in immunosuppressed individuals than in those who are immunocompetent.

Listeriosis is caused by *Listeria monocytogenes*, a facultative anaerobic gram-positive bacillus. Although *L. monocytogenes* can infect immunocompetent individuals, those with abnormalities in cellular immunity are at particular risk. The predominant source of infection is the consumption of raw milk or products (cheese) made from raw milk, although some cases have been associated with pasteurized milk as well [21, 22]. In a recent review of listeriosis, 12 of 34 patients (35 %) had an underlying lymphoid malignancy [23]. Lymphocytopenia was observed in 62 % of patients, and 76 % had received prior corticosteroid therapy. In 11 patients listeriosis complicated hematopoietic stem cell transplantation.

Bacteremia (74 %) was the most common presentation followed by meningoencephalitis (21 %). Although the overall response to antimicrobial therapy (most commonly ampicillin and gentamicin) was 79 % only, three of six patients with meningoencephalitis responded.

Capnocytophaga species are facultative anaerobic gram-negative bacilli that are part of the normal human oral flora. In one report of 28 patients with bacteremia caused by *Capnocytophaga* species, 11(21 %) had an underlying lymphoma, and 11 had CLL [24]. Ninety three percent were neutropenic at the onset of infection, and 50 % had moderate to severe mucositis. *Capnocytophaga ochracea* was the most common species isolated, and 14 % of these infections were polymicrobial. Fluoroquinolone resistance is not uncommon, but the organisms are generally susceptible to beta-lactam antimicrobial agents (penicillins, cephalosporins, and carbapenems).

2.6 Mycobacterial Infections

Cell-mediated immunity plays an essential role in the control of mycobacterial infections. T cells elaborate cytokines that are capable of activating macrophage antibacterial activities [25]. It is this cell-mediated response that is responsible for controlling primary infection with *Mycobacterium tuberculosis*. Conditions that compromise cell-mediated immunity allow the infection to spread and cause symptomatic disease [25]. Mycobacterial infection in such patients frequently becomes far advanced before it is suspected and diagnosed.

The association between tuberculosis and Hodgkin's disease [HD] or hairy cell leukemia has been well described [26–29]. Tuberculosis can precede the diagnosis of HD, occur concomitantly, or develop during treatment for HD. It can also develop after HD therapy has been completed, making it difficult to differentiate it from refractory or relapsed disease. These features were highlighted in a recent retrospective review of 70 pediatric patients with HD [26]. Fourteen of these patients (20 %) had pulmonary tuberculosis. In three, tuberculosis was diagnosed before HD, two had both entities concomitantly, in seven it occurred during treatment, and in two patients it was diagnosed post HD therapy. Cough and fever were the most common symptoms, and diffuse pulmonary infiltrates with or without mediastinal enlargement were the most common radiographic findings. Specific therapy resulted in response in all 14 patients.

Nontuberculous mycobacterial infections are less common than tuberculosis in patients with malignant lymphomas [30–33]. They produce pulmonary infections, lymphadenitis, soft-tissue infections, and disseminated disease [30]. The species isolated most often are *M. avium-intracellulare*, *M. abscessus*, *M. chelonae*, *M. fortuitum*, *M. kansasii*, and *M. marinum*. Prolonged, multiple drug therapy is usually administered for actively progressive infection. A detailed discussion of the diagnostic and therapeutic strategies for mycobacterial infections is beyond the scope of this chapter. However, specific guidelines dealing with these issues are available [34, 35].

2.7 Fungal Infections

Invasive mold infections caused primarily by *Aspergillus* species, and less frequently by the zygomycetes, *Fusarium* species, and other filamentous fungi are seen not only in patients with prolonged neutropenia but also in those with impaired cellular immunity and prolonged corticosteroid usage. Pneumonia is the most common manifestation of invasive mold infections although fungemia and dissemination to other organs, particularly the CNS, can occur. The clinical manifestations, radiographic features, and histopathologic finding of infections caused by these fungi are often indistinguishable from each other. The diagnosis and management of these infections has been dealt with in detail elsewhere in this volume.

Pneumocystis pneumonia (PCP) has traditionally been associated with impaired cell-mediated immunity resulting in reactivation of a dormant infection [36]. The clinical presentation is usually subacute. Common clinical features include fever, a nonproductive cough, and progressive dyspnea. Often the presentation is subacute, and consequently a high index of suspicion is necessary in the right setting. Patients at risk for PCP who are not receiving prophylaxis and who develop elevated LDH levels often have smoldering infection and should undergo appropriate diagnostic evaluation. The most common radiographic finding is a diffuse bilateral reticulonodular pulmonary infiltrate although atypical lesions such as granulomatous pulmonary nodules have been described [37]. The diagnosis is usually made by demonstrating the organisms on respiratory specimens (including biopsy tissue) using a number of special stains (methenamine silver, Wright-Giemsa, or immunofluorescent staining). High-dose trimethoprim/sulfamethoxazole (TMP/SMX) is the agent of choice for the treatment of PCP and is also strongly recommended for prophylaxis in high-risk patients.

Rituximab is a chimeric human/murine monoclonal antibody which targets the B-cell-specific antigen CD20. It has been used effectively for the treatment of B-cell lymphoma. In recent years, several reports have documented the increasing frequency of PCP in patients with aggressive B-cell lymphoma being treated with R-CHOP 14 (biweekly rituximab, cyclophosphamide, Adriamycin, and prednisone) but not with R-CHOP 21 (the same regimen given every 3 weeks) [38]. Most of these patients were not severely immunosuppressed with CD4+ T lymphocyte counts being >200/mm^3 and immunoglobulin levels being within the normal range. It has been postulated by some investigators that the reason for the increased risk of PCP is the greater intensity of corticosteroid exposure as well as the cumulative corticosteroid dose [38]. Others have suggested that B-cell depletion caused by rituximab may play a role in increasing the risk of PCP [39]. PCP prophylaxis is now strongly recommended in this subset of patients and has been shown to be effective [40].

Cryptococcosis is caused by two sibling species, *Cryptococcus neoformans* and *Cryptococcus gattii*. The primary site of infection is the lung which follows the inhalation of cryptococcal spores [41]. Dissemination usually involving the CNS occurs in severe cases. Both species cause infection in immunocompetent and immunosuppressed individuals. Several reports have noted the association between cryptococcosis, lymphoproliferative disorders (especially lymphomas), and impaired cell-mediated immunity [42]. In recent reports chemotherapy regimens which include rituximab have been implicated as a risk factor for cryptococcosis [43–45]. Fever and meningeal symptoms are the most common manifestations of cryptococcal meningitis. Cerebrospinal fluid (CSF) abnormalities include raised CSF opening pressure, lymphocytosis, elevated proteins, and low glucose levels. The diagnosis is made by visualization of the organism in the CSF by India Ink staining and/or its recovery on culture. Cryptococcal antigen is also detected in CSF and serum in most cases. Induction therapy with amphotericin B (or its lipid formulations) plus 5-fluorocytosine, followed by maintenance therapy with fluconazole, is the current standard of care. Detailed guidelines for the management of cryptococcosis have been published [46]. Histoplasmosis is far less common than cryptococcosis in cancer patients with impaired cell-mediated immunity [47]. It can cause pulmonary, CNS, or disseminated infection and should be considered in the differential diagnosis in endemic areas of the world.

2.8 Parasitic Infections

Toxoplasmosis is one of the most common parasitic infestations in man. Most cases in immunocompetent individuals are asymptomatic [48]. Disseminated disease which can often be fulminant generally occurs in immunocompromised individuals, with the CNS, lungs, and heart being the most common sites of involvement. Toxoplasmosis has occasionally been described in patients with lymphoproliferative disorders (primarily lymphomas). Even in this setting, disseminated toxoplasmosis usually occurs after allogeneic HSCT has resulted in increased immunosuppression [49–52]. In a review of 2,574 transplant procedures performed at 16 participating centers, the Gruppo Italiano Malattie Ematologiche dell'Adulto (GIMEMA) found the incidence of toxoplasmosis to be 1.9/1,000 in autologous transplant recipients and 8/1,000 in allogeneic transplant recipients [53]. The group postulated that the relative rarity of toxoplasmosis in this setting was probably due to difficulties in establishing a diagnosis and due to the administration of prophylaxis with TMP/SMX, since such patients are also at risk for PCP.

Many cases are diagnosed postmortem. Consequently, in the right clinical setting, a high index of suspicion needs to be maintained and the appropriate battery of diagnostic tests needs to be ordered. Computerized tomography (CT) or magnetic resonance imaging (MRI) of the brain reveals multiple hypodense lesions, often with moderate contrast ring enhancement. The diagnosis can be confirmed by serological testing or biopsy, if feasible. Empiric therapy against *Toxoplasma gondii* is often administered in immunosuppressed individuals with encephalopathy and ring-enhancing CNS lesions while other diagnostic information is pending. Specific therapy consists of pyrimethamine plus sulfadiazine, or spiramycin. Alternative agents such as clindamycin, atovaquone, and TMP/SMX have also been used for treatment and/or prophylaxis.

Strongyloides stercoralis is a soil-transmitted helminth that has been estimated to infect 3–100 million people globally, primarily in tropical and subtropical regions but also in Europe and the United States. Lymphoma is the most common malignancy associated with strongyloidiasis [54]. Inhibition of cell-mediated immunity, humoral immunity, or mucosal immunity may trigger transformation from the rhabditiform to the filariform larval form of the parasite. This may be followed by migration from the small intestine to the lungs or gastrointestinal tracts (hyperinfection syndrome) or other organs (disseminated disease) [55]. Immunosuppression induced by corticosteroids often triggers the development of hyperinfection or dissemination. The most common clinical features include fever accompanied by gastrointestinal symptoms such as diarrhea and abdominal pain/cramping. Pulmonary infiltrates and pleural effusions which are often hemorrhagic can develop, followed by respiratory insufficiency/failure [56]. Concomitant bacteremia most often caused by enteric gram-negative bacilli *(E. coli*, *Klebsiella* species, *P. aeruginosa*) and anaerobes (*Bacteroides* species) occurs not infrequently and is often polymicrobial. Up to 55 % of patients with disseminated infection may develop meningitis. Diagnosis is based on demonstrating the organisms in stools, and respiratory or other appropriate samples, and by serological (ELISA) testing. Ivermectin is the therapeutic agent of choice with thiabendazole and albendazole being alternatives. Guidelines for the prevention and management of strongyloidiasis are limited and not definitive. Screening of high-risk patients (allogeneic HSCT recipients, corticosteroid usage) is recommended particularly in endemic areas.

Babesiosis is a tick-borne malaria-like illness caused by intraerythrocytic protozoa, *Babesia microti*, in endemic areas. Although asymptomatic parasitemia can persist for up to a year or more, the infection usually resolves after the administration of a single course of antiparasitic therapy (atovaquone and azithromycin or clindamycin and quinine). Clearance of the parasites is mediated through both the innate and adaptive branches of the immune system. Persistent, relapsing babesiosis, despite repeated courses of antiparasitic therapy, usually occurs in patients with B-cell lymphoid malignancies, as highlighted in a recent report [57]. Most of these patients had also received therapy with rituximab-based regimens, which leads to severe depletion of CD20-positive B cells. Additionally, approximately three-fourths of these patients were asplenic. Such patients have higher levels of parasitemia, a stormy clinical course, and poorer outcomes than patients with intact humoral immunity. Consequently, they require anti-babesial treatment (atovaquone and azithromycin) for at least 6 weeks, including 2 weeks after the parasitemia has been cleared.

2.9 Central Nervous System Infections

Although infrequent (<10 %), CNS infections present special diagnostic and therapeutic challenges [58]. Most patients with CNS infections will have mass lesions or meningeal manifestations. Meningitis and encephalitis tend to present acutely, whereas infections that cause cerebral masses generally tend to have a subacute or chronic presentation. In patients with B-cell deficits, meningitis is generally caused by encapsulated organisms (*S. pneumoniae*, *H. influenzae*, *N. meningitidis*). In contrast, patients with impaired cellular immunity develop meningitis caused by *L. monocytogenes and Cryptococcus* species. CNS mass lesions, on the other hand, are often caused by fungi (*Aspergillus* species and less often *Mucorales*, *Cryptococcus* species, or *Histoplasma capsulatum*); bacteria such as *Nocardia* species; mycobacteria, especially *M. tuberculosis*; and parasites such as *Toxoplasma gondii*. Mass lesions in the lung and brain are suggestive *of Nocardia* or mold infection rather than toxoplasmosis. Although following a symptomatic approach and taking into consideration the underlying immunologic deficit(s) are useful strategies that can guide empiric therapy, making a specific diagnosis is essential in order to provide targeted therapy. Bacterial meningitis, cryptococcal meningitis, and tuberculosis are usually not difficult to diagnose using various stains, culture techniques, and serological testing. In contrast, patients with CNS masses usually require a tissue biopsy to arrive at a specific diagnosis. In addition to the pathogens mentioned above, meningoencephalitis can result from infection with certain viruses including HSV, VZV, CMV, and HHV6. The most common noninfectious cause of mass-like lesions is CNS lymphoma.

2.10 Pulmonary Infections

The lung is a common site of infection in patients with malignant lymphomas. The etiology of pulmonary infiltrates in this setting is varied, and in a manner similar to the management of patients with CNS infections, the onus is on establishing a specific diagnosis, based on which specific or targeted therapy can be given. Not infrequently the etiology of pulmonary infiltrates is polymicrobial, and sequential infections also occur in the face of sustained immunosuppression. Common gram-positive and gram-negative organisms, multidrug-resistant bacterial pathogens, mycobacteria, *Nocardia* species, *Pneumocystis jirovecii*, filamentous fungi, viruses, and occasionally parasitic organisms can all be responsible for pulmonary infiltrates. The diagnostic approach and overall management of patients with pulmonary infiltrates is discussed in detail elsewhere in this volume.

References

1. Siegel R, Naishadham D, Jemal A. Cancer statistics, 2013. CA Cancer J Clin. 2013;63(1):11–30.
2. Bodey GP, Buckley M, Sathe YS, Freireich EJ. Quantitative relationships between circulating leukocytes and infection in patients with acute leukemia. Ann Intern Med. 1966;64(2):328–40.
3. Freifeld AG, Bow EJ, Sepkowitz KA, et al. Clinical practice guideline for the use of antimicrobial agents in neutropenic patients with cancer: 2010 update by the infectious diseases society of america. Clin Infect Dis. 2011;52(4):e56–93.
4. Wisplinghoff H, Seifert H, Wenzel RP, Edmond MB. Current trends in the epidemiology of nosocomial bloodstream infections in patients with hematological malignancies and solid neoplasms in hospitals in the United States. Clin Infect Dis. 2003;36(9):1103–10.
5. Shelburne SA, Tarrand J, Rolston KV. Review of streptococcal bloodstream infections at a comprehensive cancer care center, 2000–2011. J Infect. 2013;66(2):136–46.
6. Kumashi P, Girgawy E, Tarrand JJ, Rolston KV, Raad II, Safdar A. Streptococcus pneumoniae bacteremia in patients with cancer: disease characteristics and outcomes in the era of escalating drug resistance (1998–2002). Medicine (Baltimore). 2005;84(5):303–12.
7. Mitchell R, Trück J, Pollard AJ. Use of the 13-valent pneumococcal conjugate vaccine in children and adolescents aged 6–17 years. Expert Opin Biol Ther. 2013;13:1451–65.

8. Torres HA, Reddy BT, Raad II, et al. Nocardiosis in cancer patients. Medicine (Baltimore). 2002;81(5):388–97.
9. Sakai C, Takagi T, Satoh Y. Nocardia asteroides pneumonia, subcutaneous abscess and meningitis in a patient with advanced malignant lymphoma: successful treatment based on in vitro antimicrobial susceptibility. Intern Med. 1999;38(8):683–6.
10. Enomoto M, Yamasawa H, Sawai T, Bando M, Ohno S, Sugiyama Y. Pulmonary nocardiosis with bilateral diffuse granular lung shadows in a patient with subcutaneous panniculitic T-cell lymphoma. Intern Med. 2002;41(11):986–9.
11. Gradel KO, Nørgaard M, Dethlefsen C, et al. Increased risk of zoonotic Salmonella and Campylobacter gastroenteritis in patients with haematological malignancies: a population-based study. Ann Hematol. 2009;88(8):761–7.
12. Li CW, Chen PL, Lee NY, et al. Non-typhoidal Salmonella bacteremia among adults: an adverse prognosis in patients with malignancy. J Microbiol Immunol Infect. 2012;45(5):343–9.
13. Beyazit Y, Guven GS, Kocak T, Kekilli M. Salmonella meningitis in an adult patient with central nervous system lymphoma. Eur J Intern Med. 2005;16(5):377–8.
14. Pacanowski J, Lalande V, Lacombe K, et al. Campylobacter bacteremia: clinical features and factors associated with fatal outcome. Clin Infect Dis. 2008;47(6):790–6.
15. Hughes RA, Cornblath DR. Guillain-Barré syndrome. Lancet. 2005;366(9497):1653–66.
16. Sejvar JJ, Kohl KS, Gidudu J, et al. Guillain-Barré syndrome and Fisher syndrome: case definitions and guidelines for collection, analysis, and presentation of immunization safety data. Vaccine. 2011;29(3):599–612.
17. Mencacci A, Corbucci C, Castellani A, Furno P, Bistoni F, Vecchiarelli A. Legionella pneumophila serogroup 3 pneumonia in a patient with low-grade 4 non-Hodgkin lymphoma: a case report. J Med Case Rep. 2011;5:387.
18. Leoni E, De Luca G, Legnani PP, Sacchetti R, Stampi S, Zanetti F. Legionella waterline colonization: detection of Legionella species in domestic, hotel and hospital hot water systems. J Appl Microbiol. 2005;98(2):373–9.
19. Liu WK, Healing DE, Yeomans JT, Elliott TS. Monitoring of hospital water supplies for Legionella. J Hosp Infect. 1993;24(1):1–9.
20. Miyara T, Tokashiki K, Shimoji T, Tamaki K, Koide M, Saito A. Rapidly expanding lung abscess caused by Legionella pneumophila in immunocompromised patients: a report of two cases. Intern Med. 2002;41(2):133–7.
21. Singh J, Batish VK, Grover S. Simultaneous detection of Listeria monocytogenes and Salmonella spp. in dairy products using real time PCR-melt curve analysis. J Food Sci Technol. 2012;49(2):234–9.
22. Pricope-Ciolacu L, Nicolau AI, Wagner M, Rychli K. The effect of milk components and storage conditions on the virulence of Listeria monocytogenes as determined by a Caco-2 cell assay. Int J Food Microbiol. 2013;166(1):59–64.
23. Rivero GA, Torres HA, Rolston KV, Kontoyiannis DP. Listeria monocytogenes infection in patients with cancer. Diagn Microbiol Infect Dis. 2003;47(2):393–8.
24. Martino R, Rámila E, Capdevila JA, et al. Bacteremia caused by Capnocytophaga species in patients with neutropenia and cancer: results of a multicenter study. Clin Infect Dis. 2001;33(4):E20–2.
25. Dannenberg AM. Delayed-type hypersensitivity and cell-mediated immunity in the pathogenesis of tuberculosis. Immunol Today. 1991;12(7):228–33.
26. Karakas Z, Agaoglu L, Taravari B, et al. Pulmonary tuberculosis in children with Hodgkin's lymphoma. Hematol J. 2003;4(1):78–81.
27. Costa LJ, Gallafrio CT, França FO, del Giglio A. Simultaneous occurrence of Hodgkin disease and tuberculosis: report of three cases. South Med J. 2004;97(7):696–8.
28. Melero M, Gennaro O, Domínguez C, Sánchez Avalos JC. Tuberculosis in patients with lymphomas. Medicina (B Aires). 1992;52(4):291–5.
29. Codrich D, Monai M, Pelizzo G, et al. Primary pulmonary Hodgkin's disease and tuberculosis in an 11-year-old boy: case report and review of the literature. Pediatr Pulmonol. 2006;41(7):694–8.
30. Chen CY, Sheng WH, Lai CC, et al. Mycobacterial infections in adult patients with hematological malignancy. Eur J Clin Microbiol Infect Dis. 2012;31(6):1059–66.

31. Wei MC, Banaei N, Yakrus MA, Stoll T, Gutierrez KM, Agarwal R. Nontuberculous mycobacteria infections in immunocompromised patients: single institution experience. J Pediatr Hematol Oncol. 2009;31(8):556–60.
32. Gupta S, Cogbill CH, Gheorghe G, et al. Mycobacterium avium intracellulare infection coexistent with nodular lymphocyte predominant Hodgkin lymphoma involving the lung. J Pediatr Hematol Oncol. 2011;33(3):e127–31.
33. Han XY, Tarrand JJ, Infante R, Jacobson KL, Truong M. Clinical significance and epidemiologic analyses of Mycobacterium avium and Mycobacterium intracellulare among patients without AIDS. J Clin Microbiol. 2005;43(9):4407–12.
34. World Health Organization, Stop TB Initiative (World Health Organization). Treatment of tuberculosis: guidelines. 4th ed. Geneva: World Health Organization; 2010.
35. Blumberg HM, Burman WJ, Chaisson RE, et al. American Thoracic Society/Centers for Disease Control and Prevention/Infectious Diseases Society of America: treatment of tuberculosis. Am J Respir Crit Care Med. 2003;167(4):603–62.
36. Obeid KM, Aguilar J, Szpunar S, et al. Risk factors for Pneumocystis jirovecii pneumonia in patients with lymphoproliferative disorders. Clin Lymphoma Myeloma Leuk. 2012;12(1):66–9.
37. Kumar N, Bazari F, Rhodes A, Chua F, Tinwell B. Chronic Pneumocystis jiroveci presenting as asymptomatic granulomatous pulmonary nodules in lymphoma. J Infect. 2011;62(6):484–6.
38. Kamel S, O'Connor S, Lee N, Filshie R, Nandurkar H, Tam CS. High incidence of Pneumocystis jirovecii pneumonia in patients receiving biweekly rituximab and cyclophosphamide, adriamycin, vincristine, and prednisone. Leuk Lymphoma. 2010;51(5):797–801.
39. Tadmor T, McLaughlin P, Polliack A. A resurgence of Pneumocystis in aggressive lymphoma treated with R-CHOP-14: the price of a dose-dense regimen? Leuk Lymphoma. 2010;51(5):737–8.
40. Hardak E, Oren I, Dann EJ, et al. The increased risk for pneumocystis pneumonia in patients receiving rituximab-CHOP-14 can be prevented by the administration of trimethoprim/sulfamethoxazole: a single-center experience. Acta Haematol. 2012;127(2):110–4.
41. Rolston KV. Editorial commentary: Cryptococcosis due to Cryptococcus gattii. Clin Infect Dis. 2013;57(4):552–4.
42. Kontoyiannis DP, Peitsch WK, Reddy BT, et al. Cryptococcosis in patients with cancer. Clin Infect Dis. 2001;32(11):E145–50.
43. Hirai Y, Ainoda Y, Shoji T, et al. Disseminated cryptococcosis in a non-Hodgkin's lymphoma patient with late-onset neutropenia following rituximab-CHOP chemotherapy: a case report and literature review. Mycopathologia. 2011;172(3):227–32.
44. Marchand T, Revest M, Tattevin P, et al. Early cryptococcal meningitis following treatment with rituximab, fludarabine and cyclophosphamide in a patient with chronic lymphocytic leukemia. Leuk Lymphoma. 2013;54(3):643–5.
45. Slavin MA, Chen SC. Cryptococcosis, lymphoproliferative disorders and modern day chemotherapy regimens. Leuk Lymphoma. 2013;54(3):449–50.
46. Perfect JR, Dismukes WE, Dromer F, et al. Clinical practice guidelines for the management of cryptococcal disease: 2010 update by the infectious diseases society of america. Clin Infect Dis. 2010;50(3):291–322.
47. Jones O, Cleveland KO, Gelfand MS. A case of disseminated histoplasmosis following autologous stem cell transplantation for Hodgkin's lymphoma: an initial misdiagnosis with a false-positive serum galactomannan assay. Transpl Infect Dis. 2009;11(3):281–3.
48. Hill D, Dubey JP. Toxoplasma gondii: transmission, diagnosis and prevention. Clin Microbiol Infect. 2002;8(10):634–40.
49. de Medeiros BC, de Medeiros CR, Werner B, et al. Central nervous system infections following bone marrow transplantation: an autopsy report of 27 cases. J Hematother Stem Cell Res. 2000;9(4):535–40.
50. Maschke M, Dietrich U, Prumbaum M, et al. Opportunistic CNS infection after bone marrow transplantation. Bone Marrow Transplant. 1999;23(11):1167–76.
51. Mele A, Paterson PJ, Prentice HG, Leoni P, Kibbler CC. Toxoplasmosis in bone marrow transplantation: a report of two cases and systematic review of the literature. Bone Marrow Transplant. 2002;29(8):691–8.

52. Singh N, Husain S. Infections of the central nervous system in transplant recipients. Transpl Infect Dis. 2000;2(3):101–11.
53. Pagano L, Trapè G, Putzulu R, et al. Toxoplasma gondii infection in patients with hematological malignancies. Ann Hematol. 2004;83(9):592–5.
54. Marcos LA, Terashima A, Dupont HL, Gotuzzo E. Strongyloides hyperinfection syndrome: an emerging global infectious disease. Trans R Soc Trop Med Hyg. 2008;102(4):314–8.
55. Concha R, Harrington W, Rogers AI. Intestinal strongyloidiasis: recognition, management, and determinants of outcome. J Clin Gastroenterol. 2005;39(3):203–11.
56. Win TT, Sitiasma H, Zeehaida M. Strongyloides stercoralis induced bilateral blood stained pleural effusion in patient with recurrent non-Hodgkin lymphoma. Trop Biomed. 2011;28(1):64–7.
57. Krause PJ, Gewurz BE, Hill D, et al. Persistent and relapsing babesiosis in immunocompromised patients. Clin Infect Dis. 2008;46(3):370–6.
58. Cunha BA. Central nervous system infections in the compromised host: a diagnostic approach. Infect Dis Clin N Am. 2001;15(2):567–90.

Consequences from Specific Treatment Modalities

3

Georg Maschmeyer

Contents

While the depth and duration of granulocytopenia (neutropenia) represents the most important risk factor for infections in hematologic patients, other treatment- or disease-related aspects of immunosuppression must be taken into consideration. Without wanting to provide an exhaustive review of all these aspects, the following treatment modalities will be addressed here:

- Purine analogs (fludarabine, cladribine, pentostatin)
- Monoclonal antibodies to CD20, CD52, and TNF-alpha

Most hematologic cancer patients treated with one of these compounds typically receive a combination of these and/or a combination with classical cytostatic drugs. Thus, immunosuppression associated with these treatment modalities will in general be multifactorial, e.g., cellular immunodeficiency plus neutropenia. Moreover, the underlying hematologic malignancies by themselves frequently cause immune defects such as granulocytopenia or humoral immunodeficiency. The specific aspects addressed here therefore are mostly additive to the problem of therapy-induced myelosuppression.

G. Maschmeyer
Department of Hematology, Oncology and Palliative Care, Klinikum Ernst von Bergmann, Charlottenstrasse 72, D-14467 Potsdam, Germany
e-mail: gmaschmeyer@klinikumevb.de

G. Maschmeyer, K.V.I. Rolston (eds.), *Infections in Hematology*,
DOI 10.1007/978-3-662-44000-1_3

3.1 Purine Analogs

The two purine analogs most frequently used to treat hematologic malignancies are fludarabine and cladribine (2-chlorodeoxyadenosine). Both drugs induce a profound depletion of T cells lasting for several months [1–3] and are associated with a substantial risk of opportunistic infections typically controlled by cellular immune defense: reactivation of viral infections (cytomegalovirus (CMV), varicella zoster, and herpes simplex virus), Pneumocystis pneumonia (PcP), listeriosis, candidiasis, or mycobacteriosis. Primarily, B cell lymphomas such as chronic lymphocytic leukemia (B-CLL) or hairy cell leukemia, which also inherently induce immunosuppression due to hypogammaglobulinemia, are treated with fludarabine or cladribine. When fludarabine in combination with cyclophosphamide (FC regimen) and/or the CD20 antibody rituximab (FCR), eventually also with glucocorticoids added, is used in patients with late-stage chronic lymphocytic leukemia, an approximately 60 % incidence of infections has been reported [4]. In contrast, fludarabine-based first-line treatment of B-CLL is associated with lower infection rates of around 15–20 % [5–7], which are not different to those associated with other treatment modalities such as CAP (cyclophosphamide, adriamycin, and prednisone) or CHOP (same agents plus vincristine) [8]. Also, no difference in infection rates were observed between CLL patients with fludarabine alone and those treated with FC [9] nor between patients treated with FC and those treated with FCR [7, 10]. In patients with far advanced B-CLL or other indolent lymphoma who are at higher age and have been treated with other antineoplastic regimens before, the risk of infectious complications occurring under fludarabine-based treatment can be predicted using a multiparameter risk assessment [11].

However, in many patients treated with fludarabine or cladribine, antimicrobial prophylaxis against Pneumocystis, varicella zoster, herpes simplex, and yeast infections, i.e., trimethoprim-sulfamethoxazole (TMP-SMX), acyclovir, and fluconazole, is routinely given. As a consequence, these infections (as well as toxoplasmosis, nocardiosis, or listeriosis) do not primarily have to be taken into consideration in case of fever or clinically documented infection, provided the patient has been adherent to prophylaxis. This might be different for PcP, if sulfa resistance in *Pneumocystis jirovecii* conferred by dihydropteroate synthase mutation [12, 13] is a relevant problem in the local epidemiology.

Table 3.1 shows the list of infectious agents to be taken into account in patients with fever/infection under or within several months after purine analog treatment.

As a practical consequence, in patients with fever of unknown origin after purine analog treatment, peripheral blood should be checked for CMV reactivation (pp65 or preferably PCR); patients with fever and lung infiltrates should undergo bronchoscopy and bronchoalveolar lavage (BAL) to be examined for *P. jirovecii*, CMV, mycobacteria, and filamentous fungi in addition to conventional bacteriology. Please note that the determination of CMV copies in peripheral blood does not replace testing of respiratory secretions and that in BAL, nucleic acid amplification (PCR) alone may only exclude CMV or *P. jirovecii* infection, if negative, but does not prove these infections, if positive.

Table 3.1 Microbial pathogens to consider in lymphoma patients treated with purine analogs

Pathogen
L. monocytogenes[a]
S. pneumoniae
Staphylococcus spp.
Pseudomonas spp.
Gram-negative aerobic bacilli
N. meningitidis
Candida spp.[b]
Aspergillus spp.
Cryptococcus neoformans[b]
Varicella zoster virus[c]
Herpes simplex virus[c]
Cytomegalovirus
P. jirovecii[a]
Typical and atypical mycobacteria

Adapted from Tsiodras et al. [14]

[a]Less likely among patients under trimethoprim-sulfamethoxazole prophylaxis

[b]Less likely among patients under fluconazole prophylaxis

[c]Less likely among patients under acyclovir prophylaxis

For antimicrobial treatment in these patients, a broad-spectrum beta-lactam antibiotic with activity against *P. aeruginosa* and *S. aureus*, selected on the basis of the local in vitro susceptibility patterns, should initially be administered. Once results of microbiological analyses are available, appropriate adjustment of this initial treatment is required. In single patients without reliable TMP-SMX prophylaxis, who have typical pulmonary infiltrates sparing out subpleural spaces and a rapidly increased lactate dehydrogenase (LDH) in blood, preemptive start of high-dose intravenous TMP-SMX may be indicated before BAL results are known or even before bronchoscopy is performed. BAL samples remain positive for *P. jirovecii* several days after initiation of TMP-SMX therapy [15].

3.2 Monoclonal Antibodies

3.2.1 Anti-CD20 Antibodies

Monoclonal antibodies targeting the CD20 molecule on the surface of lymphoid cancer cells, predominantly rituximab but also ofatumumab and obinutuzumab (GA101), are routinely included in the treatment of patients with CD20-positive B cell lymphoma or, in case of rituximab, acute lymphoblastic leukemia. They cause a rapid depletion of CD20-positive B cells from peripheral blood; however, this is not associated with a significant increase in infection rates [7, 10, 16]. When rituximab is used for post-remission maintenance treatment in lymphoma patients, the risk of fever and infections is higher than in comparable patients without rituximab maintenance [17, 18], but a characteristic pattern of infectious problems, e.g., as a consequence of immunoglobulin deficiency, has not been reported. Therefore, a specific diagnostic or therapeutic approach to patients who develop fever and infection after CD20 antibody treatment cannot be recommended. Severe hypogammaglobulinemia, present in many patients with indolent B cell lymphomas independently from CD20 antibody treatment, may give reason for immunoglobulin G substitution.

Apart from opportunistic bacterial or fungal infections, the risk of hepatitis B virus (HBV) reactivation is considerably increased (approximately fivefold) in rituximab-treated patients [19, 20], as is the risk of hepatitis C virus (HCV) reactivation [21]. As a consequence, serological screening for HBV and HCV is recommended for patients to be treated with these CD20 antibodies [22], and transaminases should be monitored in patients with a positive HBV or HCV serology. Apart from HBV and HCV reactivation, also the risk of progressive multifocal leukoencephalopathy (PML) has reportedly been increased in rituximab recipients, predominantly those with lymphoproliferative disease [23], so that in patients with signs or symptoms of central nervous system, a search for JC virus replication may be considered.

3.2.2 Alemtuzumab (Anti-CD52 Antibody)

The administration of alemtuzumab (Campath), typically given for treatment of B-CLL or T cell lymphoma, results in a severe lymphocytopenia lasting for more than a year. Patients with these lymphoproliferative malignancies frequently have an inherent immune deficiency, so that the combined risk of opportunistic infections is very high; however, it has been clearly shown that patients treated early in the course of their disease with alemtuzumab have a markedly lower infection rate as compared to patients with far advanced, relapsed, or refractory lymphoma [24, 25]. When given for first-line treatment in 41 patients with B-CLL, who received antimicrobial prophylaxis with TMP-SMX, acyclovir, and fluconazole, CMV reactivation has been the predominant infectious event [25]. In contrast infectious complications were observed in 55 % of 93 patients undergoing alemtuzumab therapy for relapsed and refractory CLL [26]. TMP-SMX and acyclovir prophylaxis as well as monitoring of blood samples for CMV reactivation (weekly or every other week) is mandatory. A high incidence of infections must be expected also in patients receiving systemic antimicrobial prophylaxis. Among infectious events occurring in alemtuzumab recipients, CMV reactivation and other viral infections are predominant with 40–45 %, followed by bacterial (35–40 %) and fungal (17–21 %) infections including PcP [27]. Also protozoal infections and PML have been reported in these patients [28]. Severe and fatal infections have been observed particularly in patients with B-CLL given alemtuzumab for consolidation after successful remission induction [29, 30]. A specific guideline on the use of alemtuzumab, particularly with respect to severe infections, is available [31].

Table 3.2 shows infections and pathogens documented in patients who underwent alemtuzumab treatment.

Table 3.2 Infections and microbial pathogens to consider after alemtuzumab treatment ([27, 32])

Cytomegalovirus
Herpes simplex virus
Varicella zoster virus
Human herpesvirus 6
Epstein-Barr virus
Parvovirus
Influenza
Septicemia
Pneumonia
Meningitis
Tuberculosis
Cellulitis
Fever of unknown origin
Pneumocystis pneumonia
Aspergillosis
Systemic candidiasis
Mucormycosis
Cryptococcosis
Fusariosis
Scedosporiosis
Cryptosporidiosis
Microsporidiosis

Diagnostic procedures to be considered in patients with fever or other signs of infection after alemtuzumab treatment must take the extremely broad spectrum of potential pathogens into account. Apart from conventional microbiological procedures, applied on blood cultures or other body fluids according to the respective clinical syndrome, serologic and molecular methods to detect active viral replication or to exclude pulmonary tuberculosis will often be required. In patients with persistent fever and/or signs of infection despite broad-spectrum antimicrobial treatment, invasive procedures such as bronchoscopy, fine-needle biopsy, lumbar puncture, or colonoscopy must be considered. Similar to patients who underwent purine analog treatment, antimicrobial treatment is initiated with a broad-spectrum beta-lactam antibiotic and later modified according to diagnostic findings or preemptively with respect to the presumed causative pathogen(s).

3.2.3 Antibodies to Tumor Necrosis Factor Alpha (TNF-Alpha)

Tumor necrosis factor-alpha mediates essential inflammatory responses to microbial pathogens, including release of proinflammatory cytokines such as interleukin-1beta, interleukin-6, interleukin-8, and monocyte chemoattractant protein-1 as well as of adhesion molecules and the activation of phagocytosis, T cell activation, and stimulation of antibody production by B cells. Their immunomodulatory effects are mediated via downregulation of TNF-induced expression of pattern-recognition receptors, reduction of gamma interferon production, apoptosis of monocytes, and an impairment of TNF-mediated granuloma formation [33]. TNF antagonists such as infliximab, etanercept, adalimumab, or certolizumab pegol are mainly used in patients with severe rheumatic diseases and chronic inflammatory bowel disorders, but infliximab or etanercept are also given to allogeneic hematopoietic stem cell transplant recipients with severe graft-versus-host disease (GVHD) refractory to more routine immunosuppressive treatment [34–37]. Only the latter patient group will be addressed here. While these patients are at extremely high risk of opportunistic infections already because of their underlying conditions and all of them are treated not only with TNF antagonists but also a broad array of other immunosuppressants including high doses of glucocorticoids, it has been demonstrated that the addition of the TNF antagonist infliximab to GVHD management with cyclosporine and methotrexate resulted in a significant increase of bacterial and fungal infections [38]. Published reports and reviews suggest that the risk of bacterial, viral, and fungal infection is increased in GVHD patients treated with TNF antagonists [34], and this risk apparently was higher among patients treated with infliximab than with etanercept [33]. Gram-negative as well as gram-positive bacterial infections have been documented in these patients, and among viral infections, CMV as well as respiratory viruses play a relevant role [34]. Invasive fungal infections caused by *Candida spp.*, *Aspergillus spp.*, and *Cryptococcus neoformans*, but also endemic mycoses (in affected areas), primarily histoplasmosis and coccidioidomycosis, have been reported in these patients [33]. The risk of these infections increases at a hazard ratio of 13.6 (95 % confidence interval, 2.3–80.2) in patients with severe GVHD treated with infliximab [39].

Similar to the diagnostic recommendations given above for patients treated with alemtuzumab, a simple algorithm to be applied for the clinical workup of patients fever or other signs of infection after anti-TNF treatment for GVHD cannot be given, because the whole spectrum of viral, bacterial, fungal, and protozoal pathogens must be taken into consideration – also in patients undergoing systemic antimicrobial chemoprophylaxis. With respect to their high incidence and poor prognosis after deferred treatment, opportunistic mycoses should aggressively be addressed in these patients, and systemic antimicrobial treatment should very early include a broad-spectrum antifungal agent such as liposomal amphotericin B or voriconazole.

References

1. Takada K, Danning CL, Kuroiwa T, Schlimgen R, Tassiulas IO, Davis Jr JC, Yarboro CH, Fleisher TA, Boumpas DT, Illei GG. Lymphocyte depletion with fludarabine in patients with psoriatic arthritis: clinical and immunological effects. Ann Rheum Dis. 2003;62:1112–5.
2. Seymour JF, Kurzrock R, Freireich EJ, Estey EH. 2-Chlorodeoxyadenosine induces durable remissions and prolonged suppression of CD4+ lymphocyte counts in patients with hairy cell leukemia. Blood. 1994;83:2906–11.

3. Cheson BD. Infections and immunosuppressive complications of purine analog therapy. J Clin Oncol. 1995;13:2431–48.
4. Anaissie EJ, Kontoyiannis DP, O'Brien S, Kantarjian H, Robertson L, Lerner S, Keating MJ. Infections in patients with chronic lymphocytic leukemia treated with fludarabine. Am J Med. 1998;129:559–66.
5. Eichhorst BF, Busch R, Schweighofer C, Wendtner CM, Emmerich B, Hallek M, German CLL Study Group. Due to low infection rates no routine anti-infective prophylaxis is required in younger patients with chronic lymphocytic leukaemia during fludarabine-based first line therapy. Br J Haematol. 2007;136:63–72.
6. Hensel M, Kornacker M, Yammeni S, Egerer G, Ho AD. Disease activity and pretreatment, rather than hypogammaglobulinaemia, are major risk factors for infectious complications in patients with chronic lymphocytic leukaemia. Br J Haematol. 2003;122:600–6.
7. Tam CS, Seymour JF, Brown M, Campbell P, Scarlett J, Underhill C, Ritchie D, Bond R, Grigg AP. Early and late infectious consequences of adding rituximab to fludarabine and cyclophosphamide in patients with indolent lymphoid malignancies. Haematologica. 2005;90:700–2.
8. Leporrier M, Chevret S, Cazin B, Boudjerra N, Feugier P, Desablens B, Rapp MJ, Jaubert J, Autrand C, Divine M, Dreyfus B, Maloum K, Travade P, Dighiero G, Binet JL, Chastang C. French Cooperative Group on Chronic Lymphocytic Leukemia. Randomized comparison of fludarabine, CAP, and ChOP in 938 previously untreated stage B and C chronic lymphocytic leukemia patients. Blood. 2001;98:2319–25.
9. Eichhorst BF, Busch R, Hopfinger G, Pasold R, Hensel M, Steinbrecher C, Siehl S, Jäger U, Bergmann M, Stilgenbauer S, Schweighofer C, Wendtner CM, Döhner H, Brittinger G, Emmerich B, Hallek M German CLL Study Group. Fludarabine plus cyclophosphamide versus fludarabine alone in first-line therapy of younger patients with chronic lymphocytic leukemia. Blood. 2006;107:885–91.
10. Hallek M, Fischer K, Fingerle-Rowson G, Fink AM, Busch R, Mayer J, Hensel M, Hopfinger G, Hess G, von Grünhagen U, Bergmann M, Catalano J, Zinzani PL, Caligaris-Cappio F, Seymour JF, Berrebi A, Jäger U, Cazin B, Trneny M, Westermann A, Wendtner CM, Eichhorst BF, Staib P, Bühler A, Winkler D, Zenz T, Böttcher S, Ritgen M, Mendila M, Kneba M, Döhner H, Stilgenbauer S. International group of investigators; German chronic lymphocytic leukaemia study group. Addition of rituximab to fludarabine and cyclophosphamide in patients with chronic lymphocytic leukaemia: a randomised, open-label, phase 3 trial. Lancet. 2010;376:1164–74.
11. Tam CS, Wolf MM, Januszewicz EH, Grigg AP, Prince HM, Westerman D, Seymour JF. A new model for predicting infectious complications during fludarabine-based combination chemotherapy among patients with indolent lymphoid malignancies. Cancer. 2004;101:2042–9.
12. Nahimana A, Rabodonirina M, Zanetti G, Meneau I, Francioli P, Bille J, Hauser PM. Association between a specific Pneumocystis jiroveci dihydropteroate synthase mutation and failure of pyrimethamine/sulfadoxine prophylaxis in human immunodeficiency virus-positive and -negative patients. J Infect Dis. 2003;188:1017–23.
13. Stein CR. Sulfa use, dihydropteroate synthase mutations, and Pneumocystis jirovecii pneumonia. Emerg Infect Dis. 2004;10:1760–5.
14. Tsiodras S, Samonis G, Keating MJ, Kontoyiannis DP. Infection and immunity in chronic lymphocytic leukemia. Mayo Clin Proc. 2000;75:1039–54.
15. Colangelo G, Baughman RP, Dohn MN, Frame PT. Follow-up bronchoalveolar lavage in AIDS patients with Pneumocystis carinii pneumonia. Pneumocystis carinii burden predicts early relapse. Am Rev Respir Dis. 1991;143:1067–71.
16. Coiffier B, Lepage E, Brière J, Herbrecht R, Tilly H, Bouabdallah R, Morel P, van den Neste E, Salles G, Gaulard P, Reyes F, Gisselbrecht C. CHOP chemotherapy plus rituximab compared with CHOP alone in elderly patients with diffuse large-B-cell lymphoma. N Engl J Med. 2002;346:235–42.
17. Vidal L, Gafter-Gvili A, Leibovici L, Dreyling M, Ghielmini M, Hsu Schmitz SF, Cohen A, Shpilberg O. Rituximab maintenance for the treatment of patients with follicular lymphoma: systematic review and meta-analysis of randomized trials. J Natl Cancer Inst. 2009;101:248–55.

18. Salles G, Seymour JF, Offner F, López-Guillermo A, Belada D, Xerri L, Feugier P, Bouabdallah R, Catalano JV, Brice P, Caballero D, Haioun C, Pedersen LM, Delmer A, Simpson D, Leppa S, Soubeyran P, Hagenbeek A, Casasnovas O, Intragumtornchai T, Fermé C, da Silva MG, Sebban C, Lister A, Estell JA, Milone G, Sonet A, Mendila M, Coiffier B, Tilly H. Rituximab maintenance for 2 years in patients with high tumour burden follicular lymphoma responding to rituximab plus chemotherapy (PRIMA): a phase 3, randomised controlled trial. Lancet. 2011;377:42–51.
19. Yeo W, Chan TC, Leung NW, Lam WY, Mo FK, Chu MT, Chan HL, Hui EP, Lei KI, Mok TS, Chan PK. Hepatitis B virus reactivation in lymphoma patients with prior resolved hepatitis B undergoing anticancer therapy with or without rituximab. J Clin Oncol. 2009;27:605–11.
20. Evens AM, Jovanovic BD, Su YC, Raisch DW, Ganger D, Belknap SM, Dai MS, Chiu BC, Fintel B, Cheng Y, Chuang SS, Lee MY, Chen TY, Lin SF, Kuo CY. Rituximab-associated hepatitis B virus (HBV) reactivation in lymphoproliferative diseases: meta-analysis and examination of FDA safety reports. Ann Oncol. 2011;22:1170–80.
21. Ennishi D, Maeda Y, Niitsu N, Kojima M, Izutsu K, Takizawa J, Kusumoto S, Okamoto M, Yokoyama M, Takamatsu Y, Sunami K, Miyata A, Murayama K, Sakai A, Matsumoto M, Shinagawa K, Takaki A, Matsuo K, Kinoshita T, Tanimoto M. Hepatic toxicity and prognosis in hepatitis C virus-infected patients with diffuse large B-cell lymphoma treated with rituximab-containing chemotherapy regimens: a Japanese multicenter analysis. Blood. 2010;116:5119–25.
22. Zurawska U, Hicks LK, Woo G, Bell CM, Krahn M, Chan KK, Feld JJ. Hepatitis B virus screening before chemotherapy for lymphoma: a cost-effectiveness analysis. J Clin Oncol. 2012;30:3167–73.
23. Carson KR, Evens AM, Richey EA, Habermann TM, Focosi D, Seymour JF, Laubach J, Bawn SD, Gordon LI, Winter JN, Furman RR, Vose JM, Zelenetz AD, Mamtani R, Raisch DW, Dorshimer GW, Rosen ST, Muro K, Gottardi-Littell NR, Talley RL, Sartor O, Green D, Major EO, Bennett CL. Progressive multifocal leukoencephalopathy after rituximab therapy in HIV-negative patients: a report of 57 cases from the research on adverse drug events and reports project. Blood. 2009;113:4834–40.
24. Nosari A, Tedeschi A, Ricci F, Montillo M. Characteristics and stage of the underlying diseases could determine the risk of opportunistic infections in patients receiving alemtuzumab. Haematologica. 2008;93:e30–1.
25. Lundin J, Kimby E, Bjorkholm M, Lundin J, Kimby E, Björkholm M, Broliden PA, Celsing F, Hjalmar V, Mollgard L, Rebello P, Hale G, Waldmann H, Mellstedt H, Österborg A. Phase II trial of subcutaneous anti-CD52 monoclonal antibody alemtuzumab (Campath-1H) as first-line treatment for patients with Bcell chronic lymphocytic leukemia (B-CLL). Blood. 2002;100:768–73.
26. Keating MJ, Flinn I, Jain V, Binet JL, Hillmen P, Byrd J, Albitar M, Brettman L, Santabarbara P, Wacker B, Rai KR. Therapeutic role of alemtuzumab (Campath-1H) in patients who have failed fludarabine: results of a large international study. Blood. 2002;99:3554–61.
27. Thursky KA, Worth LJ, Seymour JF, Thursky KA, Worth LJ, Seymour JF, Miles Prince H, Slavin MA. Spectrum of infection, risk and recommendations for prophylaxis and screening among patients with lymphoproliferative disorders treated with alemtuzumab. Br J Haematol. 2006;132:3–12.
28. Martin SI, Marty FM, Fiumara K, Treon SP, Gribben JG, Baden LR. Infectious complications associated with alemtuzumab use for lymphoproliferative disorders. Clin Infect Dis. 2006;43:16–24.
29. Lin TS, Donohue KA, Byrd JC, Lucas MS, Hoke EE, Bengtson EM, Rai KR, Atkins JN, Link BK, Larson RA. Consolidation therapy with subcutaneous alemtuzumab after fludarabine and rituximab induction therapy for previously untreated chronic lymphocytic leukemia: final analysis of CALGB 10101. J Clin Oncol. 2010;28:4500–6.
30. Wendtner CM, Ritgen M, Schweighofer CD, Wendtner CM, Ritgen M, Schweighofer CD, Fingerle-Rowson G, Campe H, Jäger G, Eichhorst B, Busch R, Diem H, Engert A, Stilgenbauer S, Döhner H, Kneba M, Emmerich B, Hallek M German CLL Study Group. Consolidation with alemtuzumab in patients with chronic lymphocytic leukemia (CLL) in first remission

-experience on safety and efficacy within a randomized multicenter phase III trial of the German CLL Study Group (GCLLSG). Leukemia. 2004;18:1093–101.

31. Österborg A, Foa R, Bezares RF, Dearden C, Dyer MJ, Geisler C, Lin TS, Montillo M, van Oers MH, Wendtner CM, Rai KR. Management guidelines for the use of alemtuzumab in chronic lymphocytic leukemia. Leukemia. 2009;23:1980–8.
32. Desoubeaux G, Caumont C, Passot C, Dartigeas C, Bailly E, Chandenier J, Duong TH. Two cases of opportunistic parasite infections in patients receiving alemtuzumab. J Clin Pathol. 2012;65:92–5.
33. Tsiodras S, Samonis G, Boumpas DT, Kontoyiannis DP. Fungal infections complicating tumor necrosis factor alpha blockade therapy. Mayo Clin Proc. 2008;83:181–94.
34. Couriel D, Saliba R, Hicks K, Ippoliti C, de Lima M, Hosing C, Khouri I, Andersson B, Gajewski J, Donato M, Anderlini P, Kontoyiannis DP, Cohen A, Martin T, Giralt S, Champlin R. Tumor necrosis factor-alpha blockade for the treatment of acute GVHD. Blood. 2004;104:649–54.
35. Alousi AM, Weisdorf DJ, Logan BR, Bolaños-Meade J, Carter S, Difronzo N, Pasquini M, Goldstein SC, Ho VT, Hayes-Lattin B, Wingard JR, Horowitz MM, Levine JE. Etanercept, mycophenolate, denileukin, or pentostatin plus corticosteroids for acute graft-versus-host disease: a randomized phase 2 trial from the blood and marrow transplant clinical trials network. Blood. 2009;114:511–7.
36. Levine JE, Paczesny S, Mineishi S, Braun T, Choi SW, Hutchinson RJ, Jones D, Khaled Y, Kitko CL, Bickley D, Krijanovski O, Reddy P, Yanik G, Ferrara JL. Etanercept plus methylprednisolone as initial therapy for acute graft-versus-host disease. Blood. 2008;111:2470–5.
37. Busca A, Locatelli F, Marmont F, Ceretto C, Falda M. Recombinant human soluble tumor necrosis factor receptor fusion protein as treatment for steroid refractory graft-versus-host disease following allogeneic hematopoietic stem cell transplantation. Am J Hematol. 2007;82:45–52.
38. Hamadani M, Hofmeister CC, Jansak B, Phillips G, Elder P, Blum W, Penza S, Lin TS, Klisovic R, Marcucci G, Farag SS, Devine SM. Addition of infliximab to standard acute graft-versus-host disease prophylaxis following allogeneic peripheral blood cell transplantation. Biol Blood Marrow Transplant. 2008;14:783–9.
39. Marty FM, Lee SJ, Fahey MM, et al. Infliximab use in patients with severe graft-versus-host disease and other emerging risk factors of non-Candida invasive fungal infections in allogeneic hematopoietic stem cell transplant recipients: a cohort study. Blood. 2003;102:2768–76.

Infections After High-Dose Chemotherapy and Autologous Hematopoietic Stem Cell Transplantation

4

Marcio Nucci and Elias Anaissie

Contents

4.1 Introduction

High-dose chemotherapy and autologous hematopoietic stem cell transplantation (HSCT) is the standard treatment for some hematologic malignancies, especially multiple myeloma (MM), lymphoma (Hodgkin's and non-Hodgkin's), and acute myeloid leukemia (AML). Infection represents an important cause of morbidity after autologous HSCT, but its frequency and etiology depends on the presence of various risk factors.

The risk of infection in autologous HSCT recipients is the result of the interaction between the host, pathogens, and environmental exposure. Infections develop when an imbalance occurs between the weakened protective defense mechanisms of the host and the virulence factors of the offending pathogen. Table 4.1 presents a list of

M. Nucci
Department of Internal Medicine, University Hospital,
Universidade Federal do Rio de Janeiro, Rio de Janeiro, Brazil

E. Anaissie (✉)
Division of Hematology/Oncology, University of Cincinnati,
Cincinnati, OH, USA
e-mail: elias114@aol.com

G. Maschmeyer, K.V.I. Rolston (eds.), *Infections in Hematology*,
DOI 10.1007/978-3-662-44000-1_4

Table 4.1 Risk factors for infection after high-dose chemotherapy and autologous hematopoietic stem cell transplantation

Risk factor for infection	Risk category: Low	Risk category: High
1. Pretransplant		
General condition including organ function		
Performance status	Good	Poor
Renal failure	No	Yes
Diabetes mellitus	No	Yes
Iron stores [1]	Normal or decreased	Increased
Age	Younger (<40 years)	Older (>65 years)
Smoking [1]	No	Yes
Underlying disease and its treatment		
Tumor burden	None	Large
Disease-related immunosuppression[a]	Absent	Present
Prior chemotherapy	None or minimal	Extensive
Receipt of purine analogues (fludarabine, cladribine, clofarabine) or monoclonal antibodies (rituximab, alemtuzumab)	No	Yes
Exposure to pathogens		
Prior history of infection[b]	No	Yes
Colonization with pathogens (bacteria, fungi)	No	Yes
Immunogenetics		
Deficiency of MBL [2, 3]	No	Yes
2. Pre-engraftment period		
Duration of neutropenia [1]	Short (<7 days)	Long (>10 days)
Stem cell source	Peripheral blood	Bone marrow
Quantity of stem cells infused[c]	>5 × 106/Kg CD34+ cells	<2 × 106/Kg CD34+ cells
Severity of oral and gastrointestinal mucositis	Absent or mild	Severe
Conditioning regimen	Less intensive	Intensive
Polymorphisms of genes associated with metabolism of chemotherapeutic agents (pharmacogenetics)	Absent	Present
Renal failure[d]	Absent	Present
Exposure to pathogens		
Nosocomial exposure to potential pathogens (water and airborne pathogens such as *Legionella*, *Aspergillus* spp. and other molds, resistant bacteria, respiratory viruses)	No	Yes
3. Post-engraftment		
T cell immune reconstitution	Fast	Delayed
Prior chemotherapy [4]	Minimal	Extensive

Table 4.1 (continued)

Risk factor for infection	Risk category: Low	High
CMV serostatus [5]	Negative	Positive
Need for additional chemotherapy to control the underlying disease[e]	No	Yes
In vitro manipulation of stem cells[c] [6, 7]	No	Yes
Exposure to pathogens		
Prior history of infection[b]	No	Yes
Community-acquired infections, especially respiratory viruses	No	Yes

MBL mannose-binding lectin, *TLR* Toll-like receptors, *CMV* cytomegalovirus

[a]Most common disease-related immunosuppression include: hypogammaglobulinemia (multiple myeloma, low-grade B-cell non-Hodgkin's lymphoma, chronic lymphocytic leukemia), T-cell mediated immunodeficiency (Hodgkin's lymphoma and certain types of non-Hodgkin's lymphoma) and neutrophil dysfunction (acute myeloid leukemia with myelodysplasia)

[b]Infections with higher risk of recurrence after autologous hematopoietic stem cell transplantation include: mycobacteriosis (tuberculosis and others), aspergillosis, pneumocystosis, cytomegalovirus, herpes simplex and varicella-zoster virus, and toxoplasmosis and strongyloidiasis

[c]In vitro manipulation of stem cells decreases the content of CD34+ and T cells, increasing the duration of neutropenia in the early post-transplant period and delaying T cell immune reconstitution after transplant

[d]Renal failure increases the risk of severe mucositis in patients with multiple myeloma receiving melphalan-based conditioning regimens

[e]Need for additional chemotherapy in lymphoma and acute myeloid leukemia is usually related to relapse of the underlying disease, whereas in multiple myeloma additional chemotherapy is usually part of the treatment strategy

risk factors for infection in the different periods: pretransplant, early pre-engraftment, and post-engraftment period. Assessment of the risk of infection in each period and the identification of patients at higher risk of specific infections are critical to the appropriate management of infectious complications after autologous HSCT.

An important and difficult element of risk assessment in autologous HSCT recipients is to quantify the risk associated with the status of the underlying disease and prior therapies. For example, a patient with MM who undergoes a first autologous HSCT after having received a short course of induction therapy with dexamethasone plus thalidomide and whose disease is under control is at lower risk for certain infections compared with a patient with the same underlying disease, but who is receiving a third or fourth autologous HSCT in the setting of relapse after multiple treatment lines.

4.2 Risk for and Epidemiology of Infection

Immunodeficiency is the key risk factor for infection in autologous HSCT recipients. It is a result of interplay between the underlying disease and its therapy and may involve breakdowns in skin and mucous membrane barriers, qualitative and

Table 4.2 Immunodeficiency in autologous hematopoietic cell transplantation

	Disruption of skin and mucous membranes	Hypogamma-globulinemia	T-cell mediated immunodefi-ciency	Neutropenia and neutrophil dysfunction
Immunodeficiency associated with untreated underlying disease				
Acute lymphoid leukemia	+	+	+++	++
Acute myeloid leukemia	+	+	+	+++
Hodgkin's lymphoma	+	−/+	+++	−/+
Non-Hodgkin's lymphoma	+	−/+	+/+++	−/+
Multiple myeloma	−	+++	−/+	+
Immunodeficiency associated with the conditioning regimen				
Corticosteroids	+	−	+++	+
Cytotoxic chemotherapy	−/+++[a]	+/++	+/+++[a]	−/+++[a]
Monoclonal antibodies	−	+/++	+/+++	+/++
Use of catheters	+++	−	−	−

(−) no, (+) mild, (++) moderate, (+++) severe

[a]Severity of mucositis and neutropenia depend on the intensity of the conditioning regimen; duration of neutropenia also depends on the stem cell dose infused and the in vitro manipulation of the stem cell product

quantitative defects in various arms of the immune system including innate immunity (neutropenia, neutrophil dysfunction), impaired production of immunoglobulins, and defective cell-mediated immunity (CMI). While autologous HSCT recipients have deficits in various arms of the immune system, the nature of the pathogens causing infection is frequently determined by the immunodeficiency that is predominant at a given time (Tables 4.2 and 4.3).

Pretransplant variables that significantly impact the risk for major infection include host factors such as poor performance status and older age, comorbidities such as diabetes and renal failure [8], iron overload [1], smoking [1], and high tumor burden. In addition, the risk and pattern of infection after autologous HSCT are strongly influenced by the intensity of prior treatment for the underlying disease and the type of treatment. For example, patients who received purine analogues and monoclonal antibodies are at increased risk for specific infections post-transplant [9, 10]. Finally, some genetic polymorphisms in genes linked to the innate immunity are associated with an increased risk of infection. In a series of 113 autologous HSCT for multiple myeloma, patients homozygous for wild-type mannose-binding lectin (MBL) 2 were at lower risk to develop septicemia compared with patients carrying the variant MBL2 [2]. In another study, MBL deficiency was associated with higher risk of bacterial infections [3].

Table 4.3 Frequent pathogens causing infection according to immunodeficiency

	Disruption of skin and mucous membranes	Hypogamma-globulinemia	T-cell mediated immunode-ficiency	Neutropenia and neutrophil dysfunction
Bacteria				
Gram-positive cocci				
Coagulase-negative staphylococci	+++	–	–	++
Staphylococcus aureus	+++	–	–	++
Viridans streptococci	+++	–	–	++
Enterococci	++	–	–	++
Streptococcus pneumoniae	–	+++	–	–
Gram-positive bacilli				
Bacillus spp.	++	–	+	++
Corynebacterium jeikeium	++	–	+	++
Listeria monocytogenes	–	–	+++	–
Gram-negative bacilli				
Enterobacteriaceae[a]	++	–	–	+++
Pseudomonas aeruginosa	++	–	–	+++
Other nonfermentative bacteria[b]	++	–	–	+++
Salmonella spp.	+	+	++	+
Legionella spp.	–	++	++	–
Anaerobes				
Clostridium difficile	++	–	–	++
Clostridium septicum	++	–	–	++
Fungi				
Yeasts				
Candida spp.[c], mucosal disease	+	–	+++	–
Candida spp.[c], invasive disease	++	–	–	+++
Cryptococcus neoformans[a]	–	–	+++	–
Trichosporon spp.	++	–	+	++
Molds (mainly *Aspergillus* spp.)[d]	–	–	++	+++
Other				
Pneumocystis jirovecii	–	–	+++	–
Viruses				

(continued)

Table 4.3 (continued)

	Disruption of skin and mucous membranes	Hypogamma-globulinemia	T-cell mediated immunode-ficiency	Neutropenia and neutrophil dysfunction
Herpes simplex	++	–	+++	++
Varicella-zoster	–	–	+++	–
Cytomegalovirus	–	–	+++	–
Epstein-Barr virus	–	+	+++	–
Respiratory viruses[e]	+	+	++	–
Hepatitis A, B and C	–	+	+	–
Parvovirus B 19	–	++	++	–
Parasites				
Strongyloides stercoralis	–	–	++	–
Toxoplasma gondii	–	–	++	–
Cryptosporidium parvum	–	+	++	–
Mycobacteria				
Mycobacterium tuberculosis	–	–	+++	–
Rapid growing mycobacteria	++	–	+	–
Mycobacterium avium complex	–	–	+++	–

(–) no, (+) occasional, (++) frequent, (+++) very frequent

[a]Most frequent: *Escherichia coli*, *Klebsiella pneumoniae*, *Enterobacter* spp;

[b]Most frequent: *Acinetobacter* spp., *Stenotrophomonas maltophilia*;

[c]Most frequent: *C. albicans*, *C. glabrata*, *C. tropicalis*, *C. parapsilosis*;

[d]Most frequent: *A. fumigatus* (~90 %), *A. flavus*, *A. terreus*, *A. niger*;

[e]Most frequent: Respiratory syncytial virus, metapneumovirus, influenza A and B, parainfluenza 1–3, adenovirus, rhinovirus, coronavirus

4.2.1 Pre-Engraftment Period

The main risk factors for infection in the pre-engraftment period are neutropenia, oral and gastrointestinal mucositis, and the presence of central venous catheters. In general, infection occurs more frequently with longer periods of neutropenia [1], and a decrease in the rates of bacteremia has been observed with the utilization of peripheral blood, instead of marrow, as the source of stem cells [11]. In addition, severe mucositis is associated with increasing risk for infection [6, 12], and indwelling venous catheters, present in virtually all ASCT recipients during the early period, may predispose to certain bloodstream infections [13].

The majority of bacterial infections during neutropenia are caused by Gram-positive organisms; *Staphylococci* (coagulase-negative and *S. aureus*), viridans *Streptococci* and the *Enterococci*; Gram-negative bacteria including the Enterobacteriaceae *Escherichia coli*, *Klebsiella* spp. and *Enterobacter* spp., and the nonfermentative bacteria *Pseudomonas aeruginosa*, *Acinetobacter* spp. and *Stenotrophomonas maltophilia* [14, 15]. In addition, patients with severe mucositis are at increased risk to develop bloodstream infections caused by anaerobes [16], alpha-hemolytic streptococci [17, 18], *Stenotrophomonas maltophilia* [19], vancomycin-resistant enterococci [20], and *Candida* spp [21, 22].

Considerable shifts in the spectrum of bacterial infections have occurred over time as a result of antimicrobial prophylaxis therapy with more severely mucotoxic drugs [23] and the widespread use of intravascular catheters. Until the late 1980s, Gram-positive and Gram-negative organisms were equally distributed as causes of bloodstream infections. The introduction of quinolone prophylaxis was associated with a significant reduction in Gram-negative infections [24] but at the cost of an increase in infections caused by Gram-positive bacteria. A reemergence of bacteremia by resistant Gram-negative organisms has been recently observed [25–27] including quinolone-resistant Enterobacteriaceae [28], extended-spectrum c-lactamase (ESBL)-producing bacteria (Enterobacteriaceae, *P. aeruginosa*, *Acinetobacter* spp., others) [29], multidrug-resistant *P. aeruginosa*, and others [30]. Infections by resistant Gram-positive organisms have also been noted with vancomycin-resistant enterococci (VRE) and nosocomial and community-acquired methicillin-resistant *S. aureus* (MRSA) [31, 32]. A more serious problem in neutropenic patients with leukemia is the marked increase in *Clostridium difficile* colitis [33, 34]. In a retrospective study in 242 autologous HSCT recipients, 157 developed diarrhea between 1 week before and 30 days after HSCT, and 135 were tested for *C. difficile* toxin A. A diagnosis of *C. difficile*- associated diarrhea (CDAD) was made in 21 subjects (15.5 %) and occurred both before (4 patients) and after (17 patients) transplant. Patients receiving mobilization with paclitaxel and growth factor were at lower risk for CDAD compared with patients mobilized with growth factors with or without cyclophosphamide. Receipt of vancomycin or cephalosporins were risk factors for CDAD [35].

Great variability exists, between and within countries, in the etiology of bacterial infections and their susceptibility profiles [36], and an intimate knowledge of the local epidemiology remains critical in applying strategies of prophylaxis, empiric antibiotic therapy, and treatment of established infection. In a study of bacteremias in 519 HSCT recipients from a single institution, Gram-positive and Gram-negative bacteria accounted for 62 and 38 % of bacteremias, respectively [26]. The rates of bacteremias decreased over the 7-year study period, but were particularly more pronounced for Gram-positive bacteria, with a drop in the ratio of Gram-positive to Gram-negative organisms from 2.7 to 1.3.

In a prospective survey of 411 HSCT in 13 Brazilian centers, 91 patients developed bacteremia in the early post-transplant period: 47 % were caused by Gram-positive, 37 % due to Gram-negative, and 16 % were due to both Gram-positive and Gram-negative bacteria. *Pseudomonas aeruginosa* (22 %), *K. pneumoniae* (19 %) and *E. coli* (17 %) were the most frequent bacteria among Gram-negative; among Gram-positive bacteria, coagulase-negative staphylococci (50 %) and *S. aureus* (23 %) accounted for the majority of infections. Multi-drug-resistant (MDR) Gram-negative bacteria were isolated in 22 % of bacteremias (5 % of all transplants), and receipt of third-generation cephalosporins was an independent risk factor for infection due to MDR bacteria [37].

During the early post-transplant period, gastrointestinal mucositis and neutropenia predispose to the occurrence of invasive candidiasis, and unless patients are receiving fluconazole prophylaxis, this is the leading invasive fungal infection in this period. With the introduction of fluconazole prophylaxis, the incidence of candidiasis decreased dramatically, with a shift in species distribution; fewer infections due to *C. albicans* and *C. tropicalis*, but increased infections caused by *C. glabrata* and *C. krusei* [38]. This may be illustrated by three epidemiologic studies. A prospective study of 16,200 HSCTs (autologous and allogeneic) in 23 centers in the USA (Transnet database) reported 217 cases of invasive candidiasis (1.3 %). *C. glabrata* was the most frequent species, accounting for 32 % of cases. Invasive candidiasis was diagnosed within 30 days after autologous HSCT in 66 % of cases, and within 4 months in 74 % of cases [39]. In a retrospective study involving 11 centers in Italy, only 16 cases of invasive candidiasis were reported among 1979 autologous HSCTs (0.8 %). Eight of the 16 cases were caused by *C. glabrata* (n=5) or *C. krusei* (n=3) [40].

Invasive aspergillosis occurs typically in patients with profound (<100 neutrophils/mm^3) and prolonged (>10–15 days) neutropenia. Because the duration of neutropenia after autologous HSCT is shorter, the incidence of invasive aspergillosis is low. However, patients with concomitant severe CMI deficiency are at risk. This group is represented by patients with lymphoma previously treated with purine analogues [41] and heavily pretreated myeloma patients [42]. We recently analyzed a cohort of 113 patients with multiple myeloma who developed invasive aspergillosis (data not published). Sixty-three episodes occurred after autologous HSCT, at a median of 16 days after transplant. In 29 of the 63 episodes (46 %), invasive aspergillosis occurred in the pre-engraftment period. Most patients had relapsed myeloma, had been heavily pretreated, and had received high doses of corticosteroids (median cumulative dose in the last 60 days of 1,380 mg patients, prednisone equivalent).

In the Transnet database, a total of 80 cases of invasive aspergillosis were diagnosed in 9534 autologous HSCT recipients (0.8 %). Forty cases were diagnosed within 30 days after transplant [39]. In the Italian retrospective study, seven cases were diagnosed in 1979 autologous HSCT recipients (0.3 %) [40]. Except for candidiasis and aspergillosis, other invasive fungal infections are rare.

Viral infections in the early post-transplant period are limited to reactivation of herpes simplex virus (HSV) and respiratory viral infections (Influenza A and B, parainfluenza 1–3, respiratory syncytial virus [RSV], metapneumovirus, and adenovirus). In the absence of prophylaxis (acyclovir or valacyclovir), most autologous HSCT recipients will develop reactivation of HSV, manifested as oral ulcers [43, 44]. The occurrence of symptomatic HSV disease is particularly frequent in patients with severe oral mucositis [45]. Although in most cases the disease is self-limited, causing pain and discomfort, it may evolve to pneumonia as a result of aspiration of the oral secretions with the virus [46].

4.2.2 Post-engraftment Period

Although the frequency and mortality of infection after engraftment are much lower than in the early pre-engraftment period, infection is a significant cause of morbidity and an important cause of non-relapse mortality. In a retrospective analysis of 1,482 autologous HSCT, 32 % of non-relapse deaths occurring after day +100 post-transplant were caused by infectious complications. Sepsis and pneumonia were the most frequent infections, and viral and fungal disease were rare causes of death [47].

The risk for infection in the post-engraftment period is a function of the dynamics of immune reconstitution. Factors that delay immune reconstitution following ASCT are related to the underlying disease and/or to the stem cell product (Table 4.1). The most important factors influencing the speed of immune reconstitution are the immune status before HSCT and the need for additional immunosuppressive treatment. Heavily pretreated patients who exhibit severe immunodeficiency before HSCT are at greater risk of infectious complications. Likewise, additional chemotherapy after HSCT greatly increases the risk of infection. This is true for patients with MM, who receive consolidation and maintenance after HSCT.

The occurrence of neutropenia increases the risk for infection after engraftment. In a study, receipt of rituximab was an independent risk factor for delayed onset neutropenia [9]. Receipt of rituximab pretransplant has also been associated with an increased risk for CMV reactivation post-transplant [10].

In vitro manipulation of stem cells is usually associated with depletion of T cells from the harvest and results in delayed immune reconstitution and an increased risk for fungal, viral, and protozoal infections [48–52]. The influence of in vitro manipulation of stem cells on the risk of infection may be illustrated by a study of 148 patients, which reported that high T-cell content in the graft was associated with a lower incidence of varicella-zoster virus (VZV) reactivation [6] and another study of autologous HSCT for autoimmune disease. A 64 % CMV reactivation was observed with in vitro CD34 selection [7]. However, in a study in patients with lymphoma, MM and breast cancer, the incidence and causes of infection were not different among patients receiving unmanipulated or CD34 selected peripheral blood stem cells [53].

The frequency and etiology of infections occurring after engraftment were assessed in 244 autologous HSCT recipients with non-Hodgkin's lymphoma ($n=207$), Hodgkin's lymphoma ($n=27$), and MM ($n=43$). Infection occurred in 64 patients (26 %). The most frequent infections were VZV disease (56 %) and bronchopneumonia (25 %). By multivariate analysis, receipt of fludarabine was the only variable associated with infection [4]. In another study in 127 patients with breast cancer, among 99 patients with prolonged follow up, 32 (32 %) developed infection in the first year post-transplant. Upper respiratory infection ($n=11$) and dermatomal VZV disease ($n=9$) were the most frequent infections. Bacteremia occurred in only two patients [54].

Cytomegalovirus (CMV) reactivation is frequent in the late post-transplant period. In a retrospective study, 16 of 41 febrile episodes in CMV seropositive patients were associated with CMV reactivation. CMV infection was the sole cause of fever [55]. In a prospective study in 171 autologous HSCT recipients, weekly CMV antigenemia was performed from engraftment until day +60 post-transplant. Forty of 102 (39 %) CMV seropositive patients presented CMV reactivation at a median of 32 days after transplant. The majority of patients ($n=30$) were asymptomatic. Fever ($n=5$) and enteritis ($n=5$) were the clinical manifestations in the remaining patients [5].

In addition to VZV and CMV, respiratory viral infections are frequent in autologous HSCT recipients and may contribute to significant morbidity, especially in patients with lymphopenia [56].

Less frequent infections in the post-transplant period include hepatitis B and C [57], toxoplasmosis [58], tuberculosis [59, 60] and pneumocystosis, [61] and, in certain areas of the globe, Chagas disease [62].

4.3 Summary

Infection represents an important cause of morbidity after autologous HSCT. Infection results from an imbalance between host defenses and the pathogen, and the risk vary according to the phase of HSCT. Pretransplant variables that significantly impact the risk for major infection include host factors, genetic predisposition, comorbid conditions, tumor burden and the type, and duration and intensity of prior chemo- or radiotherapy. After HSCT and before engraftment, significant risk factors include neutropenia, mucositis, and central venous catheters. In the post-engraftment period, the risk of infection depends on the dynamics of the immune reconstitution that follows HSCT. Assessment of the risk of infection in each period and the identification of patients at higher risk of specific infections are critical to the appropriate management of infectious complications after autologous HSCT.

References

1. Miceli MH, Dong L, Grazziutti ML, et al. Iron overload is a major risk factor for severe infection after autologous stem cell transplantation: a study of 367 myeloma patients. Bone Marrow Transplant. 2006;37:857–64.
2. Molle I, Peterslund NA, Thiel S, Steffensen R. MBL2 polymorphism and risk of severe infections in multiple myeloma patients receiving high-dose melphalan and autologous stem cell transplantation. Bone Marrow Transplant. 2006;38:555–60.
3. Horiuchi T, Gondo H, Miyagawa H, et al. Association of MBL gene polymorphisms with major bacterial infection in patients treated with high-dose chemotherapy and autologous PBSCT. Genes Immun. 2005;6:162–6.
4. Ketterer N, Espinouse D, Chomarat M, et al. Infections following peripheral blood progenitor cell transplantation for lymphoproliferative malignancies: etiology and potential risk factors. Am J Med. 1999;106:191–7.
5. Rossini F, Terruzzi E, Cammarota S, et al. Cytomegalovirus infection after autologous stem cell transplantation: incidence and outcome in a group of patients undergoing a surveillance program. Transpl Infect Dis. 2005;7:122–5.
6. Zambelli A, Montagna D, Da Prada GA, et al. Evaluation of infectious complications and immune recovery following high-dose chemotherapy (HDC) and autologous peripheral blood progenitor cell transplantation (PBPC-T) in 148 breast cancer patients. Anticancer Res. 2002;22:3701–8.
7. Kohno K, Nagafuji K, Tsukamoto H, et al. Infectious complications in patients receiving autologous CD34-selected hematopoietic stem cell transplantation for severe autoimmune diseases. Transpl Infect Dis. 2009;11:318–23.

8. Sheean PM, Freels SA, Helton WS, Braunschweig CA. Adverse clinical consequences of hyperglycemia from total parenteral nutrition exposure during hematopoietic stem cell transplantation. Biol Blood Marrow Transplant. 2006;12:656–64.
9. Kato H, Yamamoto K, Matsuo K, et al. Clinical impact and predisposing factors of delayed-onset neutropenia after autologous hematopoietic stem-cell transplantation for B-cell non-Hodgkin lymphoma: association with an incremental risk of infectious events. Ann Oncol. 2010;21:1699–705.
10. Lee MY, Chiou TJ, Hsiao LT, et al. Rituximab therapy increased post-transplant cytomegalovirus complications in Non-Hodgkin's lymphoma patients receiving autologous hematopoietic stem cell transplantation. Ann Hematol. 2008;87:285–9.
11. Nosanchuk JD, Sepkowitz KA, Pearse RN, White MH, Nimer SD, Armstrong D. Infectious complications of autologous bone marrow and peripheral stem cell transplantation for refractory leukemia and lymphoma. Bone Marrow Transplant. 1996;18:355–9.
12. McCann S, Schwenkglenks M, Bacon P, et al. The Prospective Oral Mucositis Audit: relationship of severe oral mucositis with clinical and medical resource use outcomes in patients receiving high-dose melphalan or BEAM-conditioning chemotherapy and autologous SCT. Bone Marrow Transplant. 2009;43:141–7.
13. Celebi H, Akan H, Akcaglayan E, Ustun C, Arat M. Febrile neutropenia in allogeneic and autologous peripheral blood stem cell transplantation and conventional chemotherapy for malignancies. Bone Marrow Transplant. 2000;26:211–4.
14. Feld R. Bloodstream infections in cancer patients with febrile neutropenia. Int J Antimicrob Agents. 2008;32 Suppl 1:S30–3.
15. Dettenkofer M, Wenzler-Rottele S, Babikir R, et al. Surveillance of nosocomial sepsis and pneumonia in patients with a bone marrow or peripheral blood stem cell transplant: a multicenter project. Clin Infect Dis. 2005;40:926–31.
16. Lark RL, McNeil SA, VanderHyde K, Noorani Z, Uberti J, Chenoweth C. Risk factors for anaerobic bloodstream infections in bone marrow transplant recipients. Clin Infect Dis. 2001;33:338–43.
17. Ruescher TJ, Sodeifi A, Scrivani SJ, Kaban LB, Sonis ST. The impact of mucositis on alpha-hemolytic streptococcal infection in patients undergoing autologous bone marrow transplantation for hematologic malignancies. Cancer. 1998;82:2275–81.
18. Bochud PY, Eggiman P, Calandra T, Van Melle G, Saghafi L, Francioli P. Bacteremia due to viridans streptococcus in neutropenic patients with cancer: clinical spectrum and risk factors. Clin Infect Dis. 1994;18:25–31.
19. Labarca JA, Leber AL, Kern VL, et al. Outbreak of Stenotrophomonas maltophilia bacteremia in allogenic bone marrow transplant patients: role of severe neutropenia and mucositis. Clin Infect Dis. 2000;30:195–7.
20. Kuehnert MJ, Jernigan JA, Pullen AL, Rimland D, Jarvis WR. Association between mucositis severity and vancomycin-resistant enterococcal bloodstream infection in hospitalized cancer patients. Infect Control Hosp Epidemiol. 1999;20:660–3.
21. Bow EJ, Loewen R, Cheang MS, Schacter B. Invasive fungal disease in adults undergoing remission-induction therapy for acute myeloid leukemia: the pathogenetic role of the antileukemic regimen. Clin Infect Dis. 1995;21:361–9.
22. Bow EJ, Loewen R, Cheang MS, Shore TB, Rubinger M, Schacter B. Cytotoxic therapy-induced D-xylose malabsorption and invasive infection during remission-induction therapy for acute myeloid leukemia in adults. J Clin Oncol. 1997;15:2254–61.
23. Zinner SH. Changing epidemiology of infections in patients with neutropenia and cancer: emphasis on gram-positive and resistant bacteria. Clin Infect Dis. 1999;29:490–4.
24. Engels EA, Lau J, Barza M. Efficacy of quinolone prophylaxis in neutropenic cancer patients: a meta-analysis. J Clin Oncol. 1998;16:1179–87.
25. Garnica M, Maiolino A, Nucci M. Factors associated with bacteremia due to multidrug-resistant gram-negative bacilli in hematopoietic stem cell transplant recipients. Braz J Med Biol Res. 2009;42:289–93.
26. Collin BA, Leather HL, Wingard JR, Ramphal R. Evolution, incidence, and susceptibility of bacterial bloodstream isolates from 519 bone marrow transplant patients. Clin Infect Dis. 2001;33:947–53.

27. Viscoli C, Castagnola E. Treatment of febrile neutropenia: what is new? Curr Opin Infect Dis. 2002;15:377–82.
28. Cattaneo C, Quaresmini G, Casari S, et al. Recent changes in bacterial epidemiology and the emergence of fluoroquinolone-resistant Escherichia coli among patients with haematological malignancies: results of a prospective study on 823 patients at a single institution. J Antimicrob Chemother. 2008;61:721–8.
29. Trecarichi EM, Tumbarello M, Spanu T, et al. Incidence and clinical impact of extended-spectrum-beta-lactamase (ESBL) production and fluoroquinolone resistance in bloodstream infections caused by Escherichia coli in patients with hematological malignancies. J Infect. 2009;58:299–307.
30. Nouer SA, Nucci M, De-Oliveira MP, Pellegrino FL, Moreira BM. Risk factors for acquisition of multidrug-resistant Pseudomonas aeruginosa producing SPM metallo-beta-lactamase. Antimicrob Agents Chemother. 2005;49:3663–7.
31. Rolston KV. Challenges in the treatment of infections caused by gram-positive and gram-negative bacteria in patients with cancer and neutropenia. Clin Infect Dis. 2005;40 Suppl 4:S246–52.
32. Dubberke ER, Hollands JM, Georgantopoulos P, et al. Vancomycin-resistant enterococcal bloodstream infections on a hematopoietic stem cell transplant unit: are the sick getting sicker? Bone Marrow Transplant. 2006;38:813–9.
33. Dubberke ER, Reske KA, Yan Y, Olsen MA, McDonald LC, Fraser VJ. Clostridium difficile–associated disease in a setting of endemicity: identification of novel risk factors. Clin Infect Dis. 2007;45:1543–9.
34. Schalk E, Bohr UR, Konig B, Scheinpflug K, Mohren M. Clostridium difficile-associated diarrhoea, a frequent complication in patients with acute myeloid leukaemia. Ann Hematol. 2010;89:9–14.
35. Arango JI, Restrepo A, Schneider DL, et al. Incidence of Clostridium difficile-associated diarrhea before and after autologous peripheral blood stem cell transplantation for lymphoma and multiple myeloma. Bone Marrow Transplant. 2006;37:517–21.
36. Maschmeyer G, Haas A. The epidemiology and treatment of infections in cancer patients. Int J Antimicrob Agents. 2008;31:193–7.
37. Oliveira AL, De SM, Carvalho-Dias VM, et al. Epidemiology of bacteremia and factors associated with multi-drug-resistant gram-negative bacteremia in hematopoietic stem cell transplant recipients. Bone Marrow Transplant. 2007;39:775–81.
38. Abi-Said D, Anaissie E, Uzun O, Raad I, Pinzcowski H, Vartivarian S. The epidemiology of hematogenous candidiasis caused by different Candida species. Clin Infect Dis. 1997;24:1122–8.
39. Kontoyiannis DP, Marr KA, Park BJ, et al. Prospective surveillance for invasive fungal infections in hematopoietic stem cell transplant recipients, 2001–2006: overview of the Transplant-Associated Infection Surveillance Network (TRANSNET) Database. Clin Infect Dis. 2010;50:1091–100.
40. Pagano L, Caira M, Nosari A, et al. Fungal infections in recipients of hematopoietic stem cell transplants: results of the SEIFEM B-2004 study–Sorveglianza Epidemiologica Infezioni Fungine Nelle Emopatie Maligne. Clin Infect Dis. 2007;45:1161–70.
41. Gil L, Kozlowska-Skrzypczak M, Mol A, Poplawski D, Styczynski J, Komarnicki M. Increased risk for invasive aspergillosis in patients with lymphoproliferative diseases after autologous hematopoietic SCT. Bone Marrow Transplant. 2009;43:121–6.
42. Nucci M, Anaissie E. Infections in patients with multiple myeloma in the era of high-dose therapy and novel agents. Clin Infect Dis. 2009;49:1211–25.
43. Wade JC, Newton B, Flournoy N, Meyers JD. Oral acyclovir for prevention of herpes simplex virus reactivation after marrow transplantation. Ann Intern Med. 1984;100:823–8.
44. Dignani MC, Mykietiuk A, Michelet M, et al. Valacyclovir prophylaxis for the prevention of Herpes simplex virus reactivation in recipients of progenitor cells transplantation. Bone Marrow Transplant. 2002;29:263–7.
45. Ramphal R, Grant RM, Dzolganovski B, et al. Herpes simplex virus in febrile neutropenic children undergoing chemotherapy for cancer: a prospective cohort study. Pediatr Infect Dis J. 2007;26:700–4.
46. Taplitz RA, Jordan MC. Pneumonia caused by herpesviruses in recipients of hematopoietic cell transplants. Semin Respir Infect. 2002;17:121–9.

47. Jantunen E, Itala M, Siitonen T, et al. Late non-relapse mortality among adult autologous stem cell transplant recipients: a nation-wide analysis of 1,482 patients transplanted in 1990–2003. Eur J Haematol. 2006;77:114–9.
48. Nachbaur D, Fink FM, Nussbaumer W, et al. CD34+–selected autologous peripheral blood stem cell transplantation (PBSCT) in patients with poor-risk hematological malignancies and solid tumors. A single-centre experience. Bone Marrow Transplant. 1997;20:827–34.
49. Nachbaur D, Kropshofer G, Feichtinger H, Allerberger F, Niederwieser D. Cryptosporidiosis after CD34-selected autologous peripheral blood stem cell transplantation (PBSCT). Treatment with paromomycin, azithromycin and recombinant human interleukin-2. Bone Marrow Transplant. 1997;19:1261–3.
50. Miyamoto T, Gondo H, Miyoshi Y, et al. Early viral complications following CD34-selected autologous peripheral blood stem cell transplantation for non-Hodgkin's lymphoma. Br J Haematol. 1998;100:348–50.
51. Rutella S, Pierelli L, Sica S, Rumi C, Leone G. Transplantation of autologous peripheral blood progenitor cells: impact of CD34-cell selection on immunological reconstitution. Leuk Lymphoma. 2001;42:1207–20.
52. Nishio M, Koizumi K, Endo T, Fujimoto K, Koike T, Sawada K. Diminished T-cell recovery after CD34(+) selected autologous peripheral blood stem cell transplantation increases the risk of cytomegalovirus infection. Haematologica. 2001;86:667–8.
53. Frere P, Pereira M, Fillet G, Beguin Y. Infections after CD34-selected or unmanipulated autologous hematopoietic stem cell transplantation. Eur J Haematol. 2006;76:102–8.
54. Barton T, Collis T, Stadtmauer E, Schuster M. Infectious complications the year after autologous bone marrow transplantation or peripheral stem cell transplantation for treatment of breast cancer. Clin Infect Dis. 2001;32:391–5.
55. Fassas AB, Bolanos-Meade J, Buddharaju LN, et al. Cytomegalovirus infection and non-neutropenic fever after autologous stem cell transplantation: high rates of reactivation in patients with multiple myeloma and lymphoma. Br J Haematol. 2001;112:237–41.
56. Martino R, Porras RP, Rabella N, et al. Prospective study of the incidence, clinical features, and outcome of symptomatic upper and lower respiratory tract infections by respiratory viruses in adult recipients of hematopoietic stem cell transplants for hematologic malignancies. Biol Blood Marrow Transplant. 2005;11:781–96.
57. Zschiedrich S, Fischer R, Schmitt-Graff A, Blum H, Breidert M. Acute hepatitis after autologous stem cell transplantation and rapid progression to liver cirrhosis. Eur J Gastroenterol Hepatol. 2010;22:1141–4.
58. Gonzalez-Vicent M, Diaz MA, Sevilla J, Madero L. Cerebral toxoplasmosis following etanercept treatment for idiophatic pneumonia syndrome after autologous peripheral blood progenitor cell transplantation (PBPCT). Ann Hematol. 2003;82:649–53.
59. de la Camara R, Martino R, Granados E, et al. Tuberculosis after hematopoietic stem cell transplantation: incidence, clinical characteristics and outcome. Spanish Group on Infectious Complications in Hematopoietic Transplantation. Bone Marrow Transplant. 2000;26:291–8.
60. Cordonnier C, Martino R, Trabasso P, et al. Mycobacterial infection: a difficult and late diagnosis in stem cell transplant recipients. Clin Infect Dis. 2004;38:1229–36.
61. Chen CS, Boeckh M, Seidel K, et al. Incidence, risk factors, and mortality from pneumonia developing late after hematopoietic stem cell transplantation. Bone Marrow Transplant. 2003;32:515–22.
62. Altclas J, Sinagra A, Dictar M, et al. Chagas disease in bone marrow transplantation: an approach to preemptive therapy. Bone Marrow Transplant. 2005;36:123–9.

Microbiological Background 5

Murat Akova

Contents

5.1 Introduction

The epidemiology of infections in hematological cancer patients is complex and usually reflects the local characteristics. Bacterial infections are far more frequent than any other microbial infections, and among them resistance to antimicrobials is of great concern. For the last 40 years, the single most important risk factor for severe infection has been neutropenia, the highest frequency of infections occurring in those with $<100/\text{mm}^3$. The dynamics of neutropenia is also operative for the incidence of bacterial and fungal infection, so those patients undergoing intensive

M. Akova
Department of Infectious Diseases, Hacettepe University School of Medicine, Ankara, Turkey
e-mail: Akova.murat@gmail.com

G. Maschmeyer, K.V.I. Rolston (eds.), *Infections in Hematology*,
DOI 10.1007/978-3-662-44000-1_5

chemotherapy and with a decreasing neutrophil count of between 1,000 and 500/ mm^3 are considered to be at risk. The epidemiology of bacterial and fungal infections are affected by well-described, several other factors such as invasive procedures applied during hospitalization including indwelling vascular and other catheters, type and intensity of chemotherapy, presence of mucositis, use of antibacterial and antifungal prophylaxis, hematopoietic stem cell transplantation (HSCT), presence of severe graft-versus-host disease (GVHD), and environmental exposure to pathogens (e.g., diet, air filtration, hospital hygiene) [113]. Local patterns of antimicrobial usage not only in cancer patients in a given institution but in any other setting including the community may also affect the microbiology involved in hematology patients. Recently, increased use of monoclonal antibodies for therapeutic purposes has also contributed to the changing epidemiology and frequency of infections in these patient population [74].

5.2 Bacterial Infections

The epidemiology of bacterial infections shows great variability between institutions and geographic localizations [4]. Epidemiological trends have also changed during the past three decades for which International Antimicrobial Therapy Group of the European Organization for Research and Treatment of Cancer (IATG-EORTC) data can be used as an example. Since the early 1970s this group has run several trials in febrile neutropenic cancer patients and data for the epidemiology of bacterial infections including the frequency of single-agent bacteremias are available. Gram-negative enteric pathogens and *Pseudomonas aeruginosa* were dominating microorganisms in patients with bacteremia until mid-1980s when a swift change occurred that Gram-positive bacteria (GPB) have become more frequent (Fig. 5.1). During the 1970s when the earlier trials of IATG-EORTC were undertaken, 59–71 % of single-agent bacteremia were caused by Gram-negatives [114],

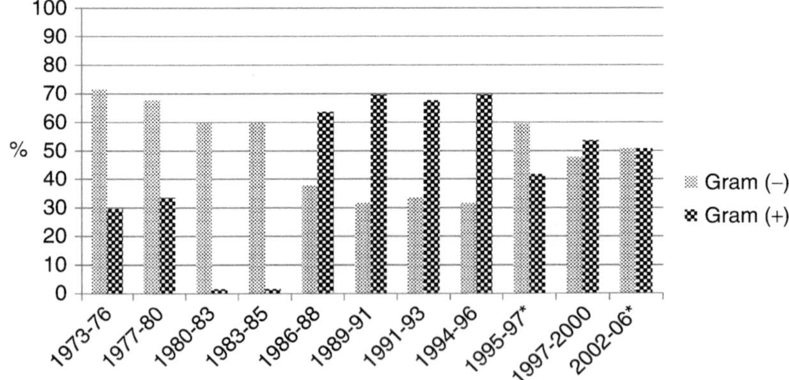

Fig. 5.1 Frequency of single-agent bacteremia in IATC-EORTC trials

whereas during the 1980s and 1990s, the same organisms were responsible for only 31–37 % of bacteremic episodes [202]. The reasons of this shift have not been studied in detail, but it was assumed that it coincided with increased use of indwelling catheters to which Gram-positives tend to adhere, introduction of more aggressive chemotherapy regimens leading to severe mucosal damage, and prophylactic and early empirical broad-spectrum antimicrobial therapy targeting mainly Gram-negative bacteria (GNB) [11, 54, 211].

Since the turn of the twenty-first century, the reports emerged indicating that GNB have gained importance again but this time with increased resistance to available broad-spectrum agents [24, 25, 29, 31, 34, 38, 41, 44, 47, 50, 67, 88, 98, 104, 105, 152, 154, 158, 198]. The latest published trial of EORTC-IATG including high-risk patients [54] found that 47 % of all bacteremic episodes were due to GNB. Whereas in the two recent EORTC trials [107, 109] in which patients were considered having low-risk neutropenia, the incidence of Gram-negative bacteremias rose to 59 and 50 %, respectively. But one should note that these trials included more patients with solid tumors and the frequencies of patients with acute leukemia were 32 and 51 %, respectively. Reemergence of Gram-negative bacterial infections has also been reported from other cancer centers [92, 152, 154]: Collin et al. [53] observed a decline in ratio of GPB/GNB from 2.7 to 2.3 between 1991 and 1997. Similarly, Mikulska et al. [139] reported from a single center in Italy with patients undergoing HSCTs that the ratio of GPB/GNB decreased from 2.4 in 2004 to 1 in 2007 ($p = .043$). Unpublished data from the most recent European Conference on Infections in Leukaemia (ECIL) group also indicated that several European cancer centers recently observed a similar increase of GNB in neutropenic cancer patients; however, GPB are still a majority in bloodstream infections (BSIs) [140].

If one compares epidemiology between different countries, in general, US centers reported that GPB are still the predominant microorganisms in cancer patients [210]. Elsewhere, many surveillance studies provided data that the incidence of GNB has become numerically higher than GPB in hematological cancer or hematopoietic stem cell transplant (HSCT) recipients [8, 41, 86, 88]. Interestingly, GNB dominance or equivalence to GPB was usually reported from outside the United States including studies from Brazil [198], Guatemala [23], Japan [50], and several southeastern Asian [25, 48, 49, 98] and Mediterranean countries [44, 86, 88, 104, 105, 158]. But similar reports from some of the Western European countries have also been available [67, 179]. The reasons for this geographical variation are not clear but may be related to the lack of widespread quinolone prophylaxis in at least some of these centers reporting more infections with GNB [86, 105], and in those still using this type of prophylaxis, emerging fluoroquinolone (FQ)-resistant *E. coli* bacteremias can be accounted for this epidemiology [44, 108]. Another theory which has originally been proposed about the spread of carbapenemase-producing enteric GNB may also be applicable to cancer patients in those countries where environmental sanitation is poor and resistant Gram-negative pathogens can be found in abundance in water and food [7]. Thus, via oral-fecal route, cancer patients may get colonized in the outpatient settings and when they become neutropenic with compromised gastrointestinal mucosa due to chemotherapy, they can acquire bacteremia with these resistant pathogens. It is also noteworthy that in some of these centers, GNB have been the leading pathogens during the last two decades [54, 55, 91, 110]. In our center in Ankara, we observed a similar picture [88, 105]. In a retrospective evaluation of bacteremic episodes in hematological cancer patients with febrile neutropenia, we analyzed 3,703 neutropenic episode in 2,098 patients between 2005 and 2009 [105]. Overall, single Gram-negative bacteremia were detected in 61 % of these episodes. Except 2005 (incidence of GNB, 48 %), GNB were the main type of microorganisms during all study years (range 58–66 %). A previous study dated back to 1997 reported similar figures [88].

Catheter-related bacteremic episodes in neutropenic patients are usually caused by coagulase-negative staphylococci (CNS) [1]. Gram-negatives, albeit much rare, can also be responsible for this picture [47].

5.2.1 Gram-Positive Bacteria and Their Antimicrobial Susceptibility

5.2.1.1 Coagulase-Negative Staphylococci (CNS)

Coagulase negative staphylococci are the most frequent GPB reported as the cause of BSIs in neutropenic cancer patients [1, 9, 113]. The rate of methicillin resistance in these microorganisms is high and varies between 33 and 100 % [38, 44, 88, 139]. In most instances CNS infections are associated with catheter-related BSI involving biofilm production [70]. There are 46 species of CNS described and at least 18 of them are human pathogens [26]. Several of them can cause bacteremia in neutropenic patients and these include *S. epidermidis*, *S. haemolyticus*, *S. warneri*, and *S. hominis* [26]. Antimicrobial susceptibility to glycopeptides and other anti-Gram-positive agents may differ between these species, thus identification into species level might be important when a CNS is isolated from blood cultures in febrile neutropenic cancer patients especially in case of failing antimicrobial therapy. *S. haemolyticus* may exhibit decreased glycopeptide susceptibility which is usually more augmented to teicoplanin than vancomycin [30, 73, 155, 168]. Decreased susceptibility is attributable to alterations in the cell wall's peptidoglycan rather than acquisition of resistance genes via horizontal gene transfer [144]. Resistance to linezolid has also been reported [22].

5.2.1.2 *Staphylococcus aureus*

This bacterium has been found responsible for up to 7 % of all bacteremic episodes in neutropenic cancer patients [84] with an overall mortality of 23–40 % [177]. Bacteremia is usually associated with skin and soft tissue infections and could also be catheter related. But in most patients, the focus of bacteremia remains undetected [199]. The incidence of methicillin resistance has been reported between 18 and 100 % in patients with hematological malignancies [38, 88, 139, 170, 199, 213]. But, the attributable hospital mortality rate was considerably low (3.5 %) as compared with Gram-negative bacteremias [199].

Staphylococcus aureus was shown to cause late bacteremia (occurring >50 days after transplant) in HSCT recipients, and the incidence was 6/100,000 patient days [137]. Eighty-four percent of bacteremias were community acquired and 85 % of patients had an indwelling central venous catheter (CVC) at presentation. Skin GVHD and length of hospital stay were found to be significant determinants for bacteremic episodes [137]. The incidence rate of methicillin-resistant *S. aureus* (MRSA) was 23 % compared to 38 % in blood isolates of non-HSCT patients in the same hospital during the same period. The mortality rate (15.4 %) was significantly higher as compared with the control cases. The case fatality rate of MRSA bacteremia was higher than that of methicillin-sensitive *S. aureus* (MSSA) bacteremia (33 % vs. 10 %).

Community-acquired MRSA isolates are frequently reported as the cause of skin and soft tissue infections in the United States, but relatively rare in Europe [60]. These strains are resistant to beta-lactam antibiotics but maintain susceptibility to many non-beta-lactam antibiotics. In Europe, there has been an increasing problem of transmission of MRSA from colonized livestock (mainly pigs) to those who are in contact with such animals [99]. Although it has not been described as a problem specifically in hematology patient population, it would be wise to advise patients with hematological cancer and immunosuppression to avoid such contacts.

Recently, heteroresistant vancomycin-intermediate *S. aureus* (hVISA) strains have gained importance. Although their incidence in hematology patients has not been clearly determined, infections with these isolates undermine the efficacy of glycopeptide antibiotics [63, 101, 102]. Those isolates are difficult to detect with routine microbiological work-up, and several reports indicated that patients infected with such strains with a vancomycin MIC >1.5 μg/mL may fail to standard-dose glycopeptide treatment [64, 101].

Fluoroquinolone resistance has become another major issue in staphylococci due to widespread prophylactic use of these agents [166]. The incidence is higher in MRSA isolates [34, 127].

5.2.1.3 Enterococci

Enterococci can colonize the gastrointestinal tract and may cause BSI in hematology patients. Risk factors for bacteremia in HSCT recipients include mismatched-related or cord-blood transplant, grade 3–4 mucositis, pharyngeal enterococci colonization, and previous cephalosporin use [138]. Vancomycin-resistant *E. faecium* (VRE) infections are among the most commonly reported causes of bacteremia from many hemato-oncology centers and these bacteria may cause epidemics [106, 112, 138, 169, 170, 211, 212]. Several risk factors described for colonization and for consequent bacteremia include use of broad-spectrum cephalosporins and vancomycin and AML as the underlying disease [12, 116, 145, 186]. Cross-contamination and cross-infection are common in closed units, thus maximum infection control practices including strict isolation of colonized/infected patients are required [178]. Vancomycin-resistant *E. faecium* colonization rates in HSCT recipients range from 5 to 27 % and the rate of VRE bacteremia in colonized patients is around 30 % [133, 169, 217]. Early VRE bacteremia after HSCT ranged from 3.6 to 22 % with mortality ranging from 0.04 to 85 % [11, 147, 207, 217]. In a recent study, VRE was detected as the leading cause of bacteremia occurring within 30 days of HSCT [103]. Fifty-three and a half percent of patients with bacteremia during this period had VRE. However, only 57 % had VRE colonization before transplantation, indicating that pre-HSCT screening may not identify all patients who are at risk for VRE bacteremia. Attributable mortality was 9 %.

5.2.1.4 Viridans Streptococci

These bacteria are frequently found in the oral flora and can colonize the respiratory and the female genital tracts. The prevalence of their infections varies from 7.8 % in neutropenic cancer patients to 48 % in those receiving high-dose cytosine arabinoside, cyclophosphamide, and idarubicin or undergoing HSCT [32, 55, 65]. Other predisposing factors include use of acid-lowering agents, FQ, or trimethoprim-sulfamethoxazole (TMP-SMX) prophylaxis [71, 167]. Mucositis leading to the breach of integrity of oral mucosa is a significant predisposing factor for streptococcal bacteremia. Other factors causing mucositis such as oral cavity irradiation and lack of *H. simplex* prophylaxis have also been described as risk factors [211]. Viridans streptococci may be related with septic shock [36]. Penicillin and 3rd-generation cephalosporin resistance may be a problem in some centers and may compromise the treatment [32, 55].

5.2.1.5 *Streptococcus pneumoniae*

Pneumococcal bacteremia is relatively rare and the incidence of non-bacteremic infections has not been clearly defined in neutropenic patients with cancer. However, in HSCT recipients with GVHD, impaired spleen function due to total body irradiation and decreased production of antipneumococcal antibodies may predispose patients to have invasive pneumococcal disease (IPD) [72, 117]. In a recent retrospective analysis, 135 patients with cancer and pneumococcal bacteremia were investigated [119]: 63 (52 %) had hematological malignancy and 29 (21 %) had HSCT of whom 11 had GVHD. Twenty-two percent of bacteremic episodes were breakthrough in nature. Sixteen (12 %) occurred nosocomially in which nine patients were neutropenic (56 %). Neutropenia was present only in 13 % of patients who acquired bacteremia in the outpatient setting ($p<0.0002$). Sixty-seven percent of patients had pneumonia, whereas in 16 % a catheter-related pneumococcal bacteremia was documented. Thirty-six percent of all isolates were non-susceptible to penicillin (MIC >2.0 μg/mL) and 7 % had intermediate susceptibility to ceftriaxone (MIC <2 and >0.5 μg/mL). Attributable mortality was 13.3 %; however, initial inappropriate antimicrobial therapy did not lead to increased mortality.

The overall incidence of IPD was reported as 7 per 1,000 HSCTs, being more prevalent in allogeneic recipients than in patients with auto allografts (9 vs. 5 per 1,000 HSCTs) [214]. Findings reported in a European survey identified more frequent IPD (8.63 per 1,000 HSCT) during >100 days post-transplant period as compared with 2.03/1,000 occurring during the first month post-transplant [72].

Since more than one type of effective vaccines are available against pneumococci and the new conjugated pneumococcal vaccines (CPVs) are more immunogenic than the classical polysaccharide one, CPVs should be used in HSCT recipients [61].

5.2.2 Gram-Negative Bacteria and Their Antimicrobial Susceptibility

5.2.2.1 Enteric Gram-Negatives

Emerging resistance to FQs and broad-spectrum cephalosporins in *E. coli* has become a significant concern recently, not only in neutropenic cancer patients but also in the community- and hospital-acquired infections worldwide [147, 216]. These trends have significant implications for empirical therapy with ecological and economical consequences: The infections caused by such resistant strains will cause increased use of carbapenems [191], and liberal use of these antibiotics carries the risk of emerging resistance due to carbapenemase production. This phenomenon has been well described worldwide in hospital- and community-acquired infections, but not investigated in hematology patients [7].

In Europe, EARS-NET data in 2010 indicate that *E. coli* isolated from invasive infections have an unimpeded increase in antimicrobial resistance [68]. The highest resistance was against aminopenicillins (54.2 %, ranged 33.8–83.6 %); increased resistance to third-generation cephalosporins (8.5 %, ranged 2.6–24.8 %) which was related with extended-spectrum beta-lactamase (ESBL) production in 65–100 % of isolates and to FQs (20.7 %, ranged 8.4–42.8 %) was also observed. Usually a north-to-south gradient is evident; more resistance was observed in southern Europe than in the northern countries. However, EARSS data do not specifically provide figures for cancer patients. But, several individual reports reflects the magnitude of the problem in this patient population.

Quinolone resistance in these bacteria is closely related with widespread prophylactic use of FQs in neutropenic patients [29, 43, 108, 110, 173, 190]. Quinolone prophylaxis reduces incidence of GNB in patients including those with acute leukemia and HSCT [37, 38, 59, 87]. Several metanalyses found that mortality is reduced and colonization and infection with FQ-resistant bacteria did not increase in patients receiving such prophylaxis [75–77, 97]. However, these studies usually did not report on baseline colonization in patients and did not take into account the delayed impact of FQs on emerging resistance not only to quinolones but also to the other antibiotics. Moreover, significant heterogeneity in studies that included these metanalyses occurred as well; studies spanned a long period of time including trials as old as 18 years, with different FQs with varying spectrum of activity.

Quinolone resistance has been on rise in the community due to extensive use of FQs for various indications, and patients previously exposed to these antibiotics may get colonized with FQ-resistant *E. coli* [123]. Thus, local epidemiological data need to be carefully considered before deciding FQ prophylaxis, and if given, the emergence of resistance in bacterial pathogens should be monitored closely. On the other hand, it has been shown that in areas with high prevalence of QR *E. coli*, FQ prophylaxis may safely be abandoned [83].

Quinolone resistance and extended-spectrum beta-lactamase production by *E. coli* and to a lesser extent by *K. pneumoniae* is usually a common occurrence in the same strain. Indeed, data in the literature indicated that use of FQs, previous hospitalization, and previous cancer chemotherapy were significant risk factors for selecting MDR *E. coli* (i.e., resistant to FQs plus to one other antimicrobial including extended-spectrum cephalosporins or penicillins and aminoglycosides) and causing breakthrough bacteremia [201]. In an analysis of data including 364 patients with 187 documented infections and 164 bacterial isolates in an Italian center, *E. coli* accounted for 20.1 % of all isolates and 86.8 % of these strains expressed resistance to FQs [44]. Multivariate analysis for identifying risk factors for FQ resistance found that FQ prophylaxis and neutropenia were independent factors.

Resistance profile in *K. pneumoniae* is similar to that of *E. coli*, although to a lesser extent. *Enterobacter cloacae* infections with resistant beta-lactam strains could pose another problem in neutropenic cancer patient population [85, 111, 158]. In our center, 50–65 % of *E. coli* and 7–25 % of *K. pneumoniae* blood isolates from neutropenic cancer patients between 2005 and 2009 were resistant to FQs. Resistance rates increased over the years during which FQ prophylaxis was solely used in patients with allogeneic HSCTs but not in others [105].

Availability of local surveillance data and identifying those patients who are likely to get colonized and infected with resistant *Enterobacteriaceae* have outmost importance for determining the empirical therapy since any delay for giving appropriate therapy would lead to a significant increase in mortality [56, 124, 192].

5.2.2.2 *Pseudomonas aeruginosa*

Currently the relative frequency of *P. aeruginosa* in BSI in febrile neutropenic cancer patients is around 10 % (reported range in the literature 0–30 %) [11, 41, 100, 139, 148, 189]. This figure represents a slight increase from prevalence in early 1990s. *Pseudomonas aeruginosa* is intrinsically resistant to many antimicrobials, but emergence of MDR strains (i.e., a strain resistant to ≥3 of the following antimicrobials: ciprofloxacin, ceftazidime, cefepime, aminoglycosides, piperacillin, or piperacillin-tazobactam) has become of a great concern. Previous exposure to FQs is a significant risk factor for MDR pattern [125]. Other risk factors include previous transplantation (solid organ or HSCT), hospital-acquired BSI, and prior admission to the ICU [100].

In a trial with 12 pediatric hematology centers in Italy, between 2000 and 2008, 127 patients with *P. aeruginosa* BSIs were analyzed: 31 % of isolates were MDR strains. Total mortality was 19.6 %, whereas mortality in patients infected with MDR *P. aeruginosa* was 35.8 %. Multivariate analysis indicated that MDR *P. aeruginosa* infection was the only significant factor associated with infection-related death [42].

The frequency of MDR strains in adult hematology patients was reported up to 71.1 % in a multicenter Italian trial, although the total number of patients was small ($n=38$) [189]. Resistance to carbapenems was also high and reported as 60 % (10 % in non-MDR vs. 80 % in MDR strains). Death within the 30 days of the first blood culture was 30.1 % (9.1 % for non-MDR vs. 40.1 % with MDR strains, $p=0.06$). A high mortality rate (67 %) was also reported in HSCT recipients. All these figures indicate that *P. aeruginosa* is responsible for a high mortality in hematological cancer patients, despite its prevalence which remains relatively low as compared with *Enterobacteriaceae*.

5.2.2.3 Other Non-fermentative Bacteria

Stenotrophomonas maltophilia is an ubiquitous Gram-negative bacterium with limited virulence. However, it may possess significant antimicrobial resistance and cause considerable morbidity and mortality in hematology patients [171]. The organism is unique to produce two different inducible beta-lactamases which can hydrolyze carbapenems, broad-spectrum penicillins, and cephalosporins, thus rendering these antibiotics ineffective for the treatment [6]. Other resistance determinants include a number of multidrug efflux pumps and aminoglycoside-inactivating enzymes [174]. Plasmid-mediated FQ resistance genes have also been described in *S. maltophilia* genome [175]. All of these mechanisms confer resistance to most available antibiotics for treatment of infections caused by this bacterium. Trimethoprim-sulfamethoxazole is the preferred agent for treating *S. maltophilia* infections. However, resistance to this agent has been increasingly reported and usually predicts multiresistance in these strains. Recent reports indicate increased incidence of *S. maltophilia* infections in cancer patients [156, 171]. The bacterium causes CVC-related bacteremia [17, 33] and also colonizes the respiratory tract and may result in consequent infections in patients with tracheostomy and prolonged ventilation [149]. Catheter-related bacteremia was reported to be frequently polymicrobial and prompt removal of catheter is an essential part of the treatment [33]. Gastrointestinal colonization in patients with diarrhea and with previous treatment of carbapenems has also been reported and was proposed to be a source of bacteremia in cancer patients [15, 16]. Other risk factors for *S. maltophilia* infections include neutropenia, mucosal damage, tracheostomy and mechanical ventilation, and graft-versus-host disease. Previous usage of broad-spectrum antimicrobials including carbapenems and FQs can select resistant *S. maltophilia.*

Acinetobacter baumannii infections have significantly increased worldwide, especially infecting patients mechanically ventilated in the ICU [66, 78]. MDR pattern is common with most isolates usually susceptible to only colistin in vitro.

In a recent analysis with 128 patients with hematological malignancies admitted to the ICU, 35 (27 %) develop infections with *A. baumannii*. Pneumonia was the most common site and older age, prior exposure to aminoglycosides, central venous catheterization, and the presence of a nasogastric tube were independent risk factors for infection. Mortality was related with low Glasgow coma score, prior immunosuppressive therapy, neutropenia, mechanical ventilation, and severe sepsis [194].

The frequency of *Acinetobacter* infections in hematology patients was reported to be 5–7 %, more frequently in non-neutropenic cases [49, 69, 79, 158, 198]. In Hacettepe University, we found that *A. baumannii* caused 8 % of all bacteremic episodes in hematology patients between 2005 and 2009 [105]. The incidence was lower in patients with acute leukemia and HSCT (6.25 %) as compared with cases with other hematological malignancies (10.4 %).

5.2.3 Anaerobic Bacteria

Although 0.5–17 % of all nosocomial bacteremias are caused by anaerobic bacteria [35, 215], these pathogens are usually underestimated and overlooked in hematological cancer patients.

Clostridium difficile is a major cause of nosocomial infectious diarrhea and can cause severe problems in patients with hematological cancer and HSCT [51, 141, 208]. One-year incidence in HSCT recipients was reported as 9.2 % [13] or 5.6

cases per 10,000 patient days [208]. Among the risk factors were previous chemotherapy, receipt of broad-spectrum antimicrobials, and acute GVHD. Higher rates of treatment failure with metronidazole or vancomycin have been reported in North America as compared with Europe and Asia [197]. Previous FQ use was found as the predominant risk factor for a *C. difficile*-related epidemic [159]. Moxifloxacin was more frequently associated with *C. difficile* diarrhea than levofloxacin in neutropenic patients [204].

5.2.4 Unusual Bacteria

Many rare microorganisms have been reported as the cause of infection in hematological cancer patients. Among these are a variety of enteric pathogens such as *Achromobacter* spp. and *Alcaligenes* spp. [2], *Kluyvera* spp., *Hafnia* spp., and *Rahnella* spp. [91]. Many bacteria have been reported to cause catheter-related infections and among them are *Bacillus* spp., diphtheroids, and nontuberculous mycobacteria [27]. *Rhodococcus equi* can cause cavitary pulmonary disease and brain abscesses [3, 27]. A detailed review for rare microorganisms in cancer patients was published [27].

5.3 Invasive Fungal Infections

The last three decades witnessed a dramatic increase in the incidence and variety of fungal infections that is concurrently followed by the advent of a series of new antifungal agents [121, 162]. In patients with hematological malignancies and HSCT recipients, invasive aspergillosis has become the most prevalent invasive fungal infection (IFI) starting from the 1990s. During this period the incidence of invasive candidiasis (IC) decreased due to mainly widespread use of fluconazole. Recently, several centers throughout the world have reported a significant increase of non-aspergillus molds including Zygomycetes, *Fusarium* spp., and *Scedosporium* spp. and non-candida yeasts such as *Trichosporon* spp. [157, 172].

A multicenter retrospective study between 1999 and 2003 in 18 hematology wards in Italy (SEIFEM-2004) included 11,802 patients with hematological malignancies of whom 35 % had acute leukemia as the underlying disease [151]. Sixty-four percent of IFIs were due to mold infections of which 90 were caused by *Aspergillus* spp. that is followed by Zygomycetes (4 %) and *Fusarium* spp. (4 %). *Candida albicans* accounted for 91 % of yeast infections; other yeasts included *Cryptococcus* spp. (4 %) and *Trichosporon* spp. (4 %). The incidence of mold infections was 2.9 % and for yeasts 1.6 %. Attributable mortality rates due to IFI were higher for non-aspergillus molds than aspergillus and yeasts and were as follows: *Aspergillus* spp. (42 %), Zygomycetes (64 %), *Fusarium* spp. (53 %), and *Candida* spp. (33 %).

A retrospective autopsy series in MD Anderson Cancer Center between 1989 and 2003 provided information about invasive fungal infections in patients with hematological malignancies over three different periods of time (1989–1993, 1994–1998, 1999–2003) [45]. Three hundred fourteen IFIs were identified in 1,017 autopsies (31 %) among which invasive mold infections increased significantly (19 %, 24 %, and 25 %, respectively, during the aforementioned three periods, $p=0.05$). Zygomycosis emerged as a significant pathogen (1, 4, and 3 %, respectively, $p=0.03$), whereas prevalence of invasive aspergillosis (IA) remained stable (16, 19, and 19 %, $p=0.36$) and that of invasive candidiasis decreased (13, 10, and 8 %, $p=0.07$). More recent epidemiological studies in the United States reported similar observations [115, 157].

5.3.1 *Candida* spp.

Non-albicans *Candida* spp. are the predominant agents of IC in hematological cancer patients [80, 90, 187, 203] in contrast to patients with solid tumors or those with non-hematological severe diseases acquiring candidiasis in the ICU in whom *C. albicans* are still the main infecting fungus [80, 89, 90, 187, 203]. We have observed a similar trend in a survey between 2001 and 2010 with 858 *Candida* isolates in Hacettepe University in Ankara [14]. There were 381 single isolates from the first episodes of candidemia of which 60 were from patients with hematological malignancies. Non-albicans *Candida* had a frequency of 67 % and *C. tropicalis* (33 %) and *C. parapsilosis* (18 %) were the most frequent isolates.

Two recent, large epidemiological studies from the United States reported very similar results in patients with HSCT [115, 142]: TRANSNET study conducted in 23 US transplant centers between 2001 and 2006 identified 983 IFIs in 875 HSCT recipients [115]. Invasive candidiasis accounted for 30 % of all IFIs with nonalbicans *Candida* as the causative agent in 81 % of episodes. *Candida glabrata* (32 %) and *C. parapsilosis* (16 %) were leading yeasts. PATH registry reported 250 IFIs in 234 patients with HSCT in 16 centers in the United States [142]. *Candida* was isolated from only 26 % of patients of which 77 % were non-albicans spp. Another PATH registry with invasive candidiasis included <13 % of patients with hematological cancer [93]. Non-albicans *Candida* spp. were responsible for >92 % of invasive infections in hematology patients including those with HSCT, with *C. krusei* and *C. tropicalis* being the most frequent ones. Candidemia with *C. krusei* was associated with neutropenia, prior antifungal use, hematological malignancy or HSCT, and steroid use. *Candida krusei* candidemia had the highest 12-week mortality rate (52, 9 %), whereas that of *C. parapsilosis* had the lowest (23.7 %).

In European surveys, antifungal resistance was low in *Candida* isolates except in *C. krusei* which is intrinsically resistant to fluconazole [121]. Previous fluconazole use has been described as a risk factor for selecting *C. krusei* or other resistant spp. [5, 118]. A recent worldwide surveillance study reported emerging resistance to azoles (fluconazole 7.7 %, posaconazole 5.1 %, and voriconazole 6.4 %) and echinocandins (anidulafungin 3.8 %, caspofungin 5.1 %, and micafungin 3.2 %) in *C. glabrata* isolates [164]. A similar observation was also reported from Europe [126].

5.3.2 Other Opportunistic Yeast-Like Fungi

There are many opportunistic yeast-like fungi which rarely cause fungemia and disseminated infections in patients with hematological malignancies. Among these the most frequently encountered ones are *Trichosporon* spp., *Rhodotorula* spp., and *Geotrichum* spp. [18, 136, 163].

Trichosporon spp. are the second most common yeast infections in hematological malignancy cases. Patients with acute leukemia are the most vulnerable ones to infection with this pathogen and the most frequent type of infection is catheter-related fungemia [81]. The agent is usually resistant to polyenes and echinocandins, with only reliable in vitro susceptibility to voriconazole.

Rhodotorula spp. cause infections worldwide but most frequently in the Asia-Pacific region with an attributable mortality of 15 % [193]. Catheter-related fungemia is the most frequent presentation in cancer patients [94]. Amphotericin B has good activity against this yeast and successful treatment can be obtained along with removal of the indwelling catheter.

Geotrichum spp. rarely causes IFIs in patients with acute leukemia. The agent is very similar to *Trichosporon* and widely distributed in nature. Related infections are fungemia or disseminated infection [81]. Amphotericin B and voriconazole are the most active in vitro agents [82].

5.3.3 *Aspergillus* spp.

Aspergillus fumigatus is the leading pathogen for IFI in hematology patients [115, 129–131, 142, 151]. However, other non-fumigatus strains have been emerging and include mainly *A. flavus* and *A. terreus* which are well known for their reduced amphotericin B susceptibility [122, 129, 196].

Patients with hematological malignancies and those undergoing HSCT are at the highest risk of developing IA [28, 115, 129, 131]. In the latter group, there is a bimodal distribution of the disease; decreased frequency has been observed during the early neutropenic phase after the first month of post-transplant and higher incidence after the first 100 days of transplantation [115, 129, 130, 195]. Possible explanations of this distribution are shortened duration of neutropenia during the early phase of HSCT and developing chronic GVHD during the late phase and exposure of patients to aspergillus spores in the outpatient settings. Several well-known risk factors have been described for predisposing patients to acquire IA and these include neutropenia, previous broad-spectrum antibiotic therapy, anticancer chemotherapy, respiratory tract colonization with *Aspergillus*, CMV or *Pneumocystis jirovecii* infection, and mismatched HSCT [58, 130, 132, 150, 195].

During the 2000s a decrease in attributable mortality, as low as 13 % [153], was observed in patients with IAs as compared with data from the 1990s [151, 195]. Possible explanations of this decline include tools allowing early diagnosis (i.e., use of HRCT, serum levels of galactomannan and beta-D glucan, and PCR-related diagnosis), availability of active antifungals (e.g., liposomal amphotericin B and voriconazole), non-myeloablative induction regimens, and use of peripheral stem cells for transplantation which led to less severe immunosuppression in patients [58, 150, 151].

Recently, *Aspergillus fumigatus* strains were described acquiring resistance to multiple azole drugs including itraconazole, voriconazole, and posaconazole, both in patients with hematological malignancies and also those with aspergilloma and chronic aspergillosis [62, 184, 196, 200]. Resistance is most commonly associated with point mutations in the Cyp51A gene and mutations can develop during treatment [40, 200]. Although the true incidence of this problem has yet to be determined, there is at least one study reporting very high (up to 55 %) resistance mutations in clinical samples from patients with chronic aspergillosis [62]. Resistance up to 12.8 % has been reported from patients with acute IA in Netherlands and elsewhere, and treatment failure with azoles was described [135, 185], although other reports did not confirm such high incidence [10]. In Dutch cases this resistance has been linked to agricultural consumption of fungicide azole drugs structurally related with triazoles used for the treatment of IA [151, 182, 183].

5.3.4 Zygomycetes

There are two distinct types of infections by these fungi: mucormycosis caused by *Mucorales* and entomophthoramycosis by *Entomophthorales*, the latter occurring infrequently and usually restricted to tropical areas causing skin infections [46, 115, 161, 176]. Mucormycosis is the third most common IFI after IA and IC in patients with hematological malignancies [115, 161]. In a recent analysis of 230 cases of mucormycosis from 13 European countries, hematological malignancy was the most common (44 %) underlying disease [181]. The incidence of mucormycosis was reported between 1 and 8 % in patients with acute leukemia and 0.9–2 % in patients with HSCT [161]. Prolonged and severe neutropenia, presence of uncontrolled diabetes mellitus, iron overload, trauma, and use of corticosteroid are among the other risk factors for developing mucormycosis [150, 161]. Prolonged use of voriconazole has been linked to increased incidence of mucormycosis [96, 146, 150, 180]. But this observation has not been confirmed in two recent studies [128, 209]. However, none of these studies involved patients with high-risk factors for developing invasive mold disease. It has also been proposed that patients receiving voriconazole might be more complicated transplant patients and therefore have higher baseline risk for mucormycosis [157].

Mucormycosis is related to very high mortality rate in patients with hematological malignancies, up to 100 %, depending on the type of infection and the underlying disease [115, 131, 151]. In the recent European survey, older age and prior use of caspofungin were found to be significantly associated with mortality [57, 181].

5.3.5 Other Rare Molds

Several hyaline (nonpigmented) molds can cause invasive infection in hematological cancer patients [163]. Among them *Fusarium* spp. [39] and *Scedosporium* spp. [157] are the most frequent ones, although their incidence is far less as compared with IA. The risk factors for these mold infections are similar to those of IA, neutropenia in hematological cancer patients and acute and chronic GVHD in HSCT recipients [150]. Mortality is higher than IA and usually between the range of 50 % and more than 90 % [131, 151, 157].

Fusarium spp. demonstrate high MIC values for fluconazole, itraconazole, and posaconazole and caspofungin [19–21, 143, 205]. These values vary between 1 and 4 μg/ml for amphotericin B and 0.25 and 4 μg/ml for voriconazole [19–21]. However, the correlation between in vitro susceptibility and clinical outcome is not straightforward. Both posaconazole and voriconazole have been successfully used for the treatment of fusariosis [160, 165]; as expected the success rates were much higher in those who recovered from neutropenia during the treatment [165].

Scedosporium spp. are ubiquitous pathogens with two species having medical importance: *Scedosporium apiospermum* (the anamorph of *Pseudallescheria boydii*) and *Scedosporium prolificans*. While the former mold is susceptible to itraconazole, voriconazole, and posaconazole [206], the latter is considered to be resistant to all available antifungal agents, voriconazole being the most active one with an MIC of 4 μg/mL [134]. Infections caused by these molds are associated with very high mortality rates in patients with hematologic malignancies [52, 95, 120, 160, 188].

References

1. Adler A, Yaniv I, Solter E, et al. Catheter-associated bloodstream infections in pediatric hematology-oncology patients: factors associated with catheter removal and recurrence. J Pediatr Hematol Oncol. 2006;28:23–8.
2. Aisenberg G, Rolston KV, Safdar A. Bacteremia caused by Achromobacter and Alcaligenes species in 46 patients with cancer (1989–2003). Cancer. 2004;101:2134–40.
3. Akan H, Akova M, Ataoglu H, et al. *Rhodococcus equi* and *Nocardia brasiliensis* infection of the brain and liver in a patient with acute nonlymphoblastic leukemia. Eur J Clin Microbiol Infect Dis. 1998;17:737–9.
4. Akova M. Emerging problem pathogens: a review of resistance patterns over time. Int J Infect Dis. 2006;10:S3–8.
5. Akova M, Akalin HE, Uzun O, Gur D. Emergence of *Candida krusei* infections after therapy of oropharyngeal candidiasis with fluconazole. Eur J Clin Microbiol Infect Dis. 1991;10: 598–9.
6. Akova M, Bonfiglio G, Livermore DM. Susceptibility to beta-lactam antibiotics of mutant strains of *Xanthomonas maltophilia* with high- and low-level constitutive expression of L1 and L2 beta-lactamases. J Med Microbiol. 1991;35:208–13.
7. Akova M, Daikos GL, Tzouvelekis L, Carmeli Y. Interventional strategies and current clinical experiences with carbapenemase producing Gram-negative bacteria. Clin Microbiol Infect. 2012;18:439–48.
8. Aksu G, Ruhi MZ, Akan H, et al. Aerobic bacterial and fungal infections in peripheral blood stem cell transplants. Bone Marrow Transplant. 2001;27:201–5.

9. Al-Tonbary YA, Soliman OE, Sarhan MM, et al. Nosocomial infections and fever of unknown origin in pediatric hematology/oncology unit: a retrospective annual study. World J Pediatr. 2011;7:60–4.
10. Alanio A, Sitterle E, Liance M, et al. Low prevalence of resistance to azoles in *Aspergillus fumigatus* in a French cohort of patients treated for haematological malignancies. J Antimicrob Chemother. 2011;66:371–4.
11. Almyroudis NG, Fuller A, Jakubowski A, et al. Pre- and post-engraftment bloodstream infection rates and associated mortality in allogeneic hematopoietic stem cell transplant recipients. Transpl Infect Dis. 2005;7:11–7.
12. Almyroudis NG, Lesse AJ, Hahn T, et al. Molecular epidemiology and risk factors for colonization by vancomycin-resistant *Enterococcus* in patients with hematologic malignancies. Infect Control Hosp Epidemiol. 2011;32:490–6.
13. Alonso CD, Treadway SB, Hanna DB, et al. Epidemiology and outcomes of *Clostridium difficile* infections in hematopoietic stem cell transplant recipients. Clin Infect Dis. 2012;54: 1053–63.
14. Alp S, Arikan-Akdagli S, Gulmez D, et al. Epidemiology of *Candida* bloodstream infections and antifungal susceptibility profiles: 10-year experience with 381 candidaemia episodes in a tertiary care university centre. 22nd European Congress of Clinical Microbiology and Infectious Diseases (ECCMID). Abst. No. 3233. European Society of Clinical Microbiology and Infectious Diseases (ESCMID), London.
15. Apisarnthanarak A, Fraser VJ, Dunne WM, et al. *Stenotrophomonas maltophilia* intestinal colonization in hospitalized oncology patients with diarrhea. Clin Infect Dis. 2003;37: 1131–5.
16. Apisarnthanarak A, Mayfield JL, Garison T, et al. Risk factors for *Stenotrophomonas maltophilia* bacteremia in oncology patients: a case-control study. Infect Control Hosp Epidemiol. 2003;24:269–74.
17. Araoka H, Baba M, Yoneyama A. Risk factors for mortality among patients with *Stenotrophomonas maltophilia* bacteremia in Tokyo, Japan, 1996–2009. Eur J Clin Microbiol Infect Dis. 2010;29:605–8.
18. Arendrup MC, et al. ESCMID and ECMM joint clinical guidelines for the diagnosis and management of rare invasive yeast infections. Clin Microbiol Infect. 2014;20 Suppl 3:76–98.
19. Arikan S, Lozano-Chiu M, Paetznick V, Nangia S, Rex JH. Microdilution susceptibility testing of amphotericin B, itraconazole, and voriconazole against clinical isolates of *Aspergillus* and *Fusarium* species. J Clin Microbiol. 1999;37:3946–51.
20. Arikan S, Lozano-Chiu M, Paetznick V, Rex JH. In vitro susceptibility testing methods for caspofungin against *Aspergillus* and *Fusarium* isolates. Antimicrob Agents Chemother. 2001;45:327–30.
21. Arikan S, Lozano-Chiu M, Paetznick V, Rex JH. In vitro synergy of caspofungin and amphotericin B against *Aspergillus* and *Fusarium* spp. Antimicrob Agents Chemother. 2002;46: 245–7.
22. Ashour HM, el-Sharif A. Microbial spectrum and antibiotic susceptibility profile of Gram-positive aerobic bacteria isolated from cancer patients. J Clin Oncol. 2007;25:5763–9.
23. Asturias EJ, Corral JE, Quezada J. Evaluation of six risk factors for the development of bacteremia in children with cancer and febrile neutropenia. Curr Oncol. 2010;17:59–63.
24. Bakhshi S, Padmanjali KS, Arya LS. Infections in childhood acute lymphoblastic leukemia: an analysis of 222 febrile neutropenic episodes. Pediatr Hematol Oncol. 2008;25:385–92.
25. Baskaran ND, Gan GG, Adeeba K, Sam IC. Bacteremia in patients with febrile neutropenia after chemotherapy at a university medical center in Malaysia. Int J Infect Dis. 2007;11:513–7.
26. Becker K, vonEiff C. Staphylococcus, micrococcus, and other catalase-positive cocci. In: Versalovic J, editor. Manual of Clinical Microbiology. 10th ed. Washington, DC: ASM Press; 2012. p. 308–30.

27. Beebe JL, Koneman EW. Recovery of uncommon bacteria from blood: association with neoplastic disease. Clin Microbiol Rev. 1995;8:336–56.
28. Bhatti Z, Shaukat A, Almyroudis NG, Segal BH. Review of epidemiology, diagnosis, and treatment of invasive mould infections in allogeneic hematopoietic stem cell transplant recipients. Mycopathologia. 2006;162:1–15.
29. Bhusal Y, Mihu CN, Tarrand JJ, Rolston KV. Incidence of fluoroquinolone-resistant and extended-spectrum beta-lactamase-producing *Escherichia coli* at a comprehensive cancer center in the United States. Chemotherapy. 2011;57:335–8.
30. Biavasco F, Vignaroli C, Varaldo PE. Glycopeptide resistance in coagulase-negative staphylococci. Eur J Clin Microbiol Infect Dis. 2000;19:403–17.
31. Blahova J, Kralikova K, Krcmery Sr V, et al. Four years of monitoring antibiotic resistance in microorganisms from bacteremic patients. J Chemother. 2007;19:665–9.
32. Blijlevens NM, Donnelly JP, de Pauw BE. Empirical therapy of febrile neutropenic patients with mucositis: challenge of risk-based therapy. Clin Microbiol Infect. 2001;7 Suppl 4:47–52.
33. Boktour M, Hanna H, Ansari S, et al. Central venous catheter and *Stenotrophomonas maltophilia* bacteremia in cancer patients. Cancer. 2006;106:1967–73.
34. Bonadio M, Morelli G, Mori S, et al. Fluoroquinolone resistance in hematopoietic stem cell transplant recipients with infectious complications. Biomed Pharmacother. 2005;59:511–6.
35. Brook I. The role of anaerobic bacteria in bacteremia. Anaerobe. 2010;16:183–9.
36. Bruckner L, Gigliotti F. Alpha-hemolytic streptococcal infections among immunocompromised hosts: increasing incidence, severity and antibiotic resistance. Pediatr Infect Dis J. 2002;21: 343–5.
37. Bucaneve G, Micozzi A, Menichetti F, et al. Levofloxacin to prevent bacterial infection in patients with cancer and neutropenia. N Engl J Med. 2005;353:977–87.
38. Busca A, Cavecchia I, Locatelli F, et al. Blood stream infections after allogeneic stem cell transplantation: a single-center experience with the use of levofloxacin prophylaxis. Transpl Infect Dis. 2012;14:40–8.
39. Campo M, Lewis RE, Kontoyiannis DP. Invasive fusariosis in patients with hematologic malignancies at a cancer center: 1998–2009. J Infect. 2010;60:331–7.
40. Camps SM, van der Linden JW, Li Y, et al. Rapid induction of multiple resistance mechanisms in *Aspergillus fumigatus* during azole therapy: a case study and review of the literature. Antimicrob Agents Chemother. 2012;56:10–6.
41. Cappellano P, Viscoli C, Bruzzi P, et al. Epidemiology and risk factors for bloodstream infections after allogeneic hematopoietic stem cell transplantation. New Microbiol. 2007;30:89–99.
42. Caselli D, Cesaro S, Ziino O, et al. Multidrug resistant *Pseudomonas aeruginosa* infection in children undergoing chemotherapy and hematopoietic stem cell transplantation. Haematologica. 2010;95:1612–5.
43. Castagnola E, Caviglia I, Pistorio A, et al. Bloodstream infections and invasive mycoses in children undergoing acute leukaemia treatment: a 13-year experience at a single Italian institution. Eur J Cancer. 2005;41:1439–45.
44. Cattaneo C, Quaresmini G, Casari S, et al. Recent changes in bacterial epidemiology and the emergence of fluoroquinolone-resistant *Escherichia coli* among patients with haematological malignancies: results of a prospective study on 823 patients at a single institution. J Antimicrob Chemother. 2008;61:721–8.
45. Chamilos G, Luna M, Lewis RE, et al. Invasive fungal infections in patients with hematologic malignancies in a tertiary care cancer center: an autopsy study over a 15-year period (1989–2003). Haematologica. 2006;91:986–9.
46. Chayakulkeeree M, Ghannoum MA, Perfect JR. Zygomycosis: the re-emerging fungal infection. Eur J Clin Microbiol Infect Dis. 2006;25:215–29.
47. Chee L, Brown M, Sasadeusz J, MacGregor L, Grigg AP. Gram-negative organisms predominate in Hickman line-related infections in non-neutropenic patients with hematological malignancies. J Infect. 2008;56:227–33.

48. Chen CY, Tang JL, Hsueh PR, et al. Trends and antimicrobial resistance of pathogens causing bloodstream infections among febrile neutropenic adults with hematological malignancy. J Formos Med Assoc. 2004;103:526–32.
49. Chen CY, Tsay W, Tang JL, et al. Epidemiology of bloodstream infections in patients with haematological malignancies with and without neutropenia. Epidemiol Infect. 2010;138:1044–51.
50. Chong Y, Yakushiji H, Ito Y, Kamimura T. Cefepime-resistant Gram-negative bacteremia in febrile neutropenic patients with hematological malignancies. Int J Infect Dis. 2010;14 Suppl 3:e171–5.
51. Chopra T, Chandrasekar P, Salimnia H, et al. Recent epidemiology of *Clostridium difficile* infection during hematopoietic stem cell transplantation. Clin Transplant. 2011;25:E82–7.
52. Chowdhary A, Meis JF, Guarro J, et al. ESCMID and ECMM joint clinical guidelines for the diagnosis and management of systemic phaeohyphomycosis: diseases caused by black fungi. Clin Microbiol Infect. 2014;20 Suppl 3:47–75.
53. Collin BA, Leather HL, Wingard JR, Ramphal R. Evolution, incidence, and susceptibility of bacterial bloodstream isolates from 519 bone marrow transplant patients. Clin Infect Dis. 2001;33:947–53.
54. Cometta A, Kern WV, De Bock R, et al. Vancomycin versus placebo for treating persistent fever in patients with neutropenic cancer receiving piperacillin-tazobactam monotherapy. Clin Infect Dis. 2003;37:382–9.
55. Cordonnier C, Buzyn A, Leverger G, et al. Epidemiology and risk factors for gram-positive coccal infections in neutropenia: toward a more targeted antibiotic strategy. Clin Infect Dis. 2003;36:149–58.
56. Cordonnier C, Herbrecht R, Buzyn A, et al. Risk factors for Gram-negative bacterial infections in febrile neutropenia. Haematologica. 2005;90:1102–9.
57. Cornely OA, Arikan-Akdagli S, Dannaoui E, et al. ESCMID and ECMM joint clinical guidelines for the diagnosis and management of mucormycosis 2013. Clin Microbiol Infect. 2014;20 Suppl 3:5–26.
58. Cornillet A, Camus C, Nimubona S, et al. Comparison of epidemiological, clinical, and biological features of invasive aspergillosis in neutropenic and nonneutropenic patients: a 6-year survey. Clin Infect Dis. 2006;43:577–84.
59. Craig M, Cumpston AD, Hobbs GR, et al. The clinical impact of antibacterial prophylaxis and cycling antibiotics for febrile neutropenia in a hematological malignancy and transplantation unit. Bone Marrow Transplant. 2007;39:477–82.
60. David MZ, Daum RS. Community-associated methicillin-resistant *Staphylococcus aureus*: epidemiology and clinical consequences of an emerging epidemic. Clin Microbiol Rev. 2010;23:616–87.
61. Debbache K, Varon E, Hicheri Y, et al. The epidemiology of invasive *Streptococcus pneumoniae* infections in onco-haematology and haematopoietic stem cell transplant patients in France. Are the serotypes covered by the available anti-pneumococcal vaccines? Clin Microbiol Infect. 2009;15:865–8.
62. Denning DW, Park S, Lass-Florl C, et al. High-frequency triazole resistance found in nonculturable *Aspergillus fumigatus* from lungs of patients with chronic fungal disease. Clin Infect Dis. 2011;52:1123–9.
63. Deresinski S. Counterpoint: Vancomycin and Staphylococcus aureus-an antibiotic enters obsolescence. Clin Infect Dis. 2007;44:1543–8.
64. Dhand A, Sakoulas G. Reduced vancomycin susceptibility among clinical *Staphylococcus aureus* isolates ('the MIC Creep'): implications for therapy. F1000 Med Rep. 2012;4:4.
65. Donnelly JP, Dompeling EC, Meis JF, de Pauw BE. Bacteremia due to oral viridans streptococci in neutropenic patients with cancer: cytostatics are a more important risk factor than antibacterial prophylaxis. Clin Infect Dis. 1995;20:469–70.
66. Durante-Mangoni E, Zarrilli R. Global spread of drug-resistant *Acinetobacter baumannii*: molecular epidemiology and management of antimicrobial resistance. Future Microbiol. 2011;6:407–22.

67. Dutronc H, Billhot M, Dupon M, et al. Management of 315 neutropenic febrile episodes in a cancer center. Med Mal Infect. 2009;39:388–93.
68. ECDC. Antimicrobial resistance surveillance in Europe 2010. Annual Report of the European Antimicrobial Resistance Surveillance Network (EARS-Net). Stockholm, ECDC. 2011. http://www.ecdc.europa.eu/en/publications/Publications/1111_SUR_AMR_data.pdf. Accessed 19 Mar 2012.
69. El-Mahallawy H, Sidhom I, El-Din NH, Zamzam M, El-Lamie MM. Clinical and microbiologic determinants of serious bloodstream infections in Egyptian pediatric cancer patients: a one-year study. Int J Infect Dis. 2005;9:43–51.
70. Elishoov H, Or R, Strauss N, Engelhard D. Nosocomial colonization, septicemia, and Hickman/Broviac catheter-related infections in bone marrow transplant recipients. A 5-year prospective study. Medicine (Baltimore). 1998;77:83–101.
71. Elting LS, Bodey GP, Keefe BH. Septicemia and shock syndrome due to viridans streptococci: a case-control study of predisposing factors. Clin Infect Dis. 1992;14:1201–7.
72. Engelhard D, Cordonnier C, Shaw PJ, et al. Early and late invasive pneumococcal infection following stem cell transplantation: a European Bone Marrow Transplantation survey. Br J Haematol. 2002;117:444–50.
73. Falcone M, Micozzi A, Pompeo ME, et al. Methicillin-resistant staphylococcal bacteremia in patients with hematologic malignancies: clinical and microbiological retrospective comparative analysis of *S. haemolyticus*, *S. epidermidis* and *S. aureus*. J Chemother. 2004;16:540–8.
74. Faraci M, Lanino E, Morreale G, et al. Bacteremias and invasive fungal diseases in children receiving etanercept for steroid-resistant acute GVHD. Bone Marrow Transplant. 2011;46:159–60.
75. Gafter-Gvili A, Fraser A, Paul M, Leibovici L. Meta-analysis: antibiotic prophylaxis reduces mortality in neutropenic patients. Ann Intern Med. 2005;142:979–95.
76. Gafter-Gvili A, Fraser A, Paul M, et al. Antibiotic prophylaxis for bacterial infections in afebrile neutropenic patients following chemotherapy. Cochrane Database Syst Rev. 2012;1:CD004386.
77. Gafter-Gvili A, Paul M, Fraser A, Leibovici L. Effect of quinolone prophylaxis in afebrile neutropenic patients on microbial resistance: systematic review and meta-analysis. J Antimicrob Chemother. 2007;59:5–22.
78. Garnacho-Montero J, Amaya-Villar R. Multiresistant *Acinetobacter baumannii* infections: epidemiology and management. Curr Opin Infect Dis. 2010;23:332–9.
79. Ghosh I, Raina V, Kumar L, et al. Profile of infections and outcome in high-risk febrile neutropenia: experience from a tertiary care cancer center in India. Med Oncol. 2011;29:1354–60.
80. Girmenia C, Martino P, De Bernardis F, et al. Rising incidence of *Candida parapsilosis* fungemia in patients with hematologic malignancies: clinical aspects, predisposing factors, and differential pathogenicity of the causative strains. Clin Infect Dis. 1996;23:506–14.
81. Girmenia C, Pagano L, Martino B, et al. Invasive infections caused by *Trichosporon species* and *Geotrichum capitatum* in patients with hematological malignancies: a retrospective multicenter study from Italy and review of the literature. J Clin Microbiol. 2005;43:1818–28.
82. Girmenia C, Pizzarelli G, D'Antonio D, Cristini F, Martino P. In vitro susceptibility testing of *Geotrichum capitatum*: comparison of the E-test, disk diffusion, and Sensititre colorimetric methods with the NCCLS M27-A2 broth microdilution reference method. Antimicrob Agents Chemother. 2003;47:3985–8.
83. Gomez L, Garau J, Estrada C, et al. Ciprofloxacin prophylaxis in patients with acute leukemia and granulocytopenia in an area with a high prevalence of ciprofloxacin-resistant *Escherichia coli*. Cancer. 2003;97:419–24.
84. Gonzalez-Barca E, Carratala J, Mykietiuk A, Fernandez-Sevilla A, Gudiol F. Predisposing factors and outcome of *Staphylococcus aureus* bacteremia in neutropenic patients with cancer. Eur J Clin Microbiol Infect Dis. 2001;20:117–9.

85. Greenberg D, Moser A, Yagupsky P, et al. Microbiological spectrum and susceptibility patterns of pathogens causing bacteraemia in paediatric febrile neutropenic oncology patients: comparison between two consecutive time periods with use of different antibiotic treatment protocols. Int J Antimicrob Agents. 2005;25:469–73.
86. Gudiol C, Tubau F, Calatayud L, et al. Bacteraemia due to multidrug-resistant Gram-negative bacilli in cancer patients: risk factors, antibiotic therapy and outcomes. J Antimicrob Chemother. 2011;66:657–63.
87. Guthrie KA, Yong M, Frieze D, Corey L, Fredricks DN. The impact of a change in antibacterial prophylaxis from ceftazidime to levofloxacin in allogeneic hematopoietic cell transplantation. Bone Marrow Transplant. 2010;45:675–81.
88. Guven GS, Uzun O, Cakir B, Akova M, Unal S. Infectious complications in patients with hematological malignancies consulted by the infectious diseases team: a retrospective cohort study (1997–2001). Support Care Cancer. 2006;14:52–5.
89. Hachem R, Hanna H, Kontoyiannis D, Jiang Y, Raad I. The changing epidemiology of invasive candidiasis: *Candida glabrata* and *Candida krusei* as the leading causes of candidemia in hematologic malignancy. Cancer. 2008;112:2493–9.
90. Hope W, Morton A, Eisen DP. Increase in prevalence of nosocomial non-*Candida albicans* candidaemia and the association of *Candida krusei* with fluconazole use. J Hosp Infect. 2002;50:56–65.
91. Hoppe JE, Herter M, Aleksic S, Klingebiel T, Niethammer D. Catheter-related *Rahnella aquatilis* bacteremia in a pediatric bone marrow transplant recipient. J Clin Microbiol. 1993;31:1911–2.
92. Horasan ES, Ersoz G, Tombak A, Tiftik N, Kaya A. Bloodstream infections and mortality-related factors in febrile neutropenic cancer patients. Med Sci Monit. 2011;17:CR304–9.
93. Horn DL, Neofytos D, Anaissie EJ, et al. Epidemiology and outcomes of candidemia in 2019 patients: data from the prospective antifungal therapy alliance registry. Clin Infect Dis. 2009;48:1695–703.
94. Hsueh PR, Teng LJ, Ho SW, Luh KT. Catheter-related sepsis due to *Rhodotorula glutinis*. J Clin Microbiol. 2003;41:857–9.
95. Husain S, Munoz P, Forrest G, et al. Infections due to *Scedosporium apiospermum* and *Scedosporium prolificans* in transplant recipients: clinical characteristics and impact of antifungal agent therapy on outcome. Clin Infect Dis. 2005;40:89–99.
96. Imhof A, Balajee SA, Fredricks DN, Englund JA, Marr KA. Breakthrough fungal infections in stem cell transplant recipients receiving voriconazole. Clin Infect Dis. 2004;39:743–6.
97. Imran H, Tleyjeh IM, Arndt CA, et al. Fluoroquinolone prophylaxis in patients with neutropenia: a meta-analysis of randomized placebo-controlled trials. Eur J Clin Microbiol Infect Dis. 2008;27:53–63.
98. Jin J, Lee YM, Ding Y, et al. Prospective audit of febrile neutropenia management at a tertiary university hospital in Singapore. Ann Acad Med Singapore. 2010;39:453–9.
99. Johnson AP. Methicillin-resistant *Staphylococcus aureus*: the European landscape. J Antimicrob Chemother. 2011;66 Suppl 4:iv43–8.
100. Johnson LE, D'Agata EM, Paterson DL, et al. *Pseudomonas aeruginosa* bacteremia over a 10-year period: multidrug resistance and outcomes in transplant recipients. Transpl Infect Dis. 2009;11:227–34.
101. Jones RN. Key considerations in the treatment of complicated staphylococcal infections. Clin Microbiol Infect. 2008;14 Suppl 2:3–9.
102. Jones RN. Microbiological features of vancomycin in the 21st century: minimum inhibitory concentration creep, bactericidal/static activity, and applied breakpoints to predict clinical outcomes or detect resistant strains. Clin Infect Dis. 2006;42 Suppl 1:S13–24.
103. Kamboj M, Chung D, Seo SK, et al. The changing epidemiology of vancomycin-resistant *Enterococcus* (VRE) bacteremia in allogeneic hematopoietic stem cell transplant (HSCT) recipients. Biol Blood Marrow Transplant. 2010;16:1576–81.

104. Kanafani ZA, Dakdouki GK, El-Chammas KI, et al. Bloodstream infections in febrile neutropenic patients at a tertiary care center in Lebanon: a view of the past decade. Int J Infect Dis. 2007;11:450–3.
105. Kara O, Zarakolu P, Ascioglu S, Buyukasik Y, Akova M. Changing epidemiology with emerging resistance of bloodstream infections due to Gram-negative bacteria in patients with hematologic malignancies. 50th Interscience Conference on Antimicrobial Agents and Chemotherapy (ICAAC). Abstract no. K-959. American Society for Microbiology: Boston.; 2010.
106. Kawalec M, Kedzierska J, Gajda A, et al. Hospital outbreak of vancomycin-resistant enterococci caused by a single clone of *Enterococcus raffinosus* and several clones of *Enterococcus faecium*. Clin Microbiol Infect. 2007;13:893–901.
107. Kern WV, Cometta A, De Bock R, et al. Oral versus intravenous empirical antimicrobial therapy for fever in patients with granulocytopenia who are receiving cancer chemotherapy. International Antimicrobial Therapy Cooperative Group of the European Organization for Research and Treatment of Cancer. N Engl J Med. 1999;341:312–8.
108. Kern WV, Klose K, Jellen-Ritter AS, et al. Fluoroquinolone resistance of *Escherichia coli* at a cancer center: epidemiologic evolution and effects of discontinuing prophylactic fluoroquinolone use in neutropenic patients with leukemia. Eur J Clin Microbiol Infect Dis. 2005;24:111–8.
109. Kern WV, Marchetti O, Drgona L, et al. Oral antibiotics for fever in low-risk neutropenic patients with cancer: a double-blind, randomized, multicenter trail comparing single daily moxifloxacin with twice daily ciprofloxacin plus amoxicillin/clavulanic acid combination therapy-EORTC infectious diseases group trial XV. J Clin Oncol. 2013;31:1149–56.
110. Kern WV, Steib-Bauert M, de With K, et al. Fluoroquinolone consumption and resistance in haematology-oncology patients: ecological analysis in two university hospitals 1999–2002. J Antimicrob Chemother. 2005;55:57–60.
111. Kirby JT, Fritsche TR, Jones RN. Influence of patient age on the frequency of occurrence and antimicrobial resistance patterns of isolates from hematology/oncology patients: report from the Chemotherapy Alliance for Neutropenics and the Control of Emerging Resistance Program (North America). Diagn Microbiol Infect Dis. 2006;56:75–82.
112. Kirdar S, Sener AG, Arslan U, Yurtsever SG. Molecular epidemiology of vancomycin-resistant *Enterococcus faecium* strains isolated from haematological malignancy patients in a research hospital in Turkey. J Med Microbiol. 2010;59:660–4.
113. Klastersky J, Ameye L, Maertens J, et al. Bacteraemia in febrile neutropenic cancer patients. Int J Antimicrob Agents. 2007;30 Suppl 1:S51–9.
114. Klastersky J, Zinner SH, Calandra T, et al. Empiric antimicrobial therapy for febrile granulocytopenic cancer patients: lessons from four EORTC trials. Eur J Cancer Clin Oncol. 1988;24 Suppl 1:S35–45.
115. Kontoyiannis DP, Marr KA, Park BJ, et al. Prospective surveillance for invasive fungal infections in hematopoietic stem cell transplant recipients, 2001–2006: overview of the Transplant-Associated Infection Surveillance Network (TRANSNET) Database. Clin Infect Dis. 2010;50:1091–100.
116. Kraft S, Mackler E, Schlickman P, Welch K, DePestel DD. Outcomes of therapy: vancomycin-resistant enterococcal bacteremia in hematology and bone marrow transplant patients. Support Care Cancer. 2011;19:1969–74.
117. Kulkarni S, Powles R, Treleaven J, et al. Chronic graft versus host disease is associated with long-term risk for pneumococcal infections in recipients of bone marrow transplants. Blood. 2000;95:3683–6.
118. Kullberg BJ, Verweij PE, Akova M, et al. European expert opinion on the management of invasive candidiasis in adults. Clin Microbiol Infect. 2011;17 Suppl 5:1–12.
119. Kumashi P, Girgawy E, Tarrand JJ, et al. *Streptococcus pneumoniae* bacteremia in patients with cancer: disease characteristics and outcomes in the era of escalating drug resistance (1998–2002). Medicine (Baltimore). 2005;84:303–12.

120. Lamaris GA, Chamilos G, Lewis RE, et al. *Scedosporium* infection in a tertiary care cancer center: a review of 25 cases from 1989–2006. Clin Infect Dis. 2006;43:1580–4.
121. Lass-Florl C. The changing face of epidemiology of invasive fungal disease in Europe. Mycoses. 2009;52:197–205.
122. Lass-Florl C, Griff K, Mayr A, et al. Epidemiology and outcome of infections due to *Aspergillus terreus*: 10-year single centre experience. Br J Haematol. 2005;131:201–7.
123. Lautenbach E, Metlay JP, Weiner MG, et al. Gastrointestinal tract colonization with fluoroquinolone-resistant *Escherichia coli* in hospitalized patients: changes over time in risk factors for resistance. Infect Control Hosp Epidemiol. 2009;30:18–24.
124. Lin MY, Weinstein RA, Hota B. Delay of active antimicrobial therapy and mortality among patients with bacteremia: impact of severe neutropenia. Antimicrob Agents Chemother. 2008;52:3188–94.
125. Lopez-Dupla M, Martinez JA, Vidal F, et al. Previous ciprofloxacin exposure is associated with resistance to beta-lactam antibiotics in subsequent Pseudomonas aeruginosa bacteremic isolates. Am J Infect Control. 2009;37:753–8.
126. Lortholary O, Dannaoui E, Raoux D, et al. In vitro susceptibility to posaconazole of 1,903 yeast isolates recovered in France from 2003 to 2006 and tested by the method of the European committee on antimicrobial susceptibility testing. Antimicrob Agents Chemother. 2007;51:3378–80.
127. MacDougall C, Powell JP, Johnson CK, Edmond MB, Polk RE. Hospital and community fluoroquinolone use and resistance in *Staphylococcus aureus* and *Escherichia coli* in 17 US hospitals. Clin Infect Dis. 2005;41:435–40.
128. Marks DI, Pagliuca A, Kibbler CC, et al. Voriconazole versus itraconazole for antifungal prophylaxis following allogeneic haematopoietic stem-cell transplantation. Br J Haematol. 2011;155:318–27.
129. Marr KA. Fungal infections in hematopoietic stem cell transplant recipients. Med Mycol. 2008;46:293–302.
130. Marr KA, Carter RA, Boeckh M, Martin P, Corey L. Invasive aspergillosis in allogeneic stem cell transplant recipients: changes in epidemiology and risk factors. Blood. 2002;100:4358–66.
131. Marr KA, Carter RA, Crippa F, Wald A, Corey L. Epidemiology and outcome of mould infections in hematopoietic stem cell transplant recipients. Clin Infect Dis. 2002;34: 909–17.
132. Martino R, Subira M, Rovira M, et al. Invasive fungal infections after allogeneic peripheral blood stem cell transplantation: incidence and risk factors in 395 patients. Br J Haematol. 2002;116:475–82.
133. Matar MJ, Safdar A, Rolston KV. Relationship of colonization with vancomycin-resistant enterococci and risk of systemic infection in patients with cancer. Clin Infect Dis. 2006;42:1506–7.
134. Meletiadis J, Meis JF, Mouton JW, et al. In vitro activities of new and conventional antifungal agents against clinical *Scedosporium* isolates. Antimicrob Agents Chemother. 2002;46:62–8.
135. Mellado E, Garcia-Effron G, Alcazar-Fuoli L, et al. A new *Aspergillus fumigatus* resistance mechanism conferring in vitro cross-resistance to azole antifungals involves a combination of cyp51A alterations. Antimicrob Agents Chemother. 2007;51:1897–904.
136. Miceli MH, Diaz JA, Lee SA. Emerging opportunistic yeast infections. Lancet Infect Dis. 2011;11:142–51.
137. Mihu CN, Schaub J, Kesh S, et al. Risk factors for late *Staphylococcus aureus* bacteremia after allogeneic hematopoietic stem cell transplantation: a single-institution, nested case-controlled study. Biol Blood Marrow Transplant. 2008;14:1429–33.
138. Mikulska M, Del Bono V, Prinapori R, et al. Risk factors for enterococcal bacteremia in allogeneic hematopoietic stem cell transplant recipients. Transpl Infect Dis. 2010;12: 505–12.

139. Mikulska M, Del Bono V, Raiola AM, et al. Blood stream infections in allogeneic hematopoietic stem cell transplant recipients: reemergence of Gram-negative rods and increasing antibiotic resistance. Biol Blood Marrow Transplant. 2009;15:47–53.
140. Mikulska M, Viscoli C, Orasch C, et al. ECIL 4: bacterial resistance in haematology. J Infect. 2014;68(4):321–31.
141. Moudgal V, Sobel JD. *Clostridium difficile* colitis: a review. Hosp Pract (Minneap). 2012; 40:139–48.
142. Neofytos D, Horn D, Anaissie E, et al. Epidemiology and outcome of invasive fungal infection in adult hematopoietic stem cell transplant recipients: analysis of Multicenter Prospective Antifungal Therapy (PATH) Alliance registry. Clin Infect Dis. 2009;48:265–73.
143. Nucci M, Marr KA, Queiroz-Telles F, et al. *Fusarium* infection in hematopoietic stem cell transplant recipients. Clin Infect Dis. 2004;38:1237–42.
144. Nunes AP, Teixeira LM, Iorio NL, et al. Heterogeneous resistance to vancomycin in *Staphylococcus epidermidis*, *Staphylococcus haemolyticus* and *Staphylococcus warneri* clinical strains: characterisation of glycopeptide susceptibility profiles and cell wall thickening. Int J Antimicrob Agents. 2006;27:307–15.
145. Oh HS, Kim EC, Oh MD, Choe KW. Outbreak of vancomycin resistant enterococcus in a hematology/oncology unit in a Korean University Hospital, and risk factors related to patients, staff, hospital care and facilities. Scand J Infect Dis. 2004;36:790–4.
146. Oren I. Breakthrough zygomycosis during empirical voriconazole therapy in febrile patients with neutropenia. Clin Infect Dis. 2005;40:770–1.
147. Ortega M, Marco F, Soriano A, et al. Analysis of 4758 *Escherichia coli* bacteraemia episodes: predictive factors for isolation of an antibiotic-resistant strain and their impact on the outcome. J Antimicrob Chemother. 2009;63:568–74.
148. Ortega M, Rovira M, Almela M, et al. Bacterial and fungal bloodstream isolates from 796 hematopoietic stem cell transplant recipients between 1991 and 2000. Ann Hematol. 2005;84:40–6.
149. Paez JI, Tengan FM, Barone AA, Levin AS, Costa SF. Factors associated with mortality in patients with bloodstream infection and pneumonia due to *Stenotrophomonas maltophilia*. Eur J Clin Microbiol Infect Dis. 2008;27:901–6.
150. Pagano L, Akova M, Dimopoulos G, et al. Risk assessment and prognostic factors for mould-related diseases in immunocompromised patients. J Antimicrob Chemother. 2011;66 Suppl 1:i5–14.
151. Pagano L, Caira M, Candoni A, et al. The epidemiology of fungal infections in patients with hematologic malignancies: the SEIFEM-2004 study. Haematologica. 2006;91:1068–75.
152. Pagano L, Caira M, Nosari A, et al. Etiology of febrile episodes in patients with acute myeloid leukemia: results from the Hema e-Chart Registry. Arch Intern Med. 2011;171:1502–3.
153. Pagano L, Caira M, Picardi M, et al. Invasive aspergillosis in patients with acute leukemia: update on morbidity and mortality—SEIFEM-C report. Clin Infect Dis. 2007;44:1524–5.
154. Pagano L, Caira M, Rossi G, et al. A prospective survey of febrile events in hematological malignancies. Ann Hematol. 2012;91:767–74.
155. Pagano L, Tacconelli E, Tumbarello M, et al. Teicoplanin-resistant coagulase-negative staphylococcal bacteraemia in patients with haematological malignancies: a problem of increasing importance. J Antimicrob Chemother. 1997;40:738–40.
156. Pakyz AL, Farr BM. Rates of Stenotrophomonas maltophilia colonization and infection in relation to antibiotic cycling protocols. Epidemiol Infect. 2009;137:1679–83.
157. Park BJ, Pappas PG, Wannemuehler KA, et al. Invasive non-*Aspergillus* mold infections in transplant recipients, United States, 2001–2006. Emerg Infect Dis. 2011;17:1855–64.
158. Paul M, Gafter-Gvili A, Leibovici L, et al. The epidemiology of bacteremia with febrile neutropenia: experience from a single center, 1988–2004. Isr Med Assoc J. 2007;9:424–9.
159. Pepin J, Saheb N, Coulombe MA, et al. Emergence of fluoroquinolones as the predominant risk factor for *Clostridium difficile*-associated diarrhea: a cohort study during an epidemic in Quebec. Clin Infect Dis. 2005;41:1254–60.
160. Perfect JR, Marr KA, Walsh TJ, et al. Voriconazole treatment for less-common, emerging, or refractory fungal infections. Clin Infect Dis. 2003;36:1122–31.

161. Petrikkos G, Skiada A, Lortholary O, et al. Epidemiology and clinical manifestations of mucormycosis. Clin Infect Dis. 2012;54 Suppl 1:S23–34.
162. Pfaller MA, Diekema DJ. Epidemiology of invasive mycoses in North America. Crit Rev Microbiol. 2010;36:1–53.
163. Pfaller MA, Diekema DJ. Rare and emerging opportunistic fungal pathogens: concern for resistance beyond *Candida albicans* and *Aspergillus fumigatus*. J Clin Microbiol. 2004;42:4419–31.
164. Pfaller MA, Messer SA, Moet GJ, Jones RN, Castanheira M. *Candida* bloodstream infections: comparison of species distribution and resistance to echinocandin and azole antifungal agents in Intensive Care Unit (ICU) and non-ICU settings in the SENTRY Antimicrobial Surveillance Program (2008–2009). Int J Antimicrob Agents. 2011;38:65–9.
165. Raad II, Hachem RY, Herbrecht R, et al. Posaconazole as salvage treatment for invasive fusariosis in patients with underlying hematologic malignancy and other conditions. Clin Infect Dis. 2006;42:1398–403.
166. Rangaraj G, Granwehr BP, Jiang Y, Hachem R, Raad I. Perils of quinolone exposure in cancer patients: breakthrough bacteremia with multidrug-resistant organisms. Cancer. 2010;116:967–73.
167. Richard P, Amador Del Valle G, Moreau P, et al. Viridans streptococcal bacteraemia in patients with neutropenia. Lancet. 1995;345:1607–9.
168. Rogers KL, Fey PD, Rupp ME. Coagulase-negative staphylococcal infections. Infect Dis Clin North Am. 2009;23:73–98.
169. Rolston KV, Jiang Y, Matar M. VRE fecal colonization/infection in cancer patients. Bone Marrow Transplant. 2007;39:567–8.
170. Rolston KV, Yadegarynia D, Kontoyiannis DP, Raad II, Ho DH. The spectrum of Gram-positive bloodstream infections in patients with hematologic malignancies, and the in vitro activity of various quinolones against Gram-positive bacteria isolated from cancer patients. Int J Infect Dis. 2006;10:223–30.
171. Safdar A, Rolston KV. *Stenotrophomonas maltophilia*: changing spectrum of a serious bacterial pathogen in patients with cancer. Clin Infect Dis. 2007;45:1602–9.
172. Sahin GO, Akova M. Treatment of invasive infections due to rare or emerging yeasts and moulds. Expert Opin Pharmacother. 2006;7:1181–90.
173. Saito T, Yoshioka S, Iinuma Y, et al. Effects on spectrum and susceptibility patterns of isolates causing bloodstream infection by restriction of fluoroquinolone prophylaxis in a hematology-oncology unit. Eur J Clin Microbiol Infect Dis. 2008;27:209–16.
174. Sanchez MB, Hernandez A, Martinez JL. *Stenotrophomonas maltophilia* drug resistance. Future Microbiol. 2009;4:655–60.
175. Sanchez MB, Hernandez A, Rodriguez-Martinez JM, Martinez-Martinez L, Martinez JL. Predictive analysis of transmissible quinolone resistance indicates *Stenotrophomonas maltophilia* as a potential source of a novel family of Qnr determinants. BMC Microbiol. 2008;8:148.
176. Sanz Alonso MA, Jarque Ramos I, Salavert Lletí M, Pemán J. Epidemiology of invasive fungal infections due to *Aspergillus* spp. and *Zygomycetes*. Clin Microbiol Infect. 2006;12:2–6.
177. Shaw BE, Boswell T, Byrne JL, Yates C, Russell NH. Clinical impact of MRSA in a stem cell transplant unit: analysis before, during and after an MRSA outbreak. Bone Marrow Transplant. 2007;39:623–9.
178. Siegel JD, Rhinehart E, Jackson M, Chiarello L. 2007 Guideline for isolation precautions: preventing transmission of infectious agents in healthcare settings. Am J Infect Control. 2007; 35:S65–164.
179. Sigurdardottir K, Digranes A, Harthug S, et al. A multi-centre prospective study of febrile neutropenia in Norway: microbiological findings and antimicrobial susceptibility. Scand J Infect Dis. 2005;37:455–64.
180. Siwek GT, Dodgson KJ, de Magalhaes-Silverman M, et al. Invasive zygomycosis in hematopoietic stem cell transplant recipients receiving voriconazole prophylaxis. Clin Infect Dis. 2004;39:584–7.

181. Skiada A, Pagano L, Groll A, et al. Zygomycosis in Europe: analysis of 230 cases accrued by the registry of the European Confederation of Medical Mycology (ECMM) Working Group on Zygomycosis between 2005 and 2007. Clin Microbiol Infect. 2011;17:1859–67.
182. Snelders E, Camps SM, Karawajczyk A, et al. Triazole fungicides can induce cross-resistance to medical triazoles in Aspergillus fumigatus. PLoS One. 2012;7:e31801.
183. Snelders E, Huis In 't Veld RA, Rijs AJ, et al. Possible environmental origin of resistance of *Aspergillus fumigatus* to medical triazoles. Appl Environ Microbiol. 2009;75:4053–7.
184. Snelders E, Melchers WJ, Verweij PE. Azole resistance in *Aspergillus fumigatus*: a new challenge in the management of invasive aspergillosis? Future Microbiol. 2011;6:335–47.
185. Snelders E, van der Lee HA, Kuijpers J, et al. Emergence of azole resistance in *Aspergillus fumigatus* and spread of a single resistance mechanism. PLoS Med. 2008;5:e219.
186. Timmers GJ, van der Zwet WC, Simoons-Smit IM, et al. Outbreak of vancomycin-resistant *Enterococcus faecium* in a haematology unit: risk factor assessment and successful control of the epidemic. Br J Haematol. 2002;116:826–33.
187. Tortorano AM, Kibbler C, Peman J, et al. Candidaemia in Europe: epidemiology and resistance. Int J Antimicrob Agents. 2006;27:359–66.
188. Tortorano AM, Richardson M, Roilides E, et al. ESCMID and ECMM joint guidelines on diagnosis and management of hyalohyphomycosis: Fusarium spp., Scedosporium spp. and others. Clin Microbiol Infect. 2014;20 Suppl 3:27–46.
189. Trecarichi EM, Tumbarello M, Caira M, et al. Multidrug resistant *Pseudomonas aeruginosa* bloodstream infection in adult patients with hematologic malignancies. Haematologica. 2011;96:e1–3. author reply e4.
190. Trecarichi EM, Tumbarello M, Spanu T, et al. Incidence and clinical impact of extended-spectrum-beta-lactamase (ESBL) production and fluoroquinolone resistance in bloodstream infections caused by *Escherichia coli* in patients with hematological malignancies. J Infect. 2009;58:299–307.
191. Tumbarello M, Spanu T, Di Bidino R, et al. Costs of bloodstream infections caused by *Escherichia coli* and influence of extended-spectrum-beta-lactamase production and inadequate initial antibiotic therapy. Antimicrob Agents Chemother. 2010;54:4085–91.
192. Tumbarello M, Trecarichi EM, Bassetti M, et al. Identifying patients harboring extended-spectrum-beta-lactamase-producing *Enterobacteriaceae* on hospital admission: derivation and validation of a scoring system. Antimicrob Agents Chemother. 2011;55:3485–90.
193. Tuon FF, Costa SF. *Rhodotorula* infection. A systematic review of 128 cases from literature. Rev Iberoam Micol. 2008;25:135–40.
194. Turkoglu M, Mirza E, Tunccan OG, et al. *Acinetobacter baumannii* infection in patients with hematologic malignancies in intensive care unit: risk factors and impact on mortality. J Crit Care. 2011;26:460–7.
195. Upton A, Kirby KA, Carpenter P, Boeckh M, Marr KA. Invasive aspergillosis following hematopoietic cell transplantation: outcomes and prognostic factors associated with mortality. Clin Infect Dis. 2007;44:531–40.
196. van der Linden JW, Warris A, Verweij PE. *Aspergillus* species intrinsically resistant to antifungal agents. Med Mycol. 2011;49 Suppl 1:S82–9.
197. Vardakas KZ, Polyzos KA, Patouni K, et al. Treatment failure and recurrence of *Clostridium difficile* infection following treatment with vancomycin or metronidazole: a systematic review of the evidence. Int J Antimicrob Agents. 2012;40:1–8.
198. Velasco E, Byington R, Martins CA, et al. Comparative study of clinical characteristics of neutropenic and non-neutropenic adult cancer patients with bloodstream infections. Eur J Clin Microbiol Infect Dis. 2006;25:1–7.
199. Venditti M, Falcone M, Micozzi A, et al. *Staphylococcus aureus* bacteremia in patients with hematologic malignancies: a retrospective case-control study. Haematologica. 2003;88:923–30.
200. Verweij PE, Mellado E, Melchers WJ. Multiple-triazole-resistant aspergillosis. N Engl J Med. 2007;356:1481–3.

201. Vigil KJ, Adachi JA, Aboufaycal H, et al. Multidrug-resistant *Escherichia coli* bacteremia in cancer patients. Am J Infect Control. 2009;37:741–5.
202. Viscoli C. Management of infection in cancer patients. studies of the EORTC International Antimicrobial Therapy Group (IATG). Eur J Cancer. 2002;38 Suppl 4:S82–7.
203. Viscoli C, Girmenia C, Marinus A, et al. Candidemia in cancer patients: a prospective, multicenter surveillance study by the Invasive Fungal Infection Group (IFIG) of the European Organization for Research and Treatment of Cancer (EORTC). Clin Infect Dis. 1999;28:1071–9.
204. von Baum H, Sigge A, Bommer M, et al. Moxifloxacin prophylaxis in neutropenic patients. J Antimicrob Chemother. 2006;58:891–4.
205. Walsh TJ, Groll A, Hiemenz J, et al. Infections due to emerging and uncommon medically important fungal pathogens. Clin Microbiol Infect. 2004;10 Suppl 1:48–66.
206. Walsh TJ, Peter J, McGough DA, et al. Activities of amphotericin B and antifungal azoles alone and in combination against *Pseudallescheria boydii*. Antimicrob Agents Chemother. 1995;39:1361–4.
207. Weinstock DM, Conlon M, Iovino C, et al. Colonization, bloodstream infection, and mortality caused by vancomycin-resistant enterococcus early after allogeneic hematopoietic stem cell transplant. Biol Blood Marrow Transplant. 2007;13:615–21.
208. Willems L, Porcher R, Lafaurie M, et al. *Clostridium difficile* infection after allogeneic hematopoietic stem cell transplantation: incidence, risk factors, and outcome. Biol Blood Marrow Transplant. 2012;18:1295–301.
209. Wingard JR, Carter SL, Walsh TJ, et al. Randomized, double-blind trial of fluconazole versus voriconazole for prevention of invasive fungal infection after allogeneic hematopoietic cell transplantation. Blood. 2010;116:5111–8.
210. Wisplinghoff H, Seifert H, Wenzel RP, Edmond MB. Current trends in the epidemiology of nosocomial bloodstream infections in patients with hematological malignancies and solid neoplasms in hospitals in the United States. Clin Infect Dis. 2003;36:1103–10.
211. Worth LJ, Slavin MA. Bloodstream infections in haematology: risks and new challenges for prevention. Blood Rev. 2009;23:113–22.
212. Yoo JH, Lee DG, Choi SM, et al. Vancomycin-resistant enterococcal bacteremia in a hematology unit: molecular epidemiology and analysis of clinical course. J Korean Med Sci. 2005;20:169–76.
213. Yoshida M, Akiyama N, Fujita H, et al. Analysis of bacteremia/fungemia and pneumonia accompanying acute myelogenous leukemia from 1987 to 2001 in the Japan Adult Leukemia Study Group. Int J Hematol. 2011;93:66–73.
214. Youssef S, Rodriguez G, Rolston KV, et al. Streptococcus pneumoniae infections in 47 hematopoietic stem cell transplantation recipients: clinical characteristics of infections and vaccine-breakthrough infections, 1989–2005. Medicine (Baltimore). 2007;86:69–77.
215. Zahar JR, Farhat H, Chachaty E, et al. Incidence and clinical significance of anaerobic bacteraemia in cancer patients: a 6-year retrospective study. Clin Microbiol Infect. 2005;11:724–9.
216. Zervos MJ, Hershberger E, Nicolau DP, et al. Relationship between fluoroquinolone use and changes in susceptibility to fluoroquinolones of selected pathogens in 10 United States teaching hospitals, 1991–2000. Clin Infect Dis. 2003;37:1643–8.
217. Zirakzadeh A, Gastineau DA, Mandrekar JN, et al. Vancomycin-resistant enterococcal colonization appears associated with increased mortality among allogeneic hematopoietic stem cell transplant recipients. Bone Marrow Transplant. 2008;41:385–92.

Part II

Diagnosis

6 The Diagnostic Approach to the Febrile Neutropenic Patient: Clinical Considerations

Eric J. Bow

Contents

6.1 Introduction

This chapter has been written from the viewpoint of the clinician who is assessing a febrile cancer patient who may be neutropenic and who may have an infection as the cause of the fever. There are a number of variables the clinician must consider at the time of presentation of a patient with a new neutropenic fever syndrome including documentation of the state of neutropenia and pyrexia. These variables listed in Table 6.1 include the diagnosis of the underlying malignancy and status of the underlying malignancy (i.e. whether the cancer is in remission, under initial assessment or treatment, persistent despite treatment, relapsed or progressive), the treatment regimen, regimen-related toxicities, the day of the treatment cycle (relative to

E.J. Bow
Departments of Medical Microbiology and Infectious Diseases, and Internal Medicine, Sections of Infectious Diseases and Haematology/Oncology, The University of Manitoba, Winnipeg, MB, Canada

Manitoba Blood and Marrow Transplant Programme, and Infection Control Services, CancerCare Manitoba, Winnipeg, MB, Canada
e-mail: EJBow@cancercare.mb.ca

G. Maschmeyer, K.V.I. Rolston (eds.), *Infections in Hematology*,
DOI 10.1007/978-3-662-44000-1_6

Table 6.1 Factors affecting risk for neutropenic fever syndromes in cancer patients receiving cytotoxic therapy

Patient-related factors
Advanced age (≥65 years) increases risk [26, 28, 108]
Performance status
ECOG ≥2 increases risk [66, 109]
Nutritional status
Low serum albumin <35 g/l is associated with increased risk [52, 66]
History of previous neutropenic fever episodes increases risk
Risk of neutropenic fever in cycles 2–6 is 4 times higher if a neutropenic fever occurred during cycle 1 than if it did not [30]
Increasing number of co-morbidities increases risk
The odds for neutropenic fever increases with the number of co-morbidities by 27, 67, and 125 % for 1, 2, and 3 or more co-morbidities [48]
Underlying malignancy-related factors
Cancer diagnosis:
Acute leukaemia/myelodysplastic syndromes (highest risk) [58]
Neutropenic fever rate 85–95 % [21, 22, 44]
Solid tissue malignancies and neutropenic fever rates (in order of risk, highest to lowest) [30, 48, 83, 84]
Soft tissue sarcomas, 26.8 %, 95 % CL 19.1–34.5 %
Non-Hodgkin's lymphoma/myeloma, 26.0 %, 95 % CL 22.2–29.3 %
Germ cell carcinomas, 22.9 %, 95 % CL 16.6–29.1 %
Hodgkin's lymphoma, 15.4 %, 95 % CL 6.6–24.2 %
Ovarian carcinoma, 12.1 %, 95 % CL 6.6–17.7 %
Lung cancers, 10.3 %, 95 % CL 9.8–10.7 %
Colorectal cancers, 5.5 %, 95 % CL 5.1–5.8 %
Head and neck carcinoma, 4.6 %, 95 % CL 1.0–8.2 %
Breast cancers, 4.4 %, 95 % CL 4.1–4.7 %
Prostate cancer, 1.0 %, 95 % CL 0.9–1.1 %
Cancer stage:
Higher risk with advanced stage of disease, ≥2 [48, 66]
Status of the cancer during the time at risk for neutropenic fever syndromes:
Remission (lower risk) versus not in remission (higher risk) [58, 98]
Response to treatment
Complete responses are at lower risk [58]
Partial responses in solid tissue malignancies are at lower risk than partial responses in acute leukaemia
Persistent, refractory, or progressive diseases despite treatment are circumstances at higher risk [19, 99]
Treatment-related factors
Choice of cytotoxic regimen:
Higher risk regimens are those containing doxorubicin or epirubicin ≥90 mg/m^2, cisplatin ≥100 mg/m^2, ifosfamide ≥9 g/m^2, cyclophosphamide ≥1 g/m^2, etoposide ≥500 mg/m^2, or cytarabine ≥1 g/m^2 [84]

Table 6.1 (continued)

Dose-dense regimens such as CHOP-14 [83]
Breast cancer regimens containing an anthracycline (doxorubicin or epirubicin) plus a taxane (docetaxel or paclitaxel) and cyclophosphamide or gemcitabine [89, 108]
Dose intensity of the anticancer regimen
Administration of >85 % of the scheduled doses of chemotherapy are associated with increased risk [83, 89]
Degree and duration of oral/gastrointestinal mucositis [21, 85]
Degree and duration of neutropenia (ANC <0.5×10^9 l) [13, 14, 49]
Degree and duration of lymphopenia (ALC <0.7×10^9 l) [8, 84]
Degree and duration of monocytopenia (AMC <0.15×10^9 l) [78]
Administration of prophylactic haematopoietic growth factors may reduce risk in selected patients [1, 92]
Administration of antimicrobial chemoprophylaxis may reduce risk in selected patients [30]

ECOG Eastern Cooperative Oncology Group, *CHOP* cyclophosphamide, hydroxydaunorubicin (doxorubicin), vincristine (Oncovin™), prednisone, *ANC* absolute neutrophil count, *ALC* absolute lymphocyte count, *AMC* absolute monocyte count

the first day of the current treatment cycle), risk factors for serious medical complications, the neutropenic fever syndrome at presentation (first fever, persistent fever, or recrudescent fever), the characterisation of the syndrome (i.e. documented or unexplained), and the presence and the clinical context in which the patient presents (initial treatment for a new diagnosis of cancer versus relapsed or persistent disease). Such considerations can be helpful in the methodological and encompassing approach to the development of a management plan.

6.2 Neutropenia and Timing of Neutropenic Fevers

The relationship between fever, infection, and the state of neutropenia was described in the seminal work by Bodey and colleagues over 40 years ago [13, 14]. The risk of invasive infection is inversely related to the circulating absolute neutrophil count (ANC) [13, 22, 90] and increases as the ANC falls below 1.0×10^9 l and, in particular, as it falls below 0.5×10^9 l (OR 2.4, 95 % CI 1.3–4.5) [87]. Accordingly, severe neutropenia, as it is related to the risk of neutropenic fevers and documented invasive infections, is defined by an ANC below 0.5×10^9 l [22]. A relationship between the risk for neutropenic fevers and an absolute lymphocyte count (ALC) of <0.7×10^9 l at day 1 of cytotoxic therapy [8, 84] has also been observed. The ANC and ALC are readily available from most automated leukocyte differential counts that are performed in routine hospital and clinic laboratories.

The nadir of cytotoxic therapy-induced myelosuppression typically occurs at the end of the second week, between day 10 and 14, from the first day of cytotoxic therapy [21]. This is, coincidentally, the time of the maximum cytotoxic effect of the anticancer chemotherapies on the intestinal mucosa [20, 21, 65] and the time of maximal oral and gastrointestinal mucositis [9, 11, 21, 85, 93, 95]. Therefore, the median time of the first neutropenic fever is typically between day 10 and 14 of the chemotherapy cycle [21, 22] which corresponds to this time of maximal cytotoxic therapy-induced intestinal epithelial mucosal damage [20, 21] and is independent of the regimen [18, 74, 95, 110].

The majority of first neutropenic fevers tend to occur during the first of a multicycle regimen of systemic cytotoxic therapy [28, 30]. Moreover, a neutropenic fever episode occurring in cycle 1 tends to predispose to further episodes during subsequent cycles [30]. The risk is related to the type of cancer [48] and to the chemotherapeutic regimen [1, 108].

The majority of infections in febrile neutropenic patients are due to bacteria and opportunistic yeasts that normally colonise the cytotoxic therapy-induced damaged mucosal surfaces [10, 75, 88]. It is not surprising, therefore, that the microorganisms that are most often associated with invasive bloodstream infections in neutropenic patients are derived of the normal microflora of the periodontium (viridans [alpha haemolytic] group streptococci) and the gastrointestinal tract (facultatively anaerobic gram-negative members of the family Enterobacteriaceae [e.g. *Escherichia coli*, *Klebsiella pneumoniae*, or *Enterobacter* spp], *Enterococcus* spp. [often referred to as nonhaemolytic streptococci prior to genus and species identification], *Staphylococcus* spp. [including thermonuclease-positive *S. aureus* and thermonuclease-negative *S. epidermidis*], *Candida* spp. and less commonly obligate anaerobic gram-positive [*Clostridium* spp., *Lactobacillus* spp] and gram-negative [*Bacteroides* spp.] bacteria or a fermentative obligately aerobic gram-negative bacilli [*Pseudomonas* spp., *Stenotrophomonas* spp., or *Acinetobacter* spp.]).

The duration of severe neutropenia is different among different patient groups and the respective cytotoxic regimens. The expected median duration of an ANC $<0.5 \times 10^9$ l among patients receiving remission-induction therapy with cytarabine and an anthracycline over 7 and 3 days, respectively, is of the order of 17 days [96] compared with 4 days for patients with solid tumours or lymphoma treated with intermittent cycles of chemotherapy [71]. The longer the duration of severe neutropenia, the greater the risk for opportunistic infection [13, 46].

6.3 Risks and Predictors for Neutropenic Fever

A number of factors have been observed to be associated with the risk for neutropenic fever syndromes. Of these, chemotherapy-induced neutropenia is perhaps the most important and is a common reason for anticancer treatment dose delays or dose reductions [89] that impacts upon the efficacy of the anticancer treatment regimen. These factors are listed in Table 6.1. Moreover, the degree of chemotherapy-induced oral and gastrointestinal mucositis is directly correlated with the risk of infection [94].

Various studies have identified risk factors for neutropenic fevers including older age (particularly ≥65 years), advanced underlying malignant disease, low baseline leukocyte counts, marrow myelophthisis, low serum albumin, anaemia, elevated lactate dehydrogenase, and co-morbid renal, cardiovascular, or hepatic conditions [82]. Such delays and reductions result in reduced dose intensity which, in turn, is linked to suboptimal anticancer treatment delivery [82, 83]. For example, in a 20-year follow-up to adjuvant CMF therapy for node-positive breast cancer, the overall survival of women who had received ≥85 % of the planned dose of CMF was 52 % compared to 32 %, 25 %, and 25 % for women who had received 65–84 %, <65 %, and 0 % (the untreated control group), respectively, of planned CMF therapy [15]. Patient outcomes are better when anticancer treatment delivery is optimal [17, 25].

A number of patient-driven circumstance-dependent predictors for neutropenic fevers have been identified including patient age (particularly 65 years or more) [40, 67, 102, 103], female sex [66], high body surface area [89], and pre-existing cardiovascular, renal, endocrine, or respiratory co-morbidities giving rise to poor performance status [66, 109] and poor nutritional status [52]. Disease-related predictors have included elevated lactate dehydrogenase (LDH) in lymphoreticular diseases [52], myelophthisis [52] with lymphopenia [8, 84], and advanced stage of the underlying malignancy [47, 58, 66, 103, 108]. Anticancer treatment-related predictors of neutropenic fevers have included administration of the planned dose intensity or dose density [67], administration of high-dose chemotherapy regimens [1, 83, 84, 92], and failure to administer haematopoietic growth factor support to patients receiving high-risk regimens [1, 102].

Different regimens carry varying risks for chemotherapy-induced neutropenia [1, 84, 92]. For example, prior to 1998, regimens based upon cyclophosphamide, methotrexate, and fluorouracil (CMF) were most frequently employed in the treatment of breast cancer [89]. Thereafter, anthracycline-based regimens became more common. The majority (70 %) of breast cancer patients receiving systemic chemotherapy now receive anthracycline-based regimens (such as FEC [fluorouracil, epirubicin, and cyclophosphamide]) or taxane plus anthracycline-based regimens (such as TAC [taxotere (docetaxel), doxorubicin (Adriamycin™), and cyclophosphamide]). The cycle length for such regimens is usually 21 days. The mean number of cycles is 7.9 ± 0.8 [83]. Neutropenic events (defined as neutropenia-related dose delays of ≥7 days, dose reductions of ≥15 %, or hospitalisations) have been more common among recipients of taxane-based regimens, followed by CMF-based regimens, and anthracycline-based regimens [89]. More neutropenic events occur among CMF recipients administered with increased dose density over 21 days rather than 28 days [62]. Neutropenic events occurring during cycle 1 of the treatment have tended to predict such events during the second and subsequent cycles [89]. Neutropenic fever syndromes have been uncommon among women receiving CMF-based adjuvant chemotherapy compared to those receiving anthracycline- or taxane-based chemotherapy regimens (none versus 5–6 %, respectively) [83]. Among patients treated with CHOP-like (cyclophosphamide, hydroxydaunorubicin [doxorubicin], vincristine [Oncovin™], and prednisone) regimens for non-Hodgkin's lymphoma, grade 4 neutropenia over the course of 6–8 cycles may be expected in one in two patients, but the event rate for neutropenic fevers may be expected in up to 22 % [83].

Increasing the dose density of CHOP by reducing the time in between cycles from 21 to 14 days increases the likelihood that a toxicity-driven dose reduction will be required (from approximately one in three patients to up to one in two patients, respectively) [83]. The French ELYPSE study group characterised regimens at high risk for neutropenic fevers as those containing anthracyclines (doxorubicin or epirubicin) ≥90 mg/m^2, cisplatin ≥100 mg/m^2, ifosfamide ≥9 g/m^2, cyclophosphamide ≥1 g/m^2, etoposide ≥500 mg/m^2, or cytarabine ≥100 mg/m^2 per course [84]. Choice of chemotherapeutic regimen is a key driver of cytotoxic therapy-induced complications including grade 4 neutropenia, onset of neutropenic fever syndromes, and reductions in relative dose intensity and consequent impact upon survival.

6.4 Classification of Neutropenic Fever Syndromes

There are several neutropenic fever syndromes that have been described [18]. These consist of first neutropenic fevers, persistent neutropenic fevers, and recrudescent neutropenic fevers for a given neutropenic episode. The number and severity of recrudescent fevers depends upon the duration of neutropenia [46, 76]. Further, each fever may be classified as documented, microbiologically (based upon identification of a pathogen isolated from an infectious focus) or clinically (based upon identification of an infectious focus without a putative pathogen), or as unexplained [50]. At the time of presentation, it may not be possible to accurately classify the neutropenic fever syndrome until the results of investigations and cultures are known. For example, a bacteraemic patient who presents with no obvious inflammatory focus may be misclassified as an unexplained fever until the blood culture results become available.

The ultimate classification of the neutropenic fever syndrome will depend, to some extent, upon the rigour with which a clinical focus of infection is sought. At the time of presentation, between one-fifth and one-third of neutropenic fevers will prove to be bloodstream infections [44, 80, 104]. In one American study among first neutropenic fevers, bloodstream infections accounted for 23 %, unexplained fevers 8 %, and clinically documented infections 69 % [80]. Of the bloodstream infections, *Staphylococcus* spp. accounted for 19 %, viridans group streptococci 27 %, other gram-positive organisms 16 %, and gram-negative bacilli 37 %. Of the clinically documented infections, the majority (63 %) originated in the gastrointestinal tract (oral mucositis, oesophagus, and enterocolitis), 10 % originated in the skin and soft tissues (the majority of which were central venous access device related), 10 % originated in the lower respiratory tract, and 8 % from the urinary tract. In contrast, another trial from Europe classified the neutropenic fever syndrome as microbiologically documented bloodstream infections in 40 % of cases, non-bacteraemic microbiologically documented infections in 6 % of cases, unexplained fevers in 43 % of cases, and clinically documented infection in only 11 % of cases [23]. The major differences in these reports were in the proportions of infections that were bacteraemia and clinically documented oral and gastrointestinal mucositis. Despite the known relationship between cytotoxic therapy-induced mucosal damage, translocation, and invasive infections in neutropenic patients [12, 20, 94], there remain differences of opinion regarding the classification of sites of mucositis as infectious foci [85].

6.5 Is the Patient Febrile? Measurement of Body Temperature

An elevated body temperature may be the earliest and only sign of infection in the neutropenic patient [90]. Prompt initiation of empirical systemic antibacterial therapy is important to avoid progression to a sepsis syndrome and possibly death. Accordingly, the accurate and reliable clinical recognition of a febrile state in neutropenic patients is critical.

The origins of the definition of normal body temperature are somewhat obscure [68]. The work of Carl Wunderlich in 1868 suggested that a normal body temperature was 37 °C (98.6 °F) and that the upper limit of normal was 38 °C (100.4 °F), beyond which fever was defined [111]. Indeed, a survey of 270 medical professionals noted that the majority (75 %) believed that the normal body temperature was 37 °C (98.6 °F) [69]. However, a study of 148 healthy men and women at the University of Maryland demonstrated the mean of 700 baseline oral temperatures to be 36.8±0.4 °C (98.2±0.7 °F) with a range of 35.6 °C (96.0 °F) to 38.2 °C (100.8 °F). According to these observations, the upper limit of normal would be 38.2 °C (100.8 °F). The temperature of 37 °C accounted for only 8 % of all readings and fell outside of the 99.9 % confidence limit for the sample mean [70].

Given these considerations, a number of guidelines have been published to provide some direction regarding the definition of a febrile state in neutropenic cancer patients. The Infectious Diseases Society of America has defined a febrile neutropenic episode as a single oral temperature of >38.3 °C (101 °F) or a temperature of >38.0 °C (100.4 °F) sustained for >1 h [49]. Other international guidelines from North and South America, Europe, and Asia have provided similar definitions [6, 55, 64, 86, 101]. The Japan Febrile Neutropenia Study Group and the Asia-Pacific febrile neutropenia guidelines group have recommended that a single oral temperature of ≥38.0 °C or a single axillary temperature of ≥37.5 °C be accepted as the definition of a febrile state [101]. Based upon the observations pertaining to the range of normal temperatures from the University of Maryland, most North and South American and European guidelines have adopted the standard of a single oral temperature of ≥38.3 °C as the definition of pyrexia in the setting of neutropenic cancer patients.

The next important question is how body temperature is measured. Most medical facilities measure body temperature by oral, infrared tympanic membrane, axillary, or rectal thermometry as a surrogate of core body temperature as measured by standard pulmonary artery catheter (PAC) or in situ urinary bladder thermometry. An accurate measurement is desirable since the decision to initiate an aggressive protocol of neutropenic fever management may be based upon the difference of a half degree Celsius [34].

One study from St. George's Hospital in London compared axillary chemical and infrared tympanic membrane thermometry to pulmonary artery catheter (PAC) thermometry for the estimation of core body temperature [36]. Based upon adjudication by an expert panel, false-negative rates resulting in possible delayed interventions of 15.3 and 21.1 % for axillary and tympanic thermometry, respectively, were observed. Similarly, false-positive rates possibly leading to unnecessary interventions of 28.8 and 37.8 % for axillary and tympanic thermometry, respectively, were observed. Whilst infrared tympanic membrane thermometry is non-invasive and convenient, the procedure is subject to inaccuracy due to observations obtained from the dependent ear [43], multiple user error [4], operator technique and equipment maintenance [39, 54, 77], and failure to remove cerumen in the external auditory canal [33]. Axillary temperatures have tended to be 0.2–0.4 °C higher than PAC thermometry [35, 36] thus overestimating patient temperature. Moreover, interventions such as warming blankets and haemofiltration have resulted in variances from PAC thermometric measurements by as much as 0.4 and 0.3 °C, respectively [36].

6.6 Risk for Serious Medical Complications Associated with the Neutropenic Fever Syndrome

Over 40 years ago, it was recognised that the population of neutropenic patients is very heterogeneous [13, 98, 99]. Neutropenic cancer patients are not only at risk of infection; they are at risk for a variety of medical complications of other treatments, other co-morbid diseases, and cancer-related problems that may lead to cardiorespiratory failure or bleeding [97]. The identification of co-morbidities among febrile neutropenic patients is linked to in-hospital mortality risk and cost of hospitalisation [60]. Early studies at the Dana-Farber Cancer Institute noted that on the average about one in five febrile neutropenic cancer patients would develop such problems; however, the risks for serious medical complications were about one in three for those who were inpatients or who had uncontrolled cancer at the time of the neutropenic fever and even higher, one in two, for those with coexisting active co-morbidities [98]. For those febrile neutropenic patients without these characteristics, a group that accounted for the majority of patients at risk of infection, the complication rate was only 2 % [98]. These observations suggested that these characteristics might be useful for developing a predictive rule to reliably identify a subgroup of patients for whom a different approach with transition to outpatient management may be feasible and safe [99, 100].

The Multinational Association for Supportive Care in Cancer (MASCC) has developed [58] and validated [105] a risk-index scoring system based upon characteristics easily identifiable at the onset of the episode predicting the development of potentially serious medical complications (shown in Table 6.2) during the neutropenic fever syndrome that would require hospitalisation or prolong hospitalisation for management. This risk-index score is presented in Table 6.3. A risk-index score of ≥21 in the initial development of the model predicted a group of patients at "low

Table 6.2 Neutropenic fever syndrome-associated medical complications considered serious

Medical complications
Hypotension (defined by a systolic blood pressure less than 90 mmHg or by the need for vasopressor support to maintain blood pressure)
Respiratory failure (defined by an arterial oxygen pressure less than 60 mmHg whilst breathing room air or by the need for mechanical ventilation)
Admission to a critical care service
Disseminated intravascular coagulation
Presence of confusion, delirium, or altered mental state
Development of congestive cardiac failure documented by chest imaging and that requires treatment
Bleeding diathesis sufficient to require blood cell transfusion
Arrhythmia or ECG changes requiring treatment
Renal failure sufficient to require investigation and/or treatment with IV fluids, dialysis, or any other intervention
Other complications judged serious and clinically significant by the medical care team

Table 6.3 The Multinational Association for Supportive Care in Cancer (MASSC) index score used to predict the likelihood of serious medical complications in "low-risk" versus "high-risk" febrile neutropenic cancer patients[a]

Prognostic factor	Weight
Burden of the neutropenic fever syndrome: no symptoms or only mild symptoms	5
No hypotension (systolic BP >90 mmHg)	5
No chronic obstructive lung disease	4
Solid tissue malignancy or haematological malignancy without previous history of invasive fungal infection	3
No dehydration that requires administration of parenteral fluids	3
Burden of the neutropenic fever syndrome: moderate symptoms	3
Outpatient status at the time of onset of the neutropenic fever syndrome	3
Age <60 years	2

[a]Derived from Klastersky et al. [58] and Uys et al. [105]. Weightings for *burden of the neutropenic fever syndrome* are not cumulative. Therefore, the maximum attainable score is 26

risk" for the kinds of medical complications shown in Table 6.2 with a sensitivity, specificity, and positive and negative predictive values of 71, 68, 91, and 36 %, respectively, with a misclassification rate of 30 % [58].

In a prospectively conducted additional validation study, the MASCC risk-index score correctly classified low-risk and high-risk patients in 98.3 and 86.3 % of cases, respectively, giving a sensitivity, specificity, and positive and negative predictive values of 95, 95, 98.3, and 86.4 %, respectively [105]. The model was further refined by the reclassification of patients with "complicated" infections (defined by presence of a visceral site of infection, sepsis syndrome, a non-necrotising skin or soft tissue infection [SSTI] of >5 cm diameter, a necrotising SSTI of any size, or oral mucositis [WHO grade >2]) as high risk for serious medical complications. This had the effect of increasing the sensitivity and negative predictive value to 100 % each among febrile neutropenic patients with a MASCC index score of ≥21 [31]. Table 6.4 details a review of the published performance of the MASCC risk-index scoring system for predicting patients at low risk for serious medical complications. The pooled sensitivity, specificity, and positive and negative predictive values were 85, 68, 83, and 68 %, respectively. The rate of misclassification was one in five (20 %, 95 % CI 10–29 %).

The concept of identifying risk at the onset of a febrile neutropenic episode has been accepted into standard practice [41, 49, 64]. The accurate identification of such low-risk patients at the onset of the episode has important significance for the choice of the empirical antibacterial therapy regimen (monotherapy versus combination therapy), route of administration (oral versus intravenous), and venue of administration (outpatient versus inpatient). In a subsequent study, Klastersky and colleagues followed 611 febrile neutropenic patient episodes classified using the MASCC risk-index score as low or high risk for the primary outcome of resolution of fever without serious medical complications [57]. A total of 178 of 383 episodes of first neutropenic fever were deemed eligible (defined by ability to swallow oral medications, no allergy to penicillin or fluoroquinolones, and no use of antibacterial chemoprophylaxis) to receive oral empirical antibacterial therapy (ciprofloxacin 500 mg tid and amoxicillin/clavulanate 500/125 mg tid) and early (within 48 h) hospital discharge. Of these 178 subjects, 79 (44 %) underwent early discharge at a median of 26 h following initiation of treatment with overall strategy success for the outpatient oral therapy in 76 (96 %, 95 % CI 92–100 %). Whilst no serious medical complications were observed in this group, three patients required readmission for intravenous antibiotics (2) or persistent fever (1). For the 99 subjects remaining in the hospital, there were 9 serious medical complications with overall strategy success in 90 subjects (91 %, 95 % CI 85–97 %). These results demonstrated the safety and feasibility of using the MASCC risk-index score to identify low-risk patients eligible for oral empirical antibacterial therapy and early hospital discharge [57].

Bacteraemia in neutropenic patients is associated with greater serious medical complications and higher overall mortality [56]. Factors at presentation of the neutropenic fever episode such as shock, temperature of >40 °C, or severe thrombocytopenia have been associated with gram-negative bloodstream infections [59] but have not been sufficiently discriminatory for use in a practical model [107]. MASCC-predicted high-risk patients have a significantly higher likelihood of having bacteraemia than low-risk patients: almost 1 in 3 (209/654, 32 %) compared to 1 in 5 (290/1,488, 19.5 %) [79]. High-risk bacteraemic patients had significantly higher rates of serious complications and death than low-risk patients for gram-positive (39 % and 9 % versus 16 % and 2 %, respectively) and gram-negative bacteraemia (60 % and 29 % versus 20 % and 6 %, respectively). The MASCC risk-index score of ≥21 had similar predictive value for successful outcome among non-bacteraemic patients (OR 6.06, 95 % CI

Table 6.4 Review of clinical trials examining the performance of the Multinational Association for the Supportive Care in Cancer (MASCC) risk-index score for identifying febrile neutropenic patients at low risk for serious medical complications

Reference	True positive	False positive	False negative	True negative	SENS	SPEC	PPV	NPV	Misclassification rate
Klastersky et al. [58]	221	22	90	50	0.71	0.69	0.91	0.36	0.29
Uys et al. [105]	57	1	3	19	0.95	0.95	0.98	0.86	0.05
Cherif et al. [24]	89	16	63	111	0.59	0.87	0.85	0.64	0.28
Innes et al. [51]	87	3	8	2	0.92	0.40	0.97	0.20	0.11
Baskaran et al. [7]	68	14	5	29	0.93	0.67	0.83	0.85	0.16
de Sousa-Viana et al. [31]	17	4	3	29	0.85	0.88	0.81	0.91	0.13
Gayol Mdel et al. [45]	19	32	3	26	0.86	0.45	0.37	0.90	0.44
Ahn et al. [2]	308	35	15	38	0.95	0.52	0.90	0.72	0.13
Mean (95 % CI)					0.85 (0.75–0.94)	0.68 (0.52–0.84)	0.83 (0.68–0.97)	0.68 (0.48–0.88)	0.20 (0.10–0.29)

SENS sensitivity, *SPEC* specificity, *PPV* positive predictive value, *NPV* negative predictive value

4.51–8.15) as for those with single gram-positive (OR 3.42, 95 % CI 1.95–5.98) or single gram-negative (OR 6.04, 95 % CI 3.01–12.09) bacteraemias [79]. The MASCC risk-index score predicts high-risk circumstances wherein bloodstream infections are more likely to occur, but does not discriminate which high-risk patients with bacteraemia.

6.7 Presentation to the Outpatient Clinic or to the Emergency Department

The signs and symptoms of inflammation and infection in neutropenic cancer patient such as swelling, local warmth, fluctuance, ulceration, or exudate may be muted [90, 91]. Pyrexia is almost invariably present in neutropenic patients with systemic infection [90]. Accordingly, the presentation of a cancer patient with a history of a febrile illness should prompt a full investigation to establish the likelihood whether the patient is neutropenic and has objective evidence of infection. A summary of this approach based upon the 2010 guideline update from the Infectious Diseases Society of America [42] is illustrated in Fig. 6.1.

The likelihood of being neutropenic is greater with a history of a syndrome or diagnosis associated with disease-related bone marrow failure such as acute leukaemia or myelodysplasia or with treatment-related bone marrow failure such as recent receipt of cytotoxic therapy or haematopoietic stem cell transplantation. These clues together with a history that suggests fever should compel the health care team to obtain a full set of vital signs (heart rate, blood pressure, respiratory rate, and arterial oxygen saturation), basic laboratory investigations including a complete blood count, at least two sets of blood cultures from separate sites, and an assessment of renal function. Such an approach should establish whether the patient is neutropenic and the presence of a systemic inflammatory response syndrome.

The term "systemic inflammatory response syndrome" (SIRS) was brought into common usage in a 1992 statement from the ACCP/SCCM consensus conference to describe the activation of the innate immune response triggered by localised or systemic infection, trauma, thermal injury, or non-infectious processes such as acute pancreatitis [63]. *SIRS* is defined by the presence of more than one of the following: body temperature higher than 38 °C or lower than 36 °C, heart rate greater than 90 beats per minute, hyperventilation defined by a respiratory rate of greater than 20 breaths per minute or $PaCO_2$ of less than 32 mmHg, or a circulating leukocyte count of greater than 12.0×10^9 l or lower than 4.0×10^9 l. Investigators have argued that these clinical criteria are non-specific and that other biochemical evidence for inflammation should be considered in the definition including increased circulating levels of interleukin 6, C-reactive protein, or procalcitonin [63, 106].

Sepsis has been defined as SIRS with evidence of infection [16] wherein infection is itself defined as a pathological process induced by a microorganism. According to the revised definitions designed to codify the clinical impression of "sepsis", this state may be documented or suspected by the presence of fever (core temperature ≥38.3 °C), hypothermia (core temperature <36 °C), tachycardia (heart

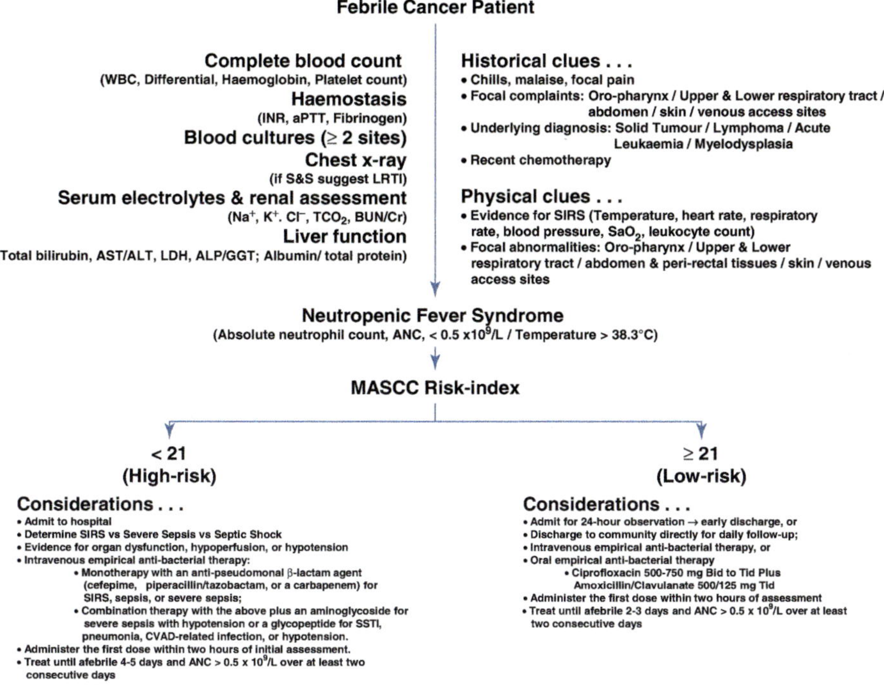

Fig. 6.1 Approach to the cancer presenting to an outpatient assessment service with suspected infection and possible neutropenic fever syndrome. Abbreviations: *INR* international normalised ratio, *apt* activated partial thromboplastin time, *Na+* sodium, *K+* potassium, *Cl−* chloride, *TCO2* total carbon dioxide, *BUN* blood urea nitrogen, *Cr* serum creatinine, *AST* aspartate transaminase, *ALT* alanine transferase, *LDH* lactate dehydrogenase, *ALP* alkaline phosphatase, *GGT* gamma glutamyl transferase, *SaO2* arterial oxygen saturation, *ANC* absolute neutrophil count, *MASCC* Multinational Association for Supportive Care in Cancer; SIRS, systemic inflammatory response syndrome, *CVAD* central venous access device, *SSTI* skin and soft tissue infection, *Bid* twice daily, *Tid* thrice daily

rate >90 min or 2 standard deviations above the age mean), tachypnea (respiratory rate >30 min), altered mental status, significant oedema or positive fluid balance (>20 ml/kg over 24 h), hyperglycaemia (blood glucose >7.7 mmol L in the absence of a diagnosis of diabetes mellitus), leukocytosis (total leukocyte count $>12.0\times10^9$ l), leukopenia (total leukocyte count $<4.0\times10^9$ l), or a normal leukocyte count with >10 % immature neutrophils in the leukocyte differential count [63].

Severe sepsis has been defined as sepsis with evidence of organ dysfunction, hypoperfusion, or hypotension. In the revised definitions, organ dysfunction may be articulated as arterial hypoxaemia (PaO_2/FIO_2 <300), acute oliguria (urine output <0.5 ml/kg/h for at least 2 h), creatinine increase ≥0.5 mg/dl, coagulation abnormalities (international normalised ratio >1.5 or activated partial thromboplastin time >60 s), ileus (absent bowel sounds), thrombocytopenia (platelet count <100,000 μl), and hyperbilirubinaemia (plasma total bilirubin >4 mg/dl or 70 mmol/l) [37, 72]. Evidence for hypoperfusion includes hyperlactataemia (>3 mmol/l), decreased capillary refill, or mottling.

Arterial hypotension is defined by systolic blood pressure <90 mmHg, a mean arterial pressure of <70 mmHg, or a systolic blood pressure decrease of >40 mmHg in adults or >2 standard deviations below the normal for age [63]. *Septic shock* is defined as sepsis with arterial hypotension despite adequate fluid resuscitation [16].

The frequency of severe sepsis or septic shock as a feature in the presentation of neutropenic fever syndromes is not well described. Almost half (45.2 %, 95 % CI 38.2–52.1 %) of febrile neutropenic cancer patients presenting to emergency rooms in France had evidence of sepsis syndrome in one review in which 56 % of subjects had solid tissue malignancies and 44 % had haematological cancers [5]. In another report of patients with acute leukaemia, 22 of 94 (23.4 %) neutropenic fever episodes were associated with severe sepsis [53]. Yet another report focusing upon low-risk patients described an event rate for the sepsis syndrome of only 2 % [29]. Septic shock in older European studies has been reported to be of the order of 2.2 % (95 % CI 1.3–3.7 %) [87]. There appears to be several predictors that contribute to the risk for evolution from SIRS to severe sepsis or septic shock that include, but are not limited to, disease-related variables such as the state of the underlying cancer (e.g., remission versus not in remission); patient-related factors such as age, sex, or the presence of pre-existing co-morbid conditions (such as lung, kidney, or heart disease); treatment-related variables such as the duration and severity of neutropenia and mucositis; and infection-related factors such as the classification of the neutropenic fever syndrome as unexplained or clinically or microbiologically documented, the appropriateness of the initial management, or pathogens involved (for example, gram-negative bacteria versus gram-positive bacteria versus fungi).

The definitions for the sepsis syndrome, developed [16] and refined [32] previously, were modified for clinical use in febrile neutropenic patients, that is, a blood lactate of >4 mmol/l, or hypotension before fluid challenge (systolic pressure of <90 mmHg or <40 mmHg below the patient's usual systolic blood pressure), or evidence of at least one organ system dysfunction (such as a serum creatinine >176 umol/l, a total bilirubin of >78 umol/l, an international normalised scale >2, or a Glasgow coma scale of <15) [5].

French guidelines [5, 73] recommend that for febrile neutropenic patients presenting with a severe sepsis syndrome, the following should occur within 90 min of presentation: at least one blood culture and a lactic acid measurement should be obtained, a fluid challenge of at least 500 ml for those with a mean arterial pressure of <65 mmHg and a dose of appropriate broad-spectrum empirical antibacterial therapy should be administered, and the patient should be admitted to the hospital. Those presenting with a "non-severe" sepsis syndrome and who are classified as "high risk" by the MASCC risk-index scoring system should have at least two blood culture from separate sites [49], receive a dose of an appropriate empirical intravenous antibacterial regimen, and be admitted to hospital. The empirical administration of haematopoietic growth factors as part of the management of the neutropenic fever syndrome is not indicated in these circumstances [92]. Patients presenting with a "non-severe" sepsis syndrome who are classified as "low risk" by the MASCC risk-index scoring system should have at least two blood cultures from separate sites [49], receive an oral empirical antibacterial regimen (such as ciprofloxacin plus amoxicillin/clavulanate), and be discharged from hospital. Similarly, the empirical addition of haematopoietic growth factors are not indicated [92].

Timeliness of empirical antibacterial treatment is important. Despite the availability of guidelines such as these, the time from assessment to treatment has been variable. In one study, the time from initial triage in the emergency department until administration of empirical antimicrobial therapy for neutropenic fever was as long as 170 min [81]. Since time to treatment is critically related to survival in patients with severe sepsis, recommendations for timely administration of empirical antibacterial therapy in such patients has been recommended [3, 61]. Even educational interventions have not produced sustained results [38]. Whilst methodological difficulties confound the ability to empirically demonstrate a time-delay effect upon survival, some investigators have suggested that such short timelines from assessment to antibiotic administration are reasonable benchmarks [27]. In one study from Brazil, the inclusion of a broad-spectrum antibiotic at the initial point of assessment for febrile neutropenic paediatric patients reduced the time from assessment to antibiotic administration by two-thirds from a median of 164 to 55 min [3]. In this example, accessibility of the antibacterial therapy seemed to be the factor most useful to achieving timely intervention. Such a score card chronicling the time from assessment to antibacterial administration seems an appropriate performance measure for medical facilities having the responsibility of providing service to febrile neutropenic patients.

References

1. Aapro MS, Cameron DA, Pettengell R, Bohlius J, Crawford J, Ellis M, Kearney N, Lyman GH, Tjan-Heijnen VC, Walewski J, Weber DC, Zielinski C. EORTC guidelines for the use of granulocyte-colony stimulating factor to reduce the incidence of chemotherapy-induced febrile neutropenia in adult patients with lymphomas and solid tumours. Eur J Cancer. 2006;42:2433–53.
2. Ahn S, Lee YS, Chun YH, et al. Predictive factors of poor prognosis in cancer patients with chemotherapy-induced febrile neutropenia. Support Care Cancer. 2011;19(8):1151–8.
3. Amado VM, Vilela GP, Queiroz Jr A, Amaral AC. Effect of a quality improvement intervention to decrease delays in antibiotic delivery in pediatric febrile neutropenia: a pilot study. J Crit Care. 2011;26(1):103.e9–12.
4. Amoateng-Adjepong Y, Del Mundo J, Manthous CA. Accuracy of an infrared tympanic thermometer. Chest. 1999;115:1002–5.
5. Andre S, Taboulet P, Elie C, Milpied N, Nahon M, Kierzek G, Billemont M, Perruche F, Charpentier S, Clement H, Pourriat JL, Claessens YE. Febrile neutropenia in French emergency departments: results of a prospective multicentre survey. Crit Care. 2010;14:R68.
6. Baden LR, Bensinger W, Angarone M, et al. NCCN Guidelines Version 2. Prevention and treatment of cancer-related infections. 2014. Available at: http://www.nccn.org/professionals/physician_gls/pdf/infections.pdf. Accessed 23 Aug 2014.
7. Baskaran ND, Gan GG, Adeeba K. Applying the multinational association for supportive care in cancer risk scoring in predicting outcome of febrile neutropenia patients in a cohort of patients. Ann hematolo. 2008;87(7):563–9.
8. Blay JY, Chauvin F, Le Cesne A, Anglaret B, Bouhour D, Lasset C, Freyer G, Philip T, Biron P. Early lymphopenia after cytotoxic chemotherapy as a risk factor for febrile neutropenia. J Clin Oncol. 1996;14:636–43.

9. Blijlevens N, Schwenkglenks M, Bacon P, D'Addio A, Einsele H, Maertens J, Niederwieser D, Rabitsch W, Roosaar A, Ruutu T, Schouten H, Stone R, Vokurka S, Quinn B, McCann S. Prospective oral mucositis audit: oral mucositis in patients receiving high-dose melphalan or BEAM conditioning chemotherapy–European Blood and Marrow Transplantation Mucositis Advisory Group. J Clin Oncol. 2008;26:1519–25.
10. Blijlevens NM, Donnelly JP, De Pauw BE. Impaired gut function as risk factor for invasive candidiasis in neutropenic patients. Br J Haematol. 2002;117:259–64.
11. Blijlevens NM, van't Land B, Donnelly JP, M'Rabet L, de Pauw BE. Measuring mucosal damage induced by cytotoxic therapy. Support Care Cancer. 2004;12:227–33.
12. Bochud PY, Eggiman P, Calandra T, Van Melle G, Saghafi L, Francioli P. Bacteremia due to viridans streptococcus in neutropenic patients with cancer: clinical spectrum and risk factors. Clin Infect Dis. 1994;18:25–31.
13. Bodey GP, Buckley M, Sathe YS, Freireich EJ. Quantitative relationships between circulating leukocytes and infection in patients with acute leukemia. Ann Intern Med. 1966;64:328–40.
14. Bodey GP, Rodriguez V, Chang HY, Narboni G. Fever and infection in leukemic patients: a study of 494 consecutive patients. Cancer. 1978;41:1610–22.
15. Bonadonna G, Valagussa P, Moliterni A, Zambetti M, Brambilla C. Adjuvant cyclophosphamide, methotrexate, and fluorouracil in node-positive breast cancer: the results of 20 years of follow-up. N Engl J Med. 1995;332:901–6.
16. Bone RC, Balk RA, Cerra FB, Dellinger RP, Fein AM, Knaus WA, Schein RM, Sibbald WJ. Definitions for sepsis and organ failure and guidelines for the use of innovative therapies in sepsis. The ACCP/SCCM Consensus Conference Committee. American College of Chest Physicians/Society of Critical Care Medicine. Chest. 1992;101:1644–55.
17. Bosly A, Bron D, Van Hoof A, De Bock R, Berneman Z, Ferrant A, Kaufman L, Dauwe M, Verhoef G. Achievement of optimal average relative dose intensity and correlation with survival in diffuse large B-cell lymphoma patients treated with CHOP. Ann Hematol. 2008;87:277–83.
18. Bow EJ. Neutropenic fever syndromes in patients undergoing cytotoxic therapy for acute leukemia and myelodysplastic syndromes. Semin Hematol. 2009;46:259–68.
19. Bow EJ, Kilpatrick MG, Scott BA, Clinch JJ, Cheang MS. Acute myeloid leukemia in Manitoba. The consequences of standard "7 + 3" remission-induction therapy followed by high dose cytarabine postremission consolidation for myelosuppression, infectious morbidity, and outcome. Cancer. 1994;74:52–60.
20. Bow EJ, Loewen R, Cheang MS, Shore TB, Rubinger M, Schacter B. Cytotoxic therapy-induced D-xylose malabsorption and invasive infection during remission-induction therapy for acute myeloid leukemia in adults. J Clin Oncol. 1997;15:2254–61.
21. Bow EJ, Meddings JB. Intestinal mucosal dysfunction and infection during remission-induction therapy for acute myeloid leukaemia. Leukemia. 2006;20:2087–92.
22. Bow EJ, Wngard JR, Bowden RA. Infectious complications in patients receiving cytotoxic therapy for acute leukemia: history, background and approaches to management. In: Management of infections in oncology patients. London: Martin Dunitz; 2003. p. 71–128.
23. Bucaneve G, Micozzi A, Menichetti F, Martino P, Dionisi MS, Martinelli G, Allione B, D'Antonio D, Buelli M, Nosari AM, Cilloni D, Zuffa E, Cantaffa R, Specchia G, Amadori S, Fabbiano F, Deliliers GL, Lauria F, Foa R, Del FA. Levofloxacin to prevent bacterial infection in patients with cancer and neutropenia. N Engl J Med. 2005;353:977–87.
24. Cherif H, Johansson E, Bjorkholm M, Kalin M. The feasibility of early hospital discharge with oral antimicrobial therapy in low risk patients with febrile neutropenia following chemotherapy for hematologic malignancies. Haematologica. 2006;91(2):215–22.
25. Chirivella I, Bermejo B, Insa A, Perez-Fidalgo A, Magro A, Rosello S, Garcia-Garre E, Martin P, Bosch A, Lluch A. Impact of chemotherapy dose-related factors on survival in breast cancer patients treated with adjuvant anthracycline-based chemotherapy. J Clin Oncol (Meet Abstr). 2006;24:668.
26. Chrischilles E, Delgado DJ, Stolshek BS, Lawless G, Fridman M, Carter WB. Impact of age and colony-stimulating factor use on hospital length of stay for febrile neutropenia in CHOP-treated non-Hodgkin's lymphoma. Cancer Control. 2002;9:203–11.

27. Corey AL, Snyder S. Antibiotics in 30 minutes or less for febrile neutropenic patients: a quality control measure in a new hospital. J Pediatr Oncol Nurs. 2008;25:208–12.
28. Crawford J, Dale DC, Lyman GH. Chemotherapy-induced neutropenia: risks, consequences, and new directions for its management. Cancer. 2004;100:228–37.
29. Cullen M, Steven N, Billingham L, Gaunt C, Hastings M, Simmonds P, Stuart N, Rea D, Bower M, Fernando I, Huddart R, Gollins S, Stanley A. Antibacterial prophylaxis after chemotherapy for solid tumors and lymphomas. N Engl J Med. 2005;353:988–98.
30. Cullen MH, Billingham LJ, Gaunt CH, Steven NM. Rational selection of patients for antibacterial prophylaxis after chemotherapy. J Clin Oncol. 2007;25:4821–8.
31. de Souza-Viana L, Serufo JC, da Costa Rocha MO, Costa RN, Duarte RC. Performance of a modified MASCC index score for identifying low-risk febrile neutropenic cancer patients. Support Care Cancer. 2008;16:841–6.
32. Dellinger RP, Carlet JM, Masur H, Gerlach H, Calandra T, Cohen J, Gea-Banacloche J, Keh D, Marshall JC, Parker MM, Ramsay G, Zimmerman JL, Vincent JL, Levy MM. Surviving sepsis campaign guidelines for management of severe sepsis and septic shock. Crit Care Med. 2004;32:858–73.
33. Doezema D, Lunt M, Tandberg D. Cerumen occlusion lowers infrared tympanic membrane temperature measurement. Acad Emerg Med. 1995;2:17–9.
34. Dzarr AA, Kamal M, Baba AA. A comparison between infrared tympanic thermometry, oral and axilla with rectal thermometry in neutropenic adults. Eur J Oncol Nurs. 2009;13:250–4.
35. Erickson RS, Meyer LT, Woo TM. Accuracy of chemical dot thermometers in critically ill adults and young children. Image J Nurs Sch. 1996;28:23–8.
36. Farnell S, Maxwell L, Tan S, Rhodes A, Philips B. Temperature measurement: comparison of non-invasive methods used in adult critical care. J Clin Nurs. 2005;14:632–9.
37. Ferreira FL, Bota DP, Bross A, Melot C, Vincent JL. Serial evaluation of the SOFA score to predict outcome in critically ill patients. JAMA. 2001;286:1754–8.
38. Ferrer R, Artigas A, Levy MM, Blanco J, Gonzalez-Diaz G, Garnacho-Montero J, Ibanez J, Palencia E, Quintana M, de la Torre-Prados MV. Improvement in process of care and outcome after a multicenter severe sepsis educational program in Spain. JAMA. 2008;299: 2294–303.
39. Fisk J, Arcona S. Tympanic membrane vs. pulmonary artery thermometry. Nurs Manag. 2001;32(42):45–8.
40. Fossa SD, Kaye SB, Mead GM, Cullen M, de Wit R, Bodrogi I, van Groeningen CJ, De Mulder PH, Stenning S, Lallemand E, De Prijck L, Collette L. Filgrastim during combination chemotherapy of patients with poor-prognosis metastatic germ cell malignancy. European Organization for Research and Treatment of Cancer, Genito-Urinary Group, and the Medical Research Council Testicular Cancer Working Party, Cambridge, United Kingdom. J Clin Oncol. 1998;16:716–24.
41. Freifeld A. Guidelines for antimicrobials in neutropenic cancer patients. In: 45th Annual Meeting of the Infectious Diseases Society of America. San Diego: IDSA; 2007.
42. Freifeld A, Bow EJ, Sepkowitz KA, Boeckh MJ, Ito JI, Mullen CA, Raad II, Roslton KV, Young JAH, Wingard JR. Clinical practice guideline for the use of antimicrobial agents in neutropenic patients with cancer: 2010 update by the Infectious Diseases Society of America. Clin Infect Dis. 2011;52(4):e46–e93.
43. Fulbrook P. Core body temperature measurement: a comparison of axilla, tympanic membrane and pulmonary artery blood temperature. Intensive Crit Care Nurs. 1997;13:266–72.
44. Gardner A, Mattiuzzi G, Faderl S, Borthakur G, Garcia-Manero G, Pierce S, Brandt M, Estey E. Randomized comparison of cooked and noncooked diets in patients undergoing remission induction therapy for acute myeloid leukemia. J Clin Oncol. 2008;26:5684–8.
45. Gayol Mdel C, Font A, Casas I, Estrada O, Dominguez MJ, Pedro-Botet ML. Usefulness of the MASCC scale in the management of neutropenic fever induced by chemotherapy in patients with solid neoplasm. Medicina clinica. 2009;133(8):296–9.
46. Gerson SL, Talbot GH, Hurwitz S, Strom BL, Lusk EJ, Cassileth PA. Prolonged granulocytopenia: the major risk factor for invasive pulmonary aspergillosis in patients with acute leukemia. Ann Intern Med. 1984;100:345–51.

47. Gianni L, Munzone E, Capri G, Fulfaro F, Tarenzi E, Villani F, Spreafico C, Laffranchi A, Caraceni A, Martini C, et al. Paclitaxel by 3-hour infusion in combination with bolus doxorubicin in women with untreated metastatic breast cancer: high antitumor efficacy and cardiac effects in a dose-finding and sequence-finding study. J Clin Oncol. 1995;13:2688–99.
48. Hosmer W, Malin J, Wong M. Development and validation of a prediction model for the risk of developing febrile neutropenia in the first cycle of chemotherapy among elderly patients with breast, lung, colorectal, and prostate cancer. Support Care Cancer. 2011;19:333–41.
49. Hughes WT, Armstrong D, Bodey GP, Bow EJ, Brown AE, Calandra T, Feld R, Pizzo PA, Rolston KVI, Shenep JL, Young LS. 2002 guidelines for the use of antimicrobial agents in neutropenic patients with cancer. Clin Infect Dis. 2002;34:730–51.
50. Immunocompromised Host S. The design, analysis, and reporting of clinical trials on the empirical antibiotic management of the neutropenic patient. J Infect Dis. 1990;161:397–401.
51. Innes H, Lim SL, Hall A, Chan SY, Bhalla N, Marshall E. Management of febrile neutropenia in solid tumours and lymphomas using the multinational association for supportive care in cancer (MASCC) risk index: feasibility and safety in routine clinical practice. Supportive care in cancer: official journal of the Multinational Association of Supportive Care in Cancer. 2008;16(5):485–91.
52. Intragumtornchai T, Sutheesophon J, Sutcharitchan P, Swasdikul D. A predictive model for life-threatening neutropenia and febrile neutropenia after the first course of CHOP chemotherapy in patients with aggressive non-Hodgkin's lymphoma. Leuk Lymphoma. 2000;37: 351–60.
53. Jeddi R, Achour M, Amor RB, Aissaoui L, Bouteraa W, Kacem K, Lakhal RB, Abid HB, BelHadjAli Z, Turki A, Meddeb B. Factors associated with severe sepsis: prospective study of 94 neutropenic febrile episodes. Hematology. 2010;15:28–32.
54. Jevon P, Jevon M. Using a tympanic thermometer. Nurs Times. 2001;97:43–4.
55. Jun HX, Zhixiang S, Chun W, Reksodiputro AH, Ranuhardy D, Tamura K, Matsumoto T, Lee DG, Purushotaman SV, Lim V, Ahmed A, Hussain Y, Chua M, Ong A, Liu CY, Hsueh PR, Lin SF, Liu YC, Suwangool P, Jootar S, Picazo JJ. Clinical guidelines for the management of cancer patients with neutropenia and unexplained fever. Int J Antimicrob Agents. 2005;26 Suppl 2:S128–32; discussion S133–40.
56. Klastersky J, Ameye L, Maertens J, Georgala A, Muanza F, Aoun M, Ferrant A, Rapoport B, Rolston K, Paesmans M. Bacteraemia in febrile neutropenic cancer patients. Int J Antimicrob Agents. 2007;30 Suppl 1:S51–9.
57. Klastersky J, Paesmans M, Georgala A, Muanza F, Plehiers B, Dubreucq L, Lalami Y, Aoun M, Barette M. Outpatient oral antibiotics for febrile neutropenic cancer patients using a score predictive for complications. J Clin Oncol. 2006;24:4129–34.
58. Klastersky J, Paesmans M, Rubenstein EB, Boyer M, Elting L, Feld R, Gallagher J, Herrstedt J, Rapoport B, Rolston K, Talcott J. The Multinational Association for Supportive Care in Cancer risk index: a multinational scoring system for identifying low-risk febrile neutropenic cancer patients. J Clin Oncol. 2000;18:3038–51.
59. Klastersky J, Zinner SH, Calandra T, Gaya H, Glauser MP, Meunier F, Rossi M, Schimpff SC, Tattersall M, Viscoli C. Empiric antimicrobial therapy for febrile granulocytopenic cancer patients: lessons from four EORTC trials. Eur J Cancer Clin Oncol. 1988;24 Suppl 1:S35–45.
60. Kuderer NM, Dale DC, Crawford J, Cosler LE, Lyman GH. Mortality, morbidity, and cost associated with febrile neutropenia in adult cancer patients. Cancer. 2006;106:2258–66.
61. Kumar A, Roberts D, Wood KE, Light B, Parrillo JE, Sharma S, Suppes R, Feinstein D, Zanotti S, Taiberg L, Gurka D, Cheang M. Duration of hypotension before initiation of effective antimicrobial therapy is the critical determinant of survival in human septic shock. Crit Care Med. 2006;34:1589–96.
62. Leonard RC, Miles D, Thomas R, Nussey F. Impact of neutropenia on delivering planned adjuvant chemotherapy: UK audit of primary breast cancer patients. Br J Cancer. 2003;89:2062–8.
63. Levy MM, Fink MP, Marshall JC, Abraham E, Angus D, Cook D, Cohen J, Opal SM, Vincent JL, Ramsay G. 2001 SCCM/ESICM/ACCP/ATS/SIS International Sepsis Definitions Conference. Intensive Care Med. 2003;29:530–8.

64. Link H, Bohme A, Cornely OA, Hoffken K, Kellner O, Kern WV, Mahlberg R, Maschmeyer G, Nowrousian MR, Ostermann H, Ruhnke M, Sezer O, Schiel X, Wilhelm M, Auner HW. Antimicrobial therapy of unexplained fever in neutropenic patients–guidelines of the Infectious Diseases Working Party (AGIHO) of the German Society of Hematology and Oncology (DGHO), Study Group Interventional Therapy of Unexplained Fever, Arbeitsgemeinschaft Supportivmassnahmen in der Onkologie (ASO) of the Deutsche Krebsgesellschaft (DKG-German Cancer Society). Ann Hematol. 2003;82 Suppl 2:S105–17.
65. Lutgens LC, Blijlevens NM, Deutz NE, Donnelly JP, Lambin P, De Pauw BE. Monitoring myeloablative therapy-induced small bowel toxicity by serum citrulline concentration: a comparison with sugar permeability tests. Cancer. 2005;103:191–9.
66. Lyman GH, Dale DC, Friedberg J, Crawford J, Fisher RI. Incidence and predictors of low chemotherapy dose-intensity in aggressive non-Hodgkin's lymphoma: a nationwide study. J Clin Oncol. 2004;22:4302–11.
67. Lyman GH, Lyman CH, Agboola O. Risk models for predicting chemotherapy-induced neutropenia. Oncologist. 2005;10:427–37.
68. Mackowiak PA, Bartlett JG, Bordon BC, et al. Concepts of fever: recent advances and lingering dogma. Clin Infect Dis. 1997;35:119–38.
69. Mackowiak PA, Wasserman SS. Physicians' perceptions regarding body temperature in health and disease. South Med J. 1995;88:934–8.
70. Mackowiak PA, Wasserman SS, Levine MM. A critical appraisal of 98.6 degrees F, the upper limit of the normal body temperature, and other legacies of Carl Reinhold August Wunderlich. JAMA. 1992;268:1578–80.
71. Maher DW, Lieschke GJ, Green M, Bishop J, Stuart-Harris R, Wolf M, Sheridan WP, Kefford RF, Cebon J, Olver I, McKendrick J, Toner G, Bradstock K, Lieschke M, Cruickshank S, Tomita DK, Hoffman EW, Fox RM, Morstyn G. Filgrastim in patients with chemotherapy-induced febrile neutropenia – a double-blind, placebo-controlled trial. Ann Intern Med. 1994;121:492–501.
72. Marshall JC, Cook DJ, Christou NV, Bernard GR, Sprung CL, Sibbald WJ. Multiple organ dysfunction score: a reliable descriptor of a complex clinical outcome. Crit Care Med. 1995;23:1638–52.
73. Martin C, Brun-Buisson C, pour les Membres du Groupe de Travail (Annane D, CJ, Dhainaut JF, Gerbeaux P, Goldstein P, Hamza J, Leclerc F, Leconte P, Montravers P, Malledant Y, Orliaguet G, Payen D, Pourriat JL, Sadik A, Sollet JP, Vallet B) Prise en charge initiale des états septiques graves de l'adulte et de l'enfant. In: Conférence de consensus 2007, vol. http://www.sfmu.org/documents/consensus/Groupe%20Transversal%20Sepsis%20Fn.doc. 2007.
74. Meropol NJ, Somer RA, Gutheil J, Pelley RJ, Modiano MR, Rowinsky EK, Rothenberg ML, Redding SW, Serdar CM, Yao B, Heard R, Rosen LS. Randomized phase I trial of recombinant human keratinocyte growth factor plus chemotherapy: potential role as mucosal protectant. J Clin Oncol. 2003;21:1452–8.
75. Nucci M, Anaissie E. Revisiting the source of candidemia: skin or gut? Clin Infect Dis. 2001;33:1959–67.
76. Nucci M, Spector N, Bueno AP, Solza C, Perecmanis T, Bacha PC, Pulcheri W. Risk factors and attributable mortality associated with superinfections in neutropenic patients with cancer. Clin Infect Dis. 1997;24:575–9.
77. O'Toole S. Alternatives to mercury thermometers. Prof Nurs. 1997;12:783–6.
78. Oguz A, Karadeniz C, Ckitak EC, Cil V. Which one is a risk factor for chemotherapy-induced febrile neutropenia in childhood solid tumors: early lymphopenia or monocytopenia? Pediatr Hematol Oncol. 2006;23:143–51.
79. Paesmans M, Klastersky J, Maertens J, Georgala A, Muanza F, Aoun M, Ferrant A, Rapoport B, Rolston K, Ameye L. Predicting febrile neutropenic patients at low risk using the MASCC score: does bacteremia matter? Support Care Cancer. 2011;19:1001–8.
80. Peacock JE, Herrington DA, Wade JC, Lazarus HM, Reed MD, Sinclair JW, Haverstock DC, Kowalsky SF, Hurd DD, Cushing DA, Harman CP, Donowitz GR. Ciprofloxacin plus piperacillin compared with tobramycin plus piperacillin as empirical therapy in febrile neutropenic patients. A randomized, double-blind trial. Ann Intern Med. 2002;137:77–87.

81. Perrone J, Hollander JE, Datner EM. Emergency department evaluation of patients with fever and chemotherapy-induced neutropenia. J Emerg Med. 2004;27:115–9.
82. Pettengell R, Bosly A, Szucs TD, Jackisch C, Leonard R, Paridaens R, Constenla M, Schwenkglenks M. Multivariate analysis of febrile neutropenia occurrence in patients with non-Hodgkin lymphoma: data from the INC-EU Prospective Observational European Neutropenia Study. Br J Haematol. 2009;144:677–85.
83. Pettengell R, Schwenkglenks M, Leonard R, Bosly A, Paridaens R, Constenla M, Szucs TD, Jackisch C. Neutropenia occurrence and predictors of reduced chemotherapy delivery: results from the INC-EU prospective observational European neutropenia study. Support Care Cancer. 2008;16(11):1299–309.
84. Ray-Coquard I, Borg C, Bachelot T, Sebban C, Philip I, Clapisson G, Le Cesne A, Biron P, Chauvin F, Blay JY. Baseline and early lymphopenia predict for the risk of febrile neutropenia after chemotherapy. Br J Cancer. 2003;88:181–6.
85. Rubenstein EB, Peterson DE, Schubert M, Keefe D, McGuire D, Epstein J, Elting LS, Fox PC, Cooksley C, Sonis ST. Clinical practice guidelines for the prevention and treatment of cancer therapy-induced oral and gastrointestinal mucositis. Cancer. 2004;100:2026–46.
86. Santolaya ME, Rabagliati R, Bidart T, Paya E, Guzman AM, Morales R, Braun S, Bronfman L, Ferres M, Flores C, Garcia P, Letelier LM, Puga B, Salgado C, Thompson L, Tordecilla J, Zubieta M. Consensus: rational approach towards the patient with cancer, fever and neutropenia. Rev Chil Infectol. 2005;22 Suppl 2:S79–113.
87. Schimpff SC, Gaya H, Klastersky J, Tattersall MH, Zinner SH. Three antibiotic regimens in the treatment of infection in febrile granulocytopenic patients with cancer. The EORTC international antimicrobial therapy project group. J Infect Dis. 1978;137:14–29.
88. Schimpff SC, Young VM, Greene WH, Vermeulen GD, Moody MR, Wiernik PH. Origin of infection in acute nonlymphocytic leukemia. Significance of hospital acquisition of potential pathogens. Ann Intern Med. 1972;77:707–14.
89. Schwenkglenks M, Jackisch C, Constenla M, Kerger JN, Paridaens R, Auerbach L, Bosly A, Pettengell R, Szucs TD, Leonard R. Neutropenic event risk and impaired chemotherapy delivery in six European audits of breast cancer treatment. Support Care Cancer. 2006;14:901–9.
90. Sickles EA, Greene WH, Wiernik PH. Clinical presentation of infection in granulocytopenic patients. Arch Intern Med. 1975;135:715–9.
91. Sickles EA, Young VM, Greene WH, Wiernik PH. Pneumonia in acute leukemia. Ann Intern Med. 1973;79:528–34.
92. Smith TJ, Khatcheressian J, Lyman GH, Ozer H, Armitage JO, Balducci L, Bennett CL, Cantor SB, Crawford J, Cross SJ, Demetri G, Desch CE, Pizzo PA, Schiffer CA, Schwartzberg L, Somerfield MR, Somlo G, Wade JC, Wade JL, Winn RJ, Wozniak AJ, Wolff AC. 2006 update of recommendations for the use of white blood cell growth factors: an evidence-based clinical practice guideline. J Clin Oncol. 2006;24:3187–205.
93. Sonis ST, Elting LS, Keefe D, Peterson DE, Schubert M, Hauer-Jensen M, Bekele BN, Raber-Durlacher J, Donnelly JP, Rubenstein EB. Perspectives on cancer therapy-induced mucosal injury: pathogenesis, measurement, epidemiology, and consequences for patients. Cancer. 2004;100:1995–2025.
94. Sonis ST, Oster G, Fuchs H, Bellm L, Bradford WZ, Edelsberg J, Hayden V, Eilers J, Epstein JB, LeVeque FG, Miller C, Peterson DE, Schubert MM, Spijkervet FK, Horowitz M. Oral mucositis and the clinical and economic outcomes of hematopoietic stem-cell transplantation. J Clin Oncol. 2001;19:2201–5.
95. Spielberger R, Stiff P, Bensinger W, Gentile T, Weisdorf D, Kewalramani T, Shea T, Yanovich S, Hansen K, Noga S, McCarty J, LeMaistre CF, Sung EC, Blazar BR, Elhardt D, Chen MG, Emmanouilides C. Palifermin for oral mucositis after intensive therapy for hematologic cancers. N Engl J Med. 2004;351:2590–8.
96. Stone RM, Berg DT, George SL, Dodge RK, Paciucci PA, Schulman P, Lee EJ, Moore JO, Powell BL, Schiffer CA. Granulocyte-macrophage colony-stimulating factor after initial chemotherapy for elderly patients with primary acute myelogenous leukemia. Cancer and Leukemia Group B. N Engl J Med. 1995;332:1671–7.

97. Talcott JA. Outpatient management of febrile neutropenia: should we change the standard of care? Oncologist. 1997;2:365–73.
98. Talcott JA, Finberg R, Mayer RJ, Goldman L. The medical course of cancer patients with fever and neutropenia. Clinical identification of a low-risk subgroup at presentation. Arch Intern Med. 1988;148:2561–8.
99. Talcott JA, Siegel RD, Finberg R, Goldman L. Risk assessment in cancer patients with fever and neutropenia: a prospective, two-center validation of a prediction rule. J Clin Oncol. 1992;10:316–22.
100. Talcott JA, Whalen A, Clark J, Rieker PP, Finberg R. Home antibiotic therapy for low-risk cancer patients with fever and neutropenia: a pilot study of 30 patients based on a validated prediction rule. J Clin Oncol. 1994;12:107–14.
101. Tamura K. Clinical guidelines for the management of neutropenic patients with unexplained fever in Japan: validation by the Japan Febrile Neutropenia Study Group. Int J Antimicrob Agents. 2005;26 Suppl 2:S123–7.
102. Timmer-Bonte JN, de Boo TM, Smit HJ, Biesma B, Wilschut FA, Cheragwandi SA, Termeer A, Hensing CA, Akkermans J, Adang EM, Bootsma GP, Tjan-Heijnen VC. Prevention of chemotherapy-induced febrile neutropenia by prophylactic antibiotics plus or minus granulocyte colony-stimulating factor in small-cell lung cancer: a Dutch randomized phase III study. J Clin Oncol. 2005;23:7974–84.
103. Tjan-Heijnen VC, Postmus PE, Ardizzoni A, Manegold CH, Burghouts J, van Meerbeeck J, Gans S, Mollers M, Buchholz E, Biesma B, Legrand C, Debruyne C, Giaccone G. Reduction of chemotherapy-induced febrile leucopenia by prophylactic use of ciprofloxacin and roxithromycin in small-cell lung cancer patients: an EORTC double-blind placebo-controlled phase III study. Ann Oncol. 2001;12:1359–68.
104. Toussaint E, Bahel-Ball E, Vekemans M, Georgala A, Al-Hakak L, Paesmans M, Aoun M. Causes of fever in cancer patients (prospective study over 477 episodes). Support Care Cancer. 2006;14:763–9.
105. Uys A, Rapoport BL, Anderson R. Febrile neutropenia: a prospective study to validate the Multinational Association of Supportive Care of Cancer (MASCC) risk-index score. Support Care Cancer. 2004;12:555–60.
106. Uys A, Rapoport BL, Fickl H, Meyer PW, Anderson R. Prediction of outcome in cancer patients with febrile neutropenia: comparison of the Multinational Association of Supportive Care in Cancer risk-index score with procalcitonin, C-reactive protein, serum amyloid A, and interleukins-1beta, -6, -8 and -10. Eur J Cancer Care (Engl). 2007;16:475–83.
107. Viscoli C, Bruzzi P, Castagnola E, Boni L, Calandra T, Gaya H, Meunier F, Feld R, Zinner S, Klastersky J, Glauser M, Glauser & Group, E.I.A.T.C.P. Factors associated with bacteremia in febrile, granulocytopenic cancer patients. Eur J Cancer. 1994;30A:430–7.
108. von Minckwitz G, Schwenkglenks M, Skacel T, Lyman GH, Pousa AL, Bacon P, Easton V, Aapro MS. Febrile neutropenia and related complications in breast cancer patients receiving pegfilgrastim primary prophylaxis versus current practice neutropaenia management: results from an integrated analysis. Eur J Cancer. 2009;45:608–17.
109. Voog E, Bienvenu J, Warzocha K, Moullet I, Dumontet C, Thieblemont C, Monneret G, Gutowski MC, Coiffier B, Salles G. Factors that predict chemotherapy-induced myelosuppression in lymphoma patients: role of the tumor necrosis factor ligand-receptor system. J Clin Oncol. 2000;18:325–31.
110. Wardley AM, Jayson GC, Swindell R, Morgenstern GR, Chang J, Bloor R, Fraser CJ, Scarffe JH. Prospective evaluation of oral mucositis in patients receiving myeloablative conditioning regimens and haemopoietic progenitor rescue. Br J Haematol. 2000;110:292–9.
111. Wunderlich CA, Seguin E. Medical thermometry and human temperature. New York: William Wood & Co.; 1871.

Diagnostic Radiology in Hematological Patients with Febrile Neutropenia

7

Claus Peter Heussel

Contents

C.P. Heussel
Diagnostic and Interventional Radiology, Chest Clinics at University Hospital Heidelberg, Amalienstrasse 5, Heidelberg 69126, Germany
e-mail: heussel@uni-heidelberg.de

G. Maschmeyer, K.V.I. Rolston (eds.), *Infections in Hematology*,
DOI 10.1007/978-3-662-44000-1_7

7.1 Early Detection of Pneumonia

The necessity for early detection of the focus of infection is based upon high fatality of infections in immunocompromised hosts, increasing within hours of delayed appropriate treatment [48]. (This paper does not refer to immunocompromised patients; maybe Greene 2007 [52] or Cornely 2010 [58] could be used), a potential negative impact of delayed diagnosis (i.e., more advanced infection) on future antineoplastic treatment, and high costs of prolonged hospitalization. This has to be compared with the costs of a non-enhanced CT scan, which is around € 230 in German hospitals. After physical examination and interpretation of laboratory findings, the search for an infectious focus starts with the identification of the most suspected organ system(s). The appropriate imaging technique has to be selected demanding for high sensitivity and clinically meaningful negative predictive value [4].

Exact proportions of organ involvement are difficult to determine and may differ from clinical and pathological findings, the latter often obtained from autopsies (i.e., negative selection). Clinically, lungs are affected in 30 % of febrile neutropenic patients and allogeneic hematopoietic stem cell transplant (aSCT) recipients, paranasal sinuses in 3 % of neutropenic patients, and 30 % in the aSCT setting (concomitant to pneumonia), while the gastrointestinal tract, liver, spleen, central nervous system, and kidneys are less frequently involved [4].

7.1.1 Conventional Chest Radiograph

Chest x-ray (CXR) is still frequently used when pneumonia is suspected or should be ruled out [14, 15]. CXR has several advantages: it is quick, widely available (even on the ward), inexpensive, and associated with a low radiation dose. CXR is occasionally done on the ward to keep neutropenic patients in protective isolation, even if performed in supine position. But CXR has the crucial disadvantage of superimposition and therefore a very limited sensitivity for the detection of pneumonia (Figs. 7.2 and 7.6) [14, 16]. Especially if performed in supine position, lung inflation is worse and lateral projection is lacking, which limits image quality besides other technical issues. In patients with fever of unknown origin (FUO) after SCT, digital CXR in supine position achieves a sensitivity for early detection of pneumonia of only 46 % [17]. While CXR provides relevant clinical information concerning central venous catheters (CVC), pleural effusion, and pulmonary congestion [17], it fails to enable early detection or exclusion of pneumonia, which is a major task in immunocompromised hosts. CXR in supine position alone is therefore not recommended for the early detection of pneumonia in these patients [5]. Also, if an infiltrate is apparent at CXR, the options for its characterization are very limited. If pneumonia is considered in these hosts, thin-section CT should be preferred at any time [18].

7.1.2 CT Technique and Terminology

The radiation dose is of limited concern in patients who eventually underwent local or total body irradiation and received cytotoxic agents, etc., considering that actual CT techniques apply 1–10 mSv per lung scan (in this diagnostic scenario: mSv = mGy) [19, 20]. The risk of developing a radiation-induced neoplasm, even after several diagnostic exposures, is low when compared to the high mortality associated to infection and disease as well as the risk of a secondary malignancy due to antineoplastic treatment.

Terms like *incremental CT*, *high-resolution CT* (HRCT), *spiral CT*, *thin-section CT*, *multislice CT* (MSCT), and *low-dose CT* are widely used and might confuse non-radiologists. To keep it simple, HRCT is an incremental scanning technique with several respiratory breath-holds resulting in inaccuracy of repositioning of the anatomical lung position. The use of 1 mm sections and gaps in between (e.g., 10 mm) results in representative, detailed images of selected lung areas; however, the noncontiguous scanning has its limitations in nodule detection, quantification, and monitoring. Volumetric techniques as used in spiral CT and MSCT, acquired without gaps, are frequently reconstructed with larger thickness (e.g., 5 mm) resulting in spatial volume effects. This results in limitations to detect inflammatory lung disease, especially ground-glass opacification [22]. Since no additional information is expected from supplemental spiral CT to HRCT, as shown in AIDS patients [23], HRCT may be used as a diagnostic standard. In contrast, thin-section MSCT provides volumetric scanning as well as detailed images [24, 25]. This technique also allows for an adequate monitoring of lung disease since the same anatomical position can be reidentified in baseline and follow-up studies [24–26]. While a rapid technical development in CT imaging is ongoing, the different techniques applied today are addressed as “CT” in this chapter.

In general, contrast enhancement is not required for detecting and characterizing pneumonia [6, 18]. Only in special situations such as suspicion of pulmonary embolism or hemoptysis caused by vessel erosion is CT angiography beneficial (Fig. 7.1) [27]. In the aSCT setting, bronchiolitis obliterans is to be considered [24, 28] where air-trapping is a relevant finding. Here, an additional expiratory CT scan is helpful [24, 28].

7.1.3 CT

The advantage of HRCT in comparison to CXR for the early detection of pneumonia was demonstrated in febrile neutropenic patients not responding to empirical antibiotic therapy [21]. In approximately 60 % of the patients with a normal CXR, HRCT showed pulmonary infiltrates (Fig. 7.2). In only 10 % of patients with a normal chest x-ray and a normal HRCT, pneumonia occurred during follow-up [21]. Exclusion of pneumonia is another clinically relevant information. Thus, CT yields

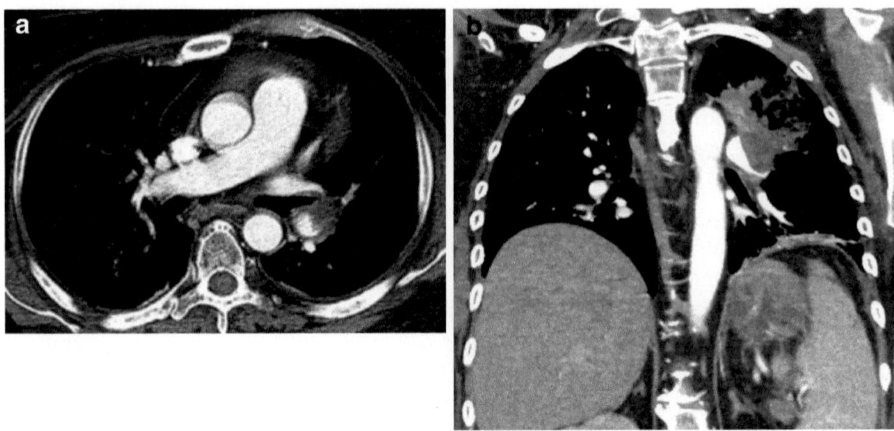

Fig. 7.1 Contract-enhanced CT demonstrates vessel erosion in a consolidating infiltrate of the left lung. An apposition thrombus can be depicted in the pulmonary artery of the left lower lobe of this 45-year-old female who underwent unrelated PBST 6 months before due to AML. She died 2 days later from brain infarction

very useful results with good sensitivity (87 %) and negative predictive value (88 %). The early use of HRCT achieves a gain of approximately 5 days during which pneumonia may be excluded [17]. In clinical practice, this may be very helpful for the management of immunocompromised hosts at high risk of life-threatening pulmonary infection [5] (Fig. 7.2).

7.1.4 Magnetic-Resonance Tomography (MRI)

MRI has been evaluated for the investigation of pulmonary disease since it has a known benefit in lesion characterization [29, 30]. Comparing CT to MRI on an intraindividual basis, MRI reveals comparable clinical results (sensitivity 95 %, specificity 88 %, positive predictive value 95 %, negative predictive value 88 %) [53]. Besides the lack of radiation, there is no clear advantage of MRI in the early detection of pneumonia (Fig. 7.3). In advanced stages, CT and MRI are comparable in the visualization of infiltrates [30]. CT is widely available, easier, and faster to perform as well as less susceptible to breathing artifacts. MRI is superior to CT in the detection of abscesses due to a clearer detection of central necrosis in T2-weighted images and rim enhancement after contrast application in T1-weighted images [29]. However, this fact has limited clinical impact and duration of MRI, and required compliance is substantially higher compared to CT. MR has problems to detect small lesions and those which are adjacent to the left ventricle due to the cardiac motion [53].

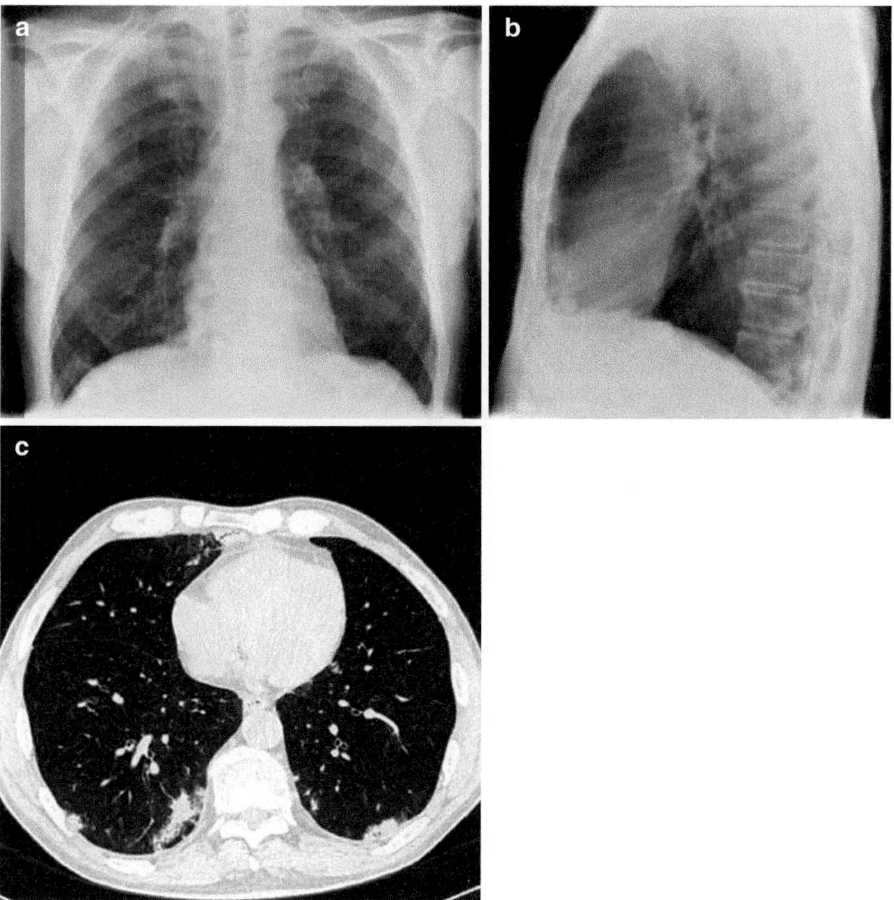

Fig. 7.2 Neutropenic febrile patient receiving broad-spectrum antibiotic therapy. CXR was normal at day 3 of fever (**a**, **b**). HRCT performed the same day demonstrates bilateral infiltrates, which were hidden behind the heart in posterior-anterior and the spine in lateral projection (**c**)

7.1.5 Recommendation for Clinical Practice

In contrast to systemic infections, identification of the underlying organism in pneumonia is more difficult and complex. Attempts to reinforce pathogen identification did not improve the clinical outcome significantly [9]. Therefore, a calculated (preemptive) decision on antimicrobial therapy in febrile immunosuppressed patients based on imaging studies is widely used.

The use of CT is recommended for the early detection of pneumonia [9]. It may serve for indication and localization of invasive diagnostic procedures such as

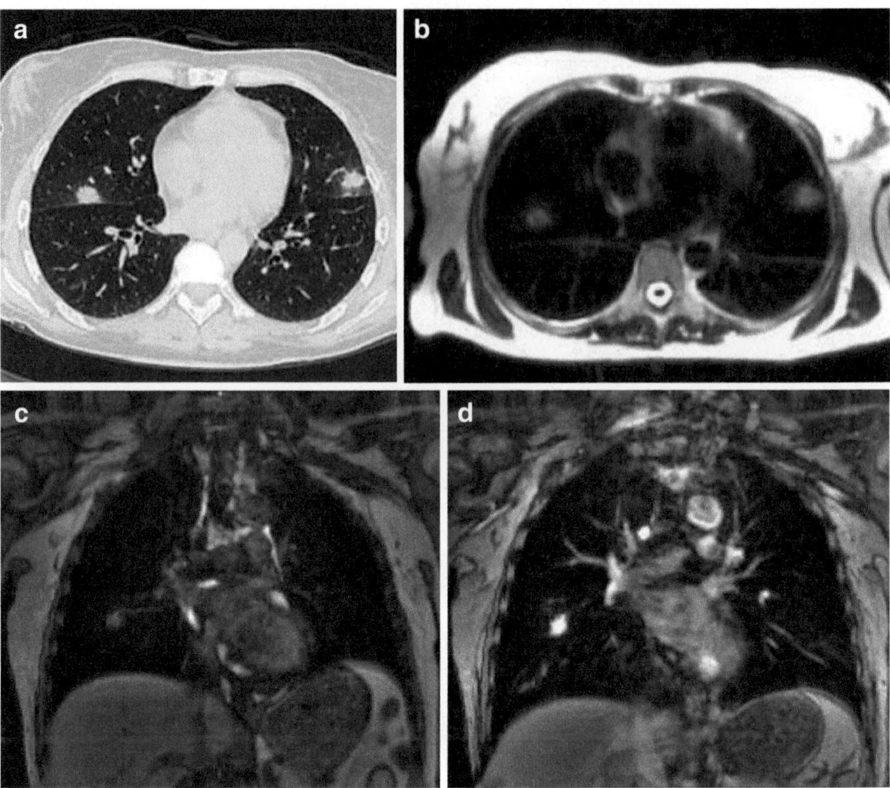

Fig. 7.3 Fungal pneumonia in HRCT (**a**), T2-weighted (**b**), non-enhanced T1-weighted GE MRI (**c**) and after Gd application performed the same day (**d**). Lesion contrast is similar in CT and contrast-enhanced MRI

bronchoscopy and bronchoalveolar lavage or CT-guided biopsy. On the other hand, the exclusion of pneumonia can be obtained with a higher reliability as compared to conventional CXR. The sequential cascade as shown in Fig. 7.4 can be modified if the local institutional CT capacity allows for the skipping of CXR.

7.2 Monitoring of Lung Infiltrates

An increasing size of pulmonary infiltrates during hematopoietic recovery has been well described by [31]. Caillot et al. evaluated HRCT in neutropenic patients with proven pulmonary aspergillosis at weekly intervals [31] and documented the time points of different radiological patterns and evaluated the size of infiltrates and documented the time points of different radiological patterns and evaluated the size of infiltrates. They frequently found a "halo sign" (Fig. 7.5) on the first CT scans and reported a low sensitivity of this pattern (68 %), which was no longer visible on follow-up scans. In contrast, the more specific "air-crescent sign" (Fig. 7.7) emerged

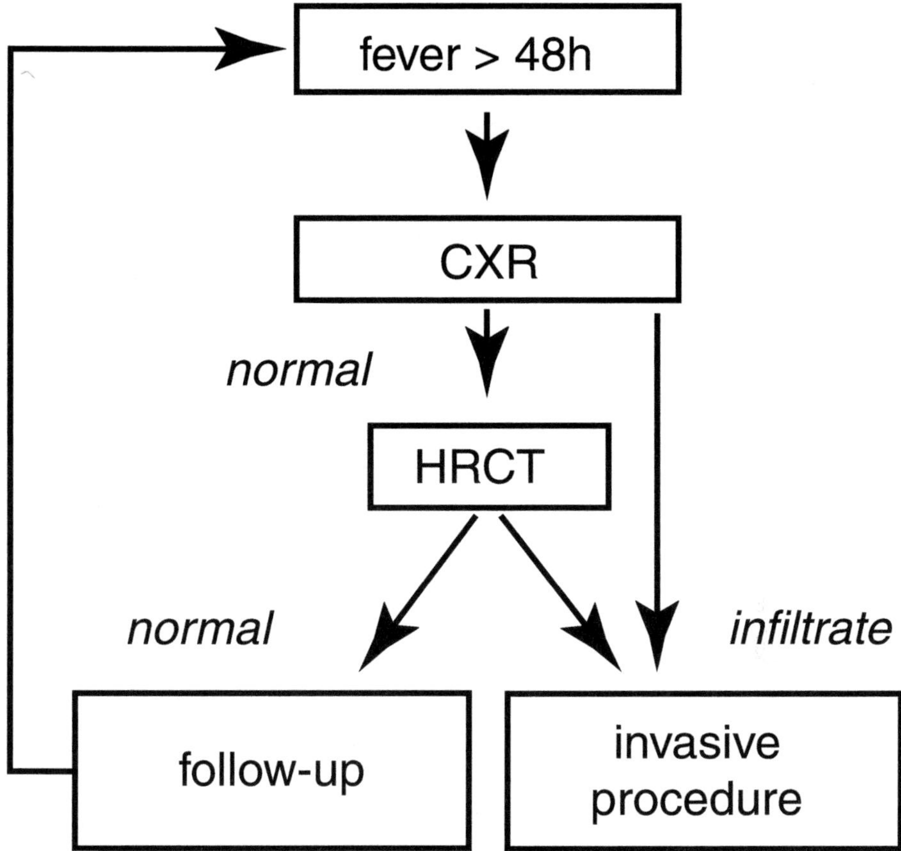

Fig. 7.4 Recommendations of the Guidelines of the Infectious Diseases Working Party (AGIHO) of the German Society of Hematology and Oncology (DGHO) [13]. Since the initial CXR is of limited use, this diagnostic step is more and more omitted and CT is performed primarily

frequently during follow-up (up to 63 %). The size of infiltrates increased by fourfold under successful antifungal treatment due to hematopoietic reconstitution. In this study, pneumonia was first detected on day 19 of neutropenia. Enlargement of infiltrates is probably caused by the invasion of newly generated neutrophil granulocytes at the beginning of bone marrow recovery. In critically ill patients, leukocyte invasion has been described as a risk factor for the development of acute respiratory distress syndrome (ARDS) [14] (Fig. 7.6 and 7.7).

7.3 Characterization of Pneumonia

Radiologists' dream is to be capable to identify the underlying microorganism in pneumonia of immunocompromised hosts with a sufficient specificity. In some cases, imaging can provide very fast useful hints, but no verification. The quality of these clues

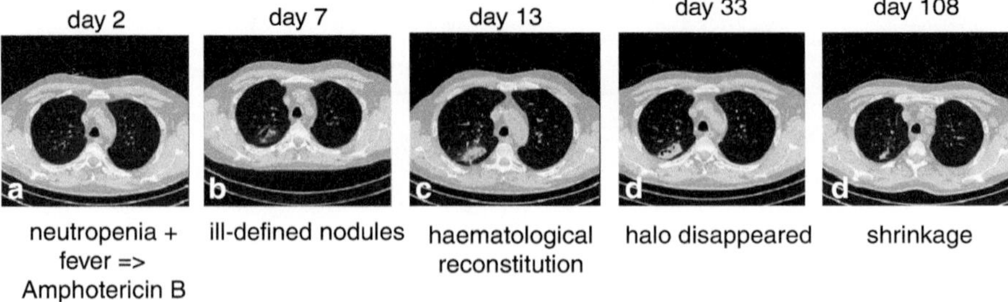

Fig. 7.5 Neutropenic febrile patient who underwent autologous peripheral blood stem cell transplantation. On day 2 after posttransplant, empirical mold-active antifungal treatment was started for neutropenic fever. Ill-defined pulmonary nodules were detected on day 7. Due to marrow recovery on day 13, the volume of lung infiltrates reached its maximum. Under continued antifungal treatment, the halo slowly disappeared and a central cavitation developed (day 33). The lesions shrinked significantly until day 108

depends on the cooperation between clinicians and radiologists and on the radiologists' experience with these complications. This requires an informational exchange concerning relevant individual patient data like severe neutropenia or allogeneic stem cell transplantation. For example, information on reactivation of cytomegalovirus (CMV) in a patient with graft-versus-host disease is very helpful for the correct interpretation of pulmonary HRCT findings. Also the chemotherapy or total body irradiation applied for conditioning before aSCT may be relevant for differential diagnostic considerations in patients who might present with clinically similar signs and symptoms [6, 7, 32, 33]. Some of the most useful clues are listed in Table 7.1.

7.3.1 Bacterial Pneumonia

Bacteria are causing approximately 90 % of infections during the early phase of neutropenia [8]. The radiological appearance of bacterial pneumonia includes consolidation, especially bronchopneumonia and positive pneumobronchogram (Fig. 7.2) [33, 34]. In contrast to immunocompetent patients, ground-glass opacification is found more often and remains nonspecific.

7.3.2 Fungal Pneumonia

Severe neutropenia lasting for more than 10–14 days is associated with an increasing risk of invasive fungal infection [3], with *Aspergillus species* being the primary pathogen, while *Candida species* very rarely cause primary pneumonia (Fig. 7.8) [5]. Typical radiological findings of fungal and non-fungal pneumonia as

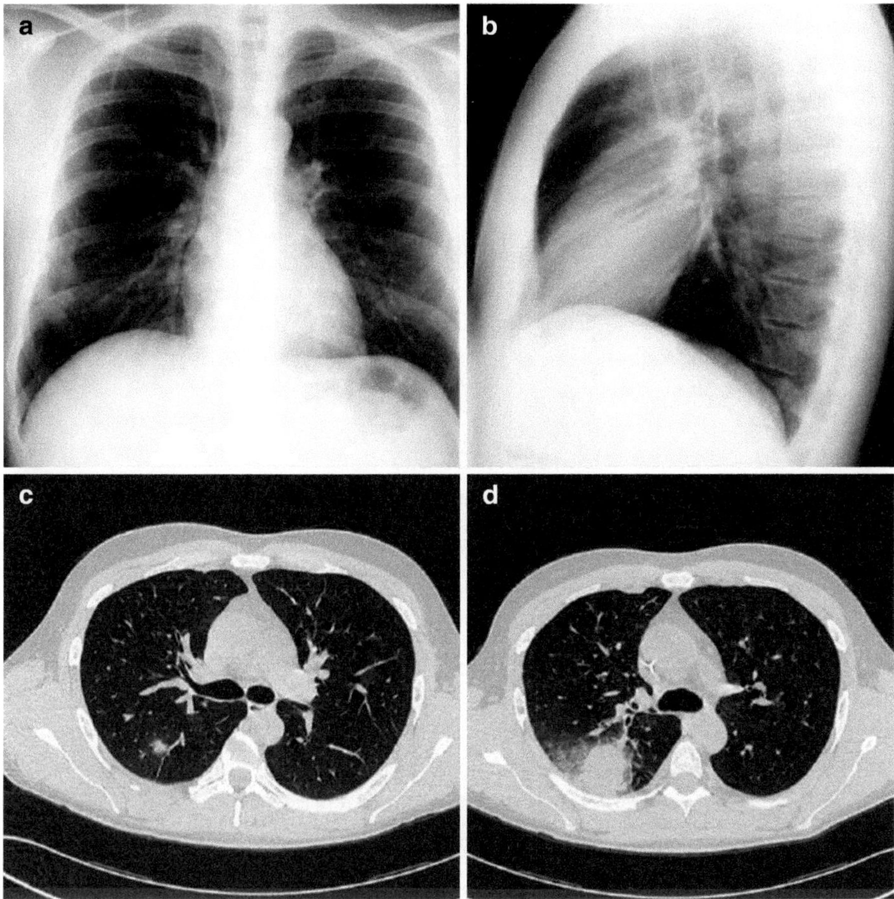

Fig. 7.6 The small ill-defined nodule in the right upper lobe (**c**) of this 34-year-old neutropenic AML patient was even retrospectively not visible on conventional chest x-ray done at the same day (**a**, **b**). Amphotericin B treatment was started due to suspicion of fungal pneumonia; however, the nodule size increased during hematopoietic reconstitution 2 weeks later (**d**). In preparation of bone marrow transplantation, the lesion was surgically resected and *Aspergillus* pneumonia was verified

well as of infiltrates from noninfectious diseases have been reviewed in detail [35]. The typical appearance of pulmonary infiltrates from fungal origin are as follows:

Early phase of fungal pneumonia:	Ill-defined nodules (Figs. 7.3, 7.5 and 7.8) [33] in combination with the Halo sign (Figs. 7.5 and 7.8) [33], which is nonspecific
Late phase:	Air-crescent sign [36]
	Cavitation (Fig. 7.8)

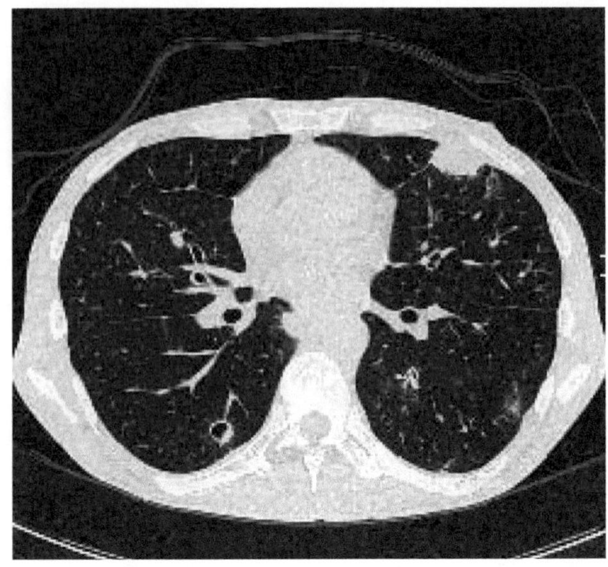

Fig. 7.7 Non-fungal lung infiltrate: ill-defined nodules with cavitation on CT scans done due to repeated febrile episodes. They appeared like fungal pneumonia and were not visible on baseline CT. After removal of a central venous port system, both the pulmonary lesions as well as the febrile episodes, disappeared

For use in the context of clinical and epidemiological research in neutropenic patients, standards for the interpretation of radiological findings in invasive fungal infections have been elaborated [10, 51]; newly emerged "typical" CT patterns (dense, well-circumscribed lesions with or without a halo sign, air-crescent sign) are classified as a clinical criterion for fungal pneumonia Figs. 7.5 and 7.8. The halo sign, first described in 1984 [49, 50], is nonspecific [33] and not a necessary part of the updated definitions [51]. A nonspecific infiltrate, rated as a minor criterion in the first version [10], was abandoned in the update [51]. In a later workup of a pharmaceutical trial investigating response rates to antifungal treatment, the evidence of the halo sign was associated with an improved response rate (52 % vs. 29 %; $p<0.001$), as well as a higher 3-month survival rate (71 % vs. 53 %; $p<0.01$) [52]. This large ($n=235$) antemortem trial suffers, however, from systemic limitations like investigation of halo which was part of inclusion criteria and technical insufficiencies like usage of thick-section CT instead of appropriate thin-section CT and evaluation of hardcopies instead of monitor reading [52]. Histopathological workup of lung biopsies verified fungal pneumonia in 56 % of cases in another study [37]. Relevant differential diagnoses for the halo sign, such as cryptogenic organizing pneumonia (COP, formerly known as bronchiolitis obliterans organizing pneumonia, BOOP), pulmonary hemorrhage, pulmonary manifestation of the underlying malignancy, lung cancer, and non-fungal infections (CMV, tuberculosis, abscesses (Fig. 7.7), etc.) or *Candida* (Fig. 7.8), have to be considered [37].

Thus, diagnostic clarification will frequently be necessary, particularly when antifungal treatment is not successful.

Table 7.1 Clinical and radiological appearance for various infectious and noninfections lung abnormalities in neutropenic hosts and after allogeneic stem cell transplantation

Diagnosis	Clinical setting	Radiological appearance
Infection bacterial	Early phase neutropenia	Consolidation, bronchopneumonia positive pneumobronchogram, GGO
Fungal	Long-term neutropenia (>10 days)	Halo = ill-defined nodules (early phase)
		Consolidations negative pneumobronchogram
		Air-crescent sign/cavitation (late phase)
Pneumocystis	Allogeneic transplantation	GGO, spared-out subpleural space
		Intralobular septae (late phase)
Tuberculosis	Each	Small ill-defined nodules/cavitations, tree in bud, homogeneous consolidation
Viral	Transplant history in graft or host	GGO – mosaic pattern
Graft versus host	Allogeneic transplantation	GGO – mosaic pattern
		Intralobular septae become visible
		Tree in bud
		Air-trapping (expiratory CT)
Radiation toxicity	Total body irradiation	GGO – paramediastinal distribution, also after TBI
		Intralobular septae become visible
Drug toxicity	Bleomycin, methotrexate, high-dose cytarabine, carmustine, etc.	GGO – mosaic pattern
		Intralobular septae become visible
		Peripheral consolidations of secondary lobule
		Traction bronchiectasis
Pulmonary congestion	Extensive hydration, renal impairment, hypoproteinosis	GGO
		Interlobular septae become visible
Leukemic infiltration	Pulmonary involvement	Thickening bronchovascular bundles thickening
		Interlobular septae become visible
		GGO
Pulmonary hemorrhage	Thrombocytopenia, post-interventional, hemoptysis	GGO – sedimentation phenomenon

GGO ground-glass opacification, *TBI* total body irradiation

Air-crescent sign and cavitation occur with hematopoietic reconstitution during the late phase of fungal infection (Fig. 7.8) [36]. Both radiological signs are known to be associated with a favorable prognosis. However, the specificities of these findings are limited, and relevant differential diagnoses have to be considered (Fig. 7.7) [37]. There are other useful patterns for the identification of fungal pneumonia, e.g.,

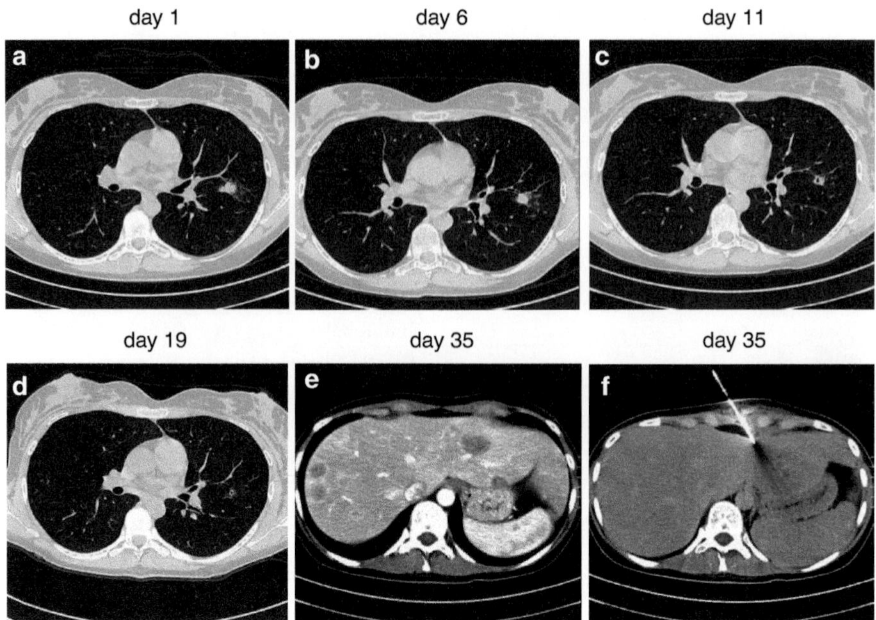

Fig. 7.8 Bilateral ill-defined nodules prompted the suspect of a fungal infection which was treated accordingly. *Candida* spp. were isolated from blood culture. Due to increasing liver enzymes, contrast-enhanced CT scan of the liver was ordered. Biopsy from the detected lesions confirmed *Candida* spp.

distribution along the bronchovascular bundle resulting in the feeding vessel sign with an angiotrophic location.

The ongoing development of antifungal therapy may have an important impact on the radiological appearance of fungal pneumonia. Thus, in the near future radiologists will not only be confronted with the question for "breakthrough fungal pneumonia," but also for fungal pneumonia caused by non-*Aspergillus* pathogens.

7.3.3 *Pneumocystis jiroveci* Pneumonia (PcP)

Pneumocystis jiroveci pneumonia (PcP) [38] is a typical finding in hematological patients affected by severe cellular (T-cell) immunosuppression and those with graft-versus-host disease after aSCT, if they are not protected by effective chemoprophylaxis [8]. Despite standard trimethoprim-sulfamethoxazole prophylaxis, 8 % of the patients develop PcP, while among patients without prophylaxis, the incidence may reach 29 % [8]. Up to 15 % of these patients will have a fatal outcome [8].

CT provides a valuable characterization for PcP [6, 7, 18, 33] and is a reliable method for discriminating it from other infectious processes [33, 39]. A combination

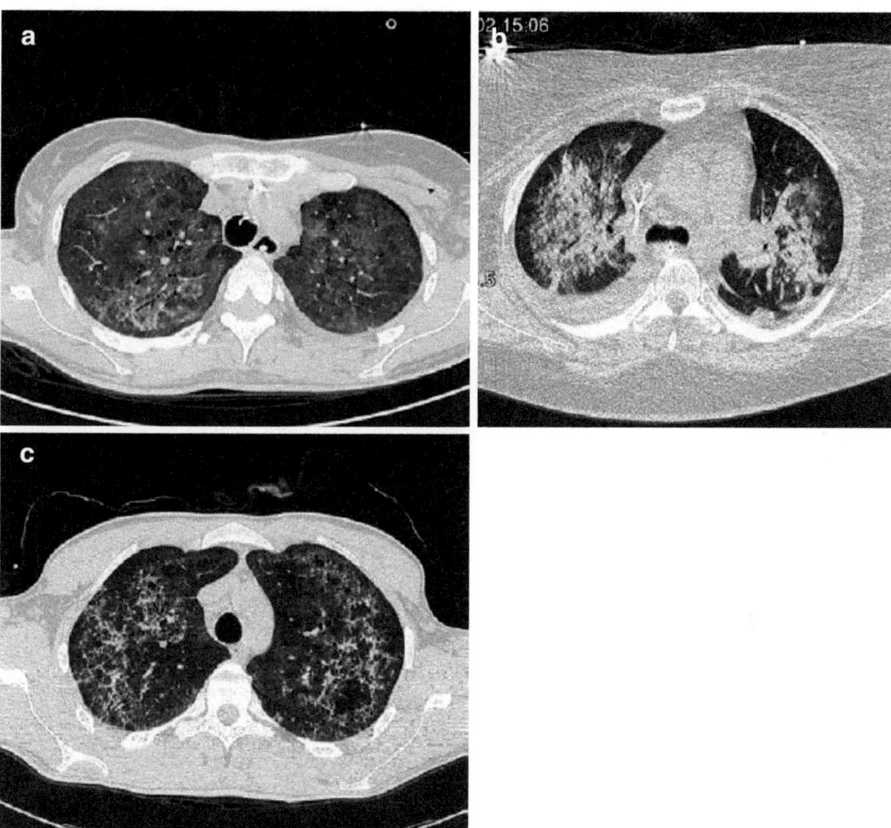

Fig. 7.9 Bilateral pneumonia caused by *Pneumocystis jiroveci* at different stages of immunosuppression. The subpleural space is typically spared out. Diffuse ground-glass opacification appears typically in the early phase of infection (**a**), while consolidations appear during a fulminant course (**b**). The predominance of intralobular linear patterns becomes visible during a later stage of PcP and under antimicrobial treatment (**c**)

of ground-glass opacities and intralobular septae sparing out the subpleural space (i.e., perihilar distribution) is very typical for PcP (Fig. 7.9) [33, 39, 40].

7.3.4 Lung Tuberculosis

Tuberculosis (TB) has to be considered as a rare but relevant differential diagnosis. In immunocompromised hosts, TB appears different compared to immunocompetent hosts (e.g., gangliopulmonary (primary) forms) [41]. More widespread lymphogenic and hematogenous dissemination can occur, and therefore, the clinical course might be fulminant [41, 42]. On the other hand, TB might mimic or come along with other infections like pulmonary aspergillosis or systemic candidiasis [42].

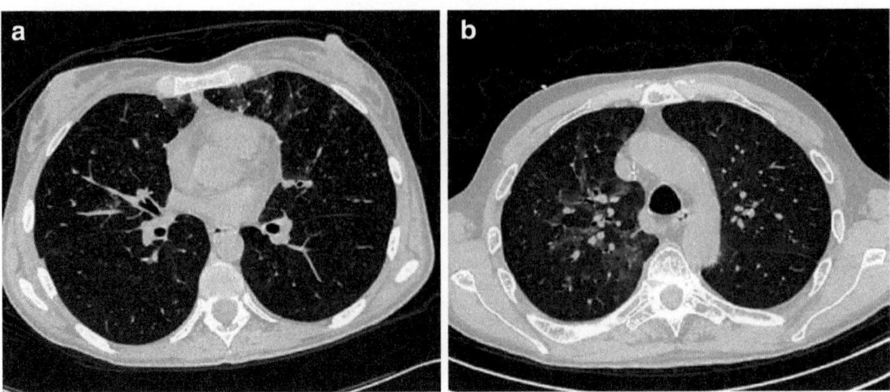

Fig. 7.10 Bilateral ground-glass opacification and mosaic pattern in both patients. However, pneumonia in patient A is caused by cytomegalovirus (*CMV*), and patient B by respiratory syncytial virus (*RSV*). Note the mosaic pattern resulting from affected and non-affected secondary lobules lying adjacent to one another

In immunocompromised hosts a segmental bronchial spread (resulting in a "tree-in-bud" sign) of small, sometimes, cavitated ill-defined nodules can be obtained as well as a miliar distribution [41, 42]. Gangliopulmonary (primary) forms, however, present with nonhomogenous consolidation and necrotizing mediastinal or hilar lymphadenopathy [41].

7.3.5 Viral Pneumonia

Interstitial pneumonia caused by viral infection may occur primarily in aSCT recipients but also in neutropenic and T-cell-immunosuppressed patients. Mortality rate may be up to 50 %. Most frequently, cytomegalovirus (CMV) is suspected; however, other herpesviruses, influenza, parainfluenza, adenovirus, or respiratory syncytial (RSV) viruses have to be considered as well. There are no specific radiological patterns available to differentiate various forms of viral pneumonia. However, confirming the suspicion of a viral pneumonia may be a clinically useful information, since effective drugs are available for some of these viruses. The typical appearance of viral pneumonia in the early stage is ground-glass opacification [33] and a mosaic pattern with affected and non-affected secondary lobules lying adjacent to one another (Fig. 7.10).

7.3.6 Noninfectious Pulmonary Lesions

Certain noninfectious diseases have to be considered in hematological patients: graft-versus-host disease (GVHD), radiation or drug toxicity, pulmonary congestion, bleeding, or progressive underlying malignancy. Fever, dyspnea, or clinical chemistry findings (c-reactive protein, elevation of liver function tests) might be

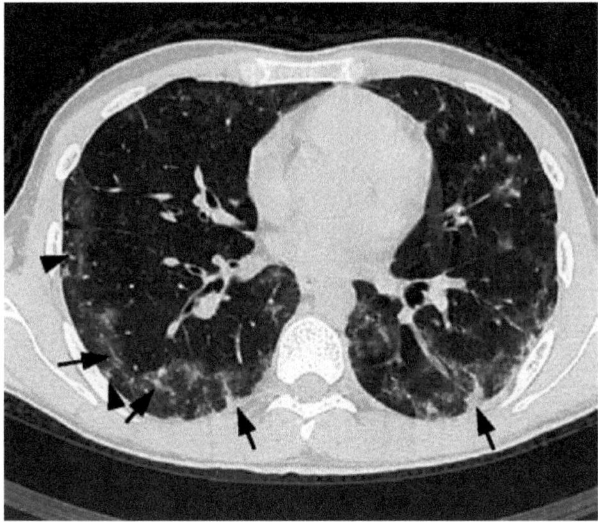

Fig. 7.11 A 28-year-old male after allogeneic retransplantation. HRCT was performed due to fever, cough, and dyspnea. Peripheral intralobular septae (*arrow*) and ground-glass opacification were seen on day 91 posttransplant. Tree-in-bud pattern (*arrowhead*) points at bronchiolitis obliterans. Acute GVHD was diagnosed from transbronchial biopsy. Under appropriate immunosuppression, clinical symptoms and radiological signs disappeared. Note the similarity to Fig. 7.13

caused by some of these processes and obscure the differentiation from infection. CT may help to detect and discriminate these diseases [6, 7, 18, 32].

7.3.7 Graft-Versus-Host Disease

Pulmonary manifestation of chronic GVHD occurs in approximately 10 % of patients after allogeneic hematopoietic stem cell transplantation (Fig. 7.11) [43]. Bronchiolitis obliterans is the pulmonary manifestation of this rejection [28]. The radiological appearance is similar to viral pneumonia, and clinical appearance and time point for both diseases are often similar (Fig. 7.11).

Ground-glass opacification and mosaic pattern, as well as signs of bronchiolitis obliterans such as air-trapping [24, 28] and bronchus wall thickening, occur during the early stage of pulmonary GVHD (Fig. 7.11), whereas intralobular septae and tree-in-bud sign follow in later stages [7, 43, 44].

7.3.8 Radiation Toxicity

An incidence of 5–25 % pulmonary radiogenic toxicity even after total body irradiation (TBI) applied for conditioning prior to stem cell transplantation is reported

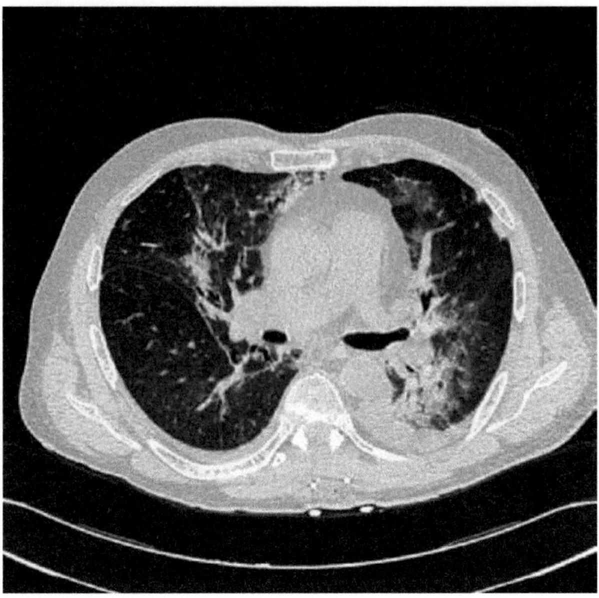

Fig. 7.12 Three weeks after radiation therapy for malignant spine destruction, this patient suffered from fever and dyspnea. Perihilar infiltrates appeared suddenly. Intralobular septae, consolidation, and ground-glass opacification were visible on HRCT. Especially the paramediastinal distribution of the infiltrates led to the differential diagnosis of radiation pneumonitis. After failure of antibiotic treatment, steroids were applied, resulting in improvement of symptoms and reduction of infiltrates

[45]. It emerges approximately 3 weeks after exposure but can also occur several months later [44, 45].

On CT scans, radiation-induced toxicity is characterized by ground-glass opacities with transition to consolidations (Fig. 7.12) [44, 45]. The key finding is the limitation of these patterns to the exposed parenchyma. For TBI, lungs are shielded, while paramediastinal and apical lung parenchyma is affected from radiation. Of note, demarcation of initially exposed from nonexposed lung parenchyma is blurred frequently due to deformation of lung parenchyma and to bridle.

7.3.9 Drug Toxicity

Chemotherapy protocols may lead to pulmonary toxicity. Some of the frequently used agents are bleomycin, high-dose methotrexate (MTX) or cytarabine (Ara-C), or carmustine (BCNU) (Fig. 7.13) [46]. Radiologists should be informed of previous exposure of patients to these agents when evaluating CT scans for pulmonary abnormalities.

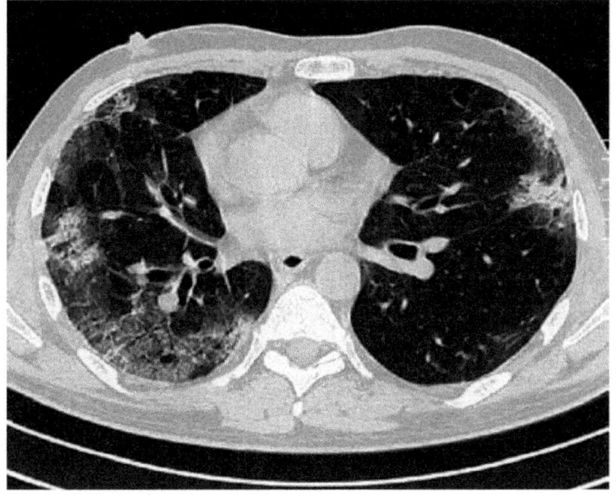

Fig. 7.13 A 40-year-old male who received chemotherapy including bleomycin for testicular cancer and had fever, cough, and dyspnea. CT revealed peripheral intralobular septae and ground-glass opacification (**a**). Bleomycin toxicity was suspected and histologically confirmed. Symptoms disappeared and findings decreased after application of steroids. Note the similarity to Fig. 7.11

The term "drug-induced pneumonitis" includes mainly nonspecific interstitial pneumonia (NSIP) and cryptogenic organizing pneumonia (COP, formerly known as bronchiolitis obliterans organizing pneumonia, BOOP) [46]. The CT appearance of NSIP consists of ground-glass opacities with transition to consolidations, intralobular septae, traction bronchiectasis, air-trapping, and in a later phase the nonspecific "crazy-paving" pattern [44, 46]. This is quite similar to radiation toxicity but without being limited to the radiation field.

7.3.10 Pulmonary Congestion

Dyspnea and infiltration are frequent in patients suffering from pulmonary congestion. Extensive hydration for renal protection during chemotherapy or to overcome renal impairment may cause pulmonary congestion also in younger patients. It is one of the most frequent disorders in patients undergoing intensive care.

At CXR, pulmonary congestion might be combined with infiltration. CT shows thickening of lymphatic vessels, corresponding to classical "Kerley lines" on conventional chest radiographs (Fig. 7.14).

7.3.11 Leukemic Infiltrates

Leukemic pulmonary infiltration is a less common clinical finding. Especially the perilymphatic pulmonary interstitium is involved [47]. This can be visualized on CT scans as thickening of bronchovascular bundles and interlobular septae. Besides

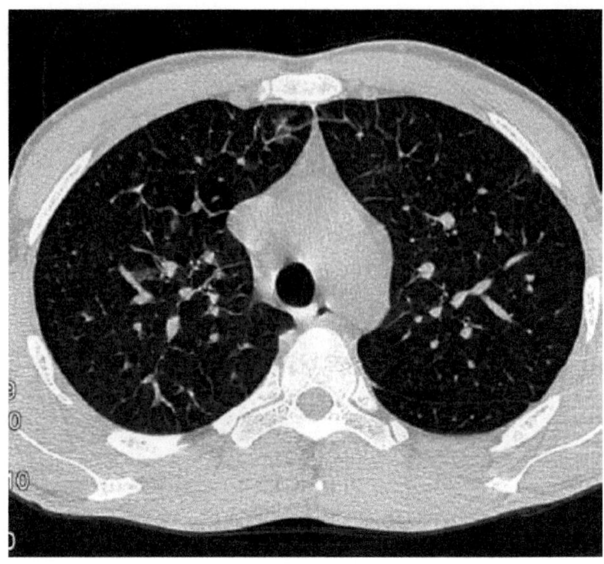

Fig. 7.14 Thickening of the intralobular septae resulting from fluid overload in lymphatic vessels

this, non-lobular and non-segmental ground-glass opacifications can be seen [32]. This pattern arrangement might mimic pulmonary congestion (Fig. 7.14).

7.3.12 Pulmonary Hemorrhage

In pancytopenia, pulmonary bleeding may occur spontaneously, secondary to invasive infections, after interventions (e.g., bronchoscopy and BAL), or during marrow recovery particularly in patients with fungal pneumonia [27].

Pulmonary bleeding might cause a focal or diffuse pattern, and the phenomenon of sedimentation within the secondary lobules can sometimes be depicted for few days (Fig. 7.15).

7.4 Extrapulmonary Focus

7.4.1 Liver and Spleen

Suspicious clinical symptoms or unexplained laboratory findings may suggest an involvement of the liver and spleen [13], particularly secondary to fungemia [54]. In addition to candidiasis, also mycobacteriosis, bacterial granulomatous hepatitis, viral hepatitis, and noninfectious organ involvement such as drug-related hepatotoxicity, GVHD, veno-occlusive disease (VOD), or relapse of the underlying disease have to be considered [12].

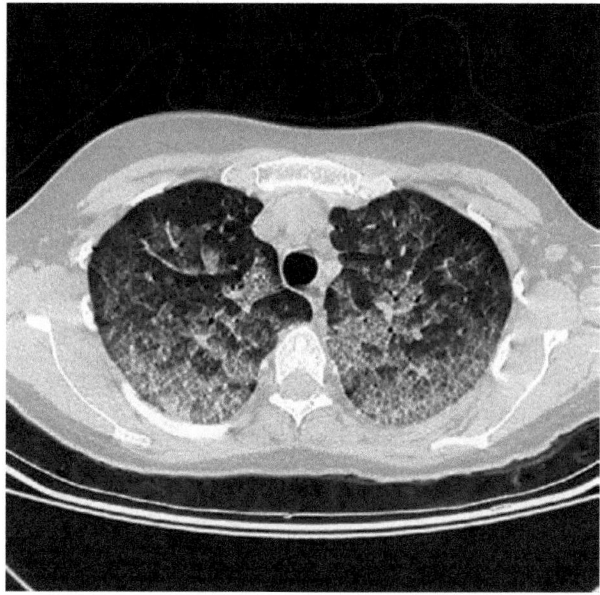

Fig. 7.15 The bilateral ground-glass opacification has an anterior-to-posterior gradient (1) over the whole lung and (2) within certain secondary lobules. This gravity-dependent sedimentation phenomenon can also occur temporarily and may be localized, e.g., after bronchoscopy and BAL

7.4.2 Gastrointestinal

Due to its microbial flora and the chemotherapy-induced mucosal injury, the gastrointestinal tract is particularly exposed to infection. However, without any history of surgical intervention, gastrointestinal involvement is rare. The main affections of the gastrointestinal tract, such as CMV colitis, pseudomembranous enterocolitis, enterocolitis in the context of rejection (GVHD), appendicitis, and diverticulitis, can be seen in CT as bowel wall thickening even without intravenous contrast after adequate oral, rectal contrast application [55].

7.4.3 Brain

Cerebral infection is a rare complication of myelosuppressive chemotherapy. It is more likely in the aSCT setting than after conventional chemotherapy [2]. Besides infectious diseases (e.g., herpesvirus group, toxoplasmosis, aspergillosis, mucormycosis, listeriosis), diagnoses such as bleeding, ischemia, drug toxicity (cyclosporine, ribavirin, voriconazole, etc.), and electrolyte disorders have to be taken into consideration. CT is helpful in emergency situations, while MRI is the method of choice in brain imaging in terms of sensitivity and specificity for detection and characterization of brain abnormalities [12].

7.4.4 Paranasal Sinuses

Since the sinuses are part of the respiratory tract, there is a coincidence of pneumonia [56]. Since the risk for sinusitis is up to 30 % in allogeneic stem cell transplant recipients, paranasal sinuses are often screened by CT prior to transplantation [57]. Bone erosion and orbital or brain invasion are classified by the 2008 EORTC guideline as clinical criteria for probable invasive fungal disease [51].

References

1. Chanock S. Evolving risk factors for infectious complications of cancer. Hematol Oncol Clin North Am. 1993;7:771–93.
2. Hiddemann W, Maschmeyer G, Runde V, Einsele H. Prevention, diagnosis and therapy of infections in patients with malignant diseases. Internist. 1996;37:1212–24.
3. Pizzo PA, Robichaud KJ, Gill FA, Witebsky FG. Empiric antibiotic and antifungal therapy for cancer patients with prolonged fever and granulocytopenia. Am J Med. 1982;72:101–11.
4. Maschmeyer G, Link H, Hiddemann W, Meyer P, Helmerking M, Eisenmann E, Schmitt J, Adam D. Pulmonary infiltrations in febrile neutropenic patients. Risk factors and outcome under empirical antimicrobial therapy in a randomized multicenter trial. Cancer. 1994;73: 2296–304.
5. Maschmeyer G. Pneumonia in febrile neutropenic patients: radiologic diagnosis. Curr Opin Oncol. 2001;13:229–35.
6. Schaefer-Prokop C, Prokop M, Fleischmann D, Herold C. High-resolution CT of diffuse interstitial lung disease: key findings in common disorders. Eur Radiol. 2001;11:373–92.
7. Tanaka N, Matsumoto T, Miura G, Emoto T, Matsunaga N. HRCT findings of chest complications in patients with leukemia. Eur Radiol. 2002;12:1512–22.
8. Einsele H, Bertz H, Beyer J, Kiehl MG, Runde V, Kolb H-J, Holler E, Beck R, Schwertfeger R, Schumacher U, Hebart H, Martin H, Kienast J, Ullmann AJ, Maschmeyer G, Krüger W, Link H, Schmidt CA, Oettle H, Klingebiel T. Epidemiologie und interventionelle Therapiestrategien infektiöser Komplikationen nach allogener Stammzelltransplantation. Dtsch Med Wochenschr. 2001;126:1278–84.
9. Maschmeyer G, Buchheidt D, Einsele H, Heußel CP, Holler E, Lorenz J, Schweigert M. Diagnostik und Therapie von Lungeninfiltraten bei febrilen neutropenischen Patienten – Leitlinien der Arbeitsgemeinschaft Infektionen in der Hämatologie und Onkologie der Deutschen Gesellschaft für Hämatologie und Onkologie. Dtsch Med Wochenschr. 1999;9:124(Suppl 1):S18–23. Update: http://www.dgho-infektionen.de/agiho/content/e125/e670/lugeninfiltrate.pdf. 26.03.03.
10. Ascioglu S, Rex JH, de Pauw B, Bennett JE, Bille J, Crokaert F, Denning DW, Donnelly JP, Edwards JE, Erjavec Z, Fiere D, Lortholary O, Maertens J, Meis JF, Patterson TF, Ritter J, Selleslag D, Shah PM, Stevens DA, Walsh TJ. Defining opportunistic invasive fungal infections in immunocompromised patients with cancer and hematopoietic stem cell transplants: an international consensus. Clin Infect Dis. 2002;34:7–14.
11. Edinburgh KJ, Jasmer RM, Huang L, Reddy GP, Chung MH, Thompson A, Halvorsen Jr RA, Webb RA. Multiple pulmonary nodules in AIDS: usefulness of CT in distinguishing among potential causes. Radiology. 2000;214:427–32.
12. Heussel CP, Kauczor H-U, Heussel G, Poguntke M, Schadmand-Fischer S, Mildenberger P, Thelen M. Magnetic resonance imaging (MRI) of liver and brain in hematologic-oncologic patients with fever of unknown origin. Rofo. 1998;169:128–34.
13. Heußel CP, Kauczor H-U, Heußel G, Derigs HG, Thelen M. Looking for the cause in neutropenic fever. Imaging diagnostics. Radiologe. 2000;40:88–101.

14. Azoulay E, Darmon M, Delclaux C, Fieux F, Bornstain C, Moreau D, Attalah H, Le Gall JR, Schlemmer B. Deterioration of previous acute lung injury during neutropenia recovery. Crit Care Med. 2002;30:781–6.
15. Navigante AH, Cerchietti LC, Costantini P, Salgado H, Castro MA, Lutteral MA, Cabalar ME. Conventional chest radiography in the initial assessment of adult cancer patients with fever and neutropenia. Cancer Control. 2002;9:346–51.
16. Barloon TJ, Galvin JR, Mori M, Stanford W, Gingrich RD. High-resolution ultrafast chest CT in the clinical management of febrile bone marrow transplant patients with normal or nonspecific chest roentgenograms. Chest. 1991;99:928–33.
17. Weber C, Maas R, Steiner P, Kramer J, Bumann D, Zander AR, Bucheler E. Importance of digital thoracic radiography in the diagnosis of pulmonary infiltrates in patients with bone marrow transplantation during aplasia. Rofo. 1999;171:294–301.
18. McLoud TC, Naidich DP. Thoracic disease in the immunocompromised patient. Radiol Clin North Am. 1992;30:525–54.
19. Cardillo I, Boal TJ, Einsiedel PF. Patient doses from chest radiography in Victoria. Australas Phys Eng Sci Med. 1997;20:92–101.
20. Schöpf UJ, Becker CXR, Obuchowski NA, Rust G-F, Ohnesorge BM, Kohl G, Schaller S, Modic MT, Reiser MF. Multi-slice computed tomography as a screening tool for colon cancer, lung cancer and coronary artery disease. Eur Radiol. 2001;11:1975–85.
21. Heussel CP, Kauczor H-U, Heussel G, Fischer B, Begrich M, Mildenberger P, Thelen M. Pneumonia in febrile neutropenic patients, bone-marrow and blood stem-cell recipients: use of high-resolution CT. J Clin Oncol. 1999;17:796–805.
22. Remy-Jardin M, Giraud F, Remy J, Copin MC, Gosselin B, Duhamel A. Computed tomography assessment of ground-glass opacity: semiology and significance. J Thorac Imaging. 1993;8:249–64.
23. Kauczor HU, Schnuetgen M, Fischer B, et al. Pulmonary manifestations in HIV patients: the role of chest films, CT and HRCT. Rofo. 1995;162:282–7.
24. Grenier PA, Beigelman-Aubry C, Fetita C, Preteux F, Brauner MW, Lenoir S. New frontiers in CT imaging of airway disease. Eur Radiol. 2002;12:1022–44.
25. Flohr T, Stierstorfer K, Bruder H, Simon J, Schaller S. New technical developments in multislice CT – part 1: approaching isotropic resolution with sub-millimeter 16-slice scanning. Rofo. 2002;174:839–45.
26. Eibel R, Ostermann H, Schiel X. Thorakale Computertomographie von Lungeninfiltraten. http://www.dgho-infektionen.de/agiho/content/e134/e619/e657. 26.03.03.
27. Heussel CP, Kauczor HU, Heussel G, Mildenberger P, Dueber C. Aneurysms complicating inflammatory diseases in immunocompromised hosts: value of contrast-enhanced CT. Eur Radiol. 1997;7:316–9.
28. Conces DJ. Noninfectious lung disease in immunocompromised patients. J Thorac Imaging. 1999;14:9–24.
29. Leutner CC, Gieseke J, Lutterbey G, Kuhl CK, Glasmacher A, Wardelmann E, Theisen A, Schild HH. MR imaging of pneumonia in immunocompromised patients: comparison with helical CT. AJR Am J Roentgenol. 2000;175:391–7.
30. Leutner C, Schild H. MRI of the lung parenchyma. Rofo. 2001;173:168–75.
31. Caillot D, Couaillier JF, Bernard A, Casasnovas O, Denning DW, Mannone L, Lopez J, Couillault G, Piard F, Vagner O, Guy H. Increasing volume and changing characteristics of invasive pulmonary aspergillosis on sequential thoracic computed tomography scans in patients with neutropenia. J Clin Oncol. 2001;19:253–9.
32. Tanaka N, Matsumoto T, Miura G, Emoto T, Matsunaga N, Satoh Y, Oka Y. CT findings of leukemic pulmonary infiltration with pathologic correlation. Eur Radiol. 2002;12:166–74.
33. Reittner P, Ward S, Heyneman L, Johkoh T, Müller NL. Pneumonia: high-resolution CT findings in 114 patients. Eur Radiol. 2003;13:515–21.
34. Conces DJ. Bacterial pneumonia in immunocompromised patients. J Thorac Imaging. 1998;13:261–70.

35. Heußel CP, Ullmann AJ, Kauczor H-U. Fungal pneumonia. Radiologe. 2000;40:518–29.
36. Kim MJ, Lee KS, Kim J, Jung KJ, Lee HG, Kim TS. Crescent sign in invasive pulmonary aspergillosis: frequency and related CT and clinical factors. J Comput Assist Tomogr. 2001;25: 305–10.
37. Kim K, Lee MH, Kim J, Lee KS, Kim SM, Jung MP, Han J, Sung KW, Kim WS, Jung CW, Yoon SS, Im YH, Kang WK, Park K, Park CH. Importance of open lung biopsy in the diagnosis of invasive pulmonary aspergillosis in patients with hematologic malignancies. Am J Hematol. 2002;71:75–9.
38. Stringer JR, Beard CB, Miller RF, Wakefield AE. A new name (Pneumocystis jiroveci) for Pneumocystis from humans. Emerg Infect Dis. 2002. http://www.cdc.gov/ncidod/EID/vol8no9/02-0096.htm. 26.03.03.
39. Hidalgo A, Falcó V, Mauleón S, Andreu J, Crespo M, Ribera E, Pahissa A, Cáceres J. Accuracy of high-resolution CT in distinguishing between Pneumocystis carinii pneumonia and non-Pneumocystis carinii pneumonia in AIDS patients. Eur Radiol. 2003. doi:10.1007/s00330-002-1641-6.
40. McGuinness G, Gruden JF. Viral and pneumocystis carinii infections of the lung in the immunocompromised host. J Thorac Imaging. 1999;14:25–36.
41. Van Dyck P, Vanhoenacker FM, Van den Brande P, De Schepper AM. Imaging of pulmonary tuberculosis. Eur Radiol. 2003. doi:10.1007/s00330-002-1612-y.
42. Goo JM, Im JG. CT of tuberculosis and nontuberculous mycobacterial infections. Radiol Clin North Am. 2002;40:73–87.
43. Leblond V, Zouabi H, Sutton L, Guillon JM, Mayaud CM, Similowski T, Beigelman C, Autran B. Late CD8+ lymphocytic alveolitis after allogeneic bone marrow transplantation and chronic graft-versus-host disease. Am J Respir Crit Care Med. 1994;150:1056–61.
44. Oikonomou A, Hansell DM. Organizing pneumonia: the many morphological faces. Eur Radiol. 2002;12:1486–96.
45. Monson JM, Stark P, Reilly JJ, Sugarbaker DJ, Strauss GM, Swanson SJ, Decamp MM, Mentzer SJ, Baldini EH. Clinical radiation pneumonitis and radiographic changes after thoracic radiation therapy for lung carcinoma. Cancer. 1998;82:842–50.
46. Erasmus JJ, McAdams HP, Rossi SE. High-resolution CT of drug-induced lung disease. Radiol Clin North Am. 2002;40:61–72.
47. Heyneman LE, Johkoh T, Ward S, Honda O, Yoshida S, Muller NL. Pulmonary leukemic infiltrates: high-resolution CT findings in 10 patients. AJR Am J Roentgenol. 2000;174: 517–21.
48. Morrell M, Fraser VJ, Kollef MH. Delaying the empiric treatment of candida bloodstream infection until positive blood culture results are obtained: a potential risk factor for hospital mortality. Antimicrob Agents Chemother. 2005;49:3640–5.
49. Gefter WB, Albelda S, Talbot G, Gerson S, Cassileth P, Miller WT. New observations on the significance of the air crescent in invasive pulmonary aspergillosis. Radiology. 1984;153:136.
50. Kuhlman JE, Fishman EK, Siegelman SS. Invasive pulmonary aspergillosis in acute leukemia: characteristic findings on CT, the CT halo sign, and the role of CT in early diagnosis. Radiology. 1985;157:611–4.
51. De Pauw B, Walsh TJ, Donnelly JP, Stevens DA, Edwards JE, Calandra T, Pappas PG, Maertens J, Lortholary O, Kauffman CA, Denning DW, Patterson TF, Maschmeyer G, Bille J, Dismukes WE, Herbrecht R, Hope WW, Kibbler CC, Kullberg BJ, Marr KA, Muñoz P, Odds FC, Perfect JR, Restrepo A, Ruhnke M, Segal BH, Sobel JD, Sorrell TC, Viscoli C, Wingard JR, Zaoutis T, Bennett JE, European Organization for Research and Treatment of Cancer/Invasive Fungal Infections Cooperative Group; National Institute of Allergy and Infectious Diseases Mycoses Study Group (EORTC/MSG) Consensus Group. Revised definitions of invasive fungal disease from the European Organization for Research and Treatment of Cancer/Invasive Fungal Infections Cooperative Group and the National Institute of Allergy and Infectious Diseases Mycoses Study Group (EORTC/MSG) Consensus Group. Clin Infect Dis. 2008;46:1813–21.

52. Greene RE, Schlamm HT, Oestmann JW, Stark P, Durand C, Lortholary O, Wingard JR, Herbrecht R, Ribaud P, Patterson TF, Troke PF, Denning DW, Bennett JE, de Pauw BE, Rubin RH. Imaging findings in acute invasive pulmonary aspergillosis: clinical significance of the halo sign. Clin Infect Dis. 2007;44:373–9.
53. Eibel R, Herzog P, Dietrich O, Rieger CT, Ostermann H, Reiser MF, Schoenberg SO. Pulmonary abnormalities in immunocompromised patients: comparative detection with parallel acquisition MR imaging and thin-section helical CT. Radiology. 2006;241:880–91.
54. Anttila VJ, Ruutu P, Bondestam S, et al. Hepatosplenic yeast infection in patients with acute leukemia: a diagnostic problem. Clin Infect Dis. 1994;18:979–81.
55. Donnelly LF, Morris CL. Acute graft-versushost disease in children: abdominal CT findings. Radiology. 1996;199:265–8.
56. Savage DG, Taylor P, Blackwell J, et al. Paranasal sinusitis following allogeneic bone marrow transplant. Bone Marrow Transplant. 1997;19:55–9.
57. Oberholzer K, Kauczor H-U, Heußel CP, Derigs HG, Thelen M. Klinische Relevanz der NNH-CT vor Knochenmarktransplantation. Rofo. 1997;166:493–7.
58. Cornely OA, Maertens J, Bresnik M, Ullmann AJ, Ebrahimi R, Herbrecht R. Treatment outcome of invasive mould disease after sequential exposure to azoles and liposomal amphotericin B. J Antimicrob Chemother. 2010;65(1):114–7.

Risk Stratification in Febrile Neutropenic Patients 8

Marianne Paesmans

Contents

8.1 Introduction

Febrile neutropenia (FN) is a common complication of antineoplastic chemotherapy especially in patients with hematologic malignancies. It can be associated with substantial morbidity and some mortality. Febrile neutropenic patients, however, represent a heterogenous group, and not all patients have the same risk of developing FN and/or related complications. A recent study [32] looked at potential factors predicting the occurrence of FN in 266 patients who received 1,017 cycles of chemotherapy. Rates of FN following the administration of a unique cycle of chemotherapy ranged from 20 % for patients with lymphoma or Hodgkin's disease to 25 % in myeloma, to more than 80 % in patients with chronic myeloid leukemia. Using patients with myeloma as reference, univariate odds ratios for the development of febrile neutropenia were 8.87 for acute myeloid leukemia and 12.11 for

M. Paesmans
Data Centre – Institut Jules Bordet, Rue Héger-Bordet, 1, Brussels B-1000, Belgium
e-mail: marianne.paesmans@bordet.be

G. Maschmeyer, K.V.I. Rolston (eds.), *Infections in Hematology*,
DOI 10.1007/978-3-662-44000-1_8

chronic myeloid leukemia. The overall risk of developing at least one febrile neutropenic episode has been reported to be >80 % in patients with hematologic malignancies [25]. A febrile neutropenic episode represents a serious and potentially lethal event, with an associated mortality of ~ 5 %. Although patients with hematologic malignancy are at higher risk of FN development, they do not appear to be at higher risk for death during the course of a febrile neutropenic episode, compared to patients with solid tumors as shown in a descriptive study by Klastersky et al. [27]: 64/1,223 episodes in patients with hematologic malignancy (5.2 %) versus 42/919 (4.6 %) in patients with solid tumors. However, aside from the risk of mortality, FN also causes serious medical complications and increased morbidity, which generate increased treatment-related costs and reduce the patients' quality of life [29, 52].

Preventing febrile neutropenia is a worthwhile goal. Colony-stimulating factors do shorten the duration of neutropenia, especially in patients with solid tumors [7]. Nevertheless, various guidelines (ASCO, EORTC) recommend their use only if the risk of febrile neutropenia exceeds 20 % [1, 43], in order to make this strategy cost-effective. This level of risk remains difficult to assess or predict. Additionally, the role of growth factors in patients with hematologic malignancies continues to be debated [31]. Another preventive strategy is to administer prophylactic antibiotics during periods of increased risk, but this strategy is associated with the emergence of resistant pathogens [50]. However, at least in patients with hematologic malignancies, neutropenic following chemotherapy administration, and afebrile, it reduces infection-related mortality and even all causes mortality as shown by meta-analyses [14, 30]. In the Gafter-Gvili meta-analysis, the relative risk for all-cause mortality is estimated to be 0.66 (95 % CI: 0.55–0.79). As all causes mortality is impacted, the benefit of prophylaxis likely outweighs the harm although only half of the studies were evaluable for the mortality outcome.

Standard management of FN patients includes hospital-based supportive care and the prompt administration of parenteral, broad-spectrum, empiric antibiotics. Although successful, this approach has some drawbacks (e.g., unnecessary hospitalization for some patients, exposure to resistant hospital microflora, increased costs), and may not be necessary in all FN patients. As previously stated, febrile neutropenic patients constitute a heterogeneous population, with a complication rate of approximately 15 % (95 % confidence interval: 12–17 %) in unselected patients [24]. In other words, 85 % of febrile episodes in neutropenic patients resolve without any complications if adequately treated with early initiation of empiric antibiotic therapy and appropriate follow-up and treatment modification, if necessary. Response rates may be even higher and the frequency of complications lower, in selected subgroups of FN patients. This knowledge has led investigators to try to identify more homogenous patient populations in terms of the risk of development of complications and to model the probability of complication development in them. The purpose of this chapter is to describe currently available risk stratification models and their predictive characteristics.

8.2 Risk Stratification

When attempting risk stratification, it is important to define the outcome one wants to study or predict. The following outcomes may be considered: response to the initial empiric antibiotic regimen, the development of bacteremia or serious medical complications before resolution of fever and neutropenia, and mortality related to the FN episode. Response to empiric antibiotic treatment has been a useful endpoint for most randomized clinical trials [6]. Although it is a fair indicator of the activity of a particular drug or regimen, the requirement for antibiotic change does not necessarily imply clinical deterioration and should not be used as a marker of worsening in risk prediction models. The same argument applies to bacteremic status, i.e., bacteremia does not necessarily represent increased clinical risk, at least in adult patients [27]. Death resulting from the febrile neutropenic episode is the most relevant endpoint. Fortunately, it is an uncommon event, making it difficult to conduct studies sufficiently powered to model for the probability of death. Consequently, the occurrence of serious medical complications appears to be the only feasible endpoint for risk assessment. It does have high clinical relevance as highlighted in a discussion of risk assessment [22].

Before developing a risk stratification rule, it is important to think about the future application of the rule and about the patient subgroup one wants to identify. Is it more meaningful to identify low-risk patients or high-risk patients? Is a binary rule satisfactory? Or does one need to be more subtle? Even, if one models the probability of the development of serious medical complications and gets a "continuous" prediction rule, the use one wants to make of the predicted probability will guide the choice of the threshold for defining low-risk, intermediate risk, or high-risk. Indeed, in clinical practice, an infectious diseases specialist needing to decide how he will treat a specific patient does not care about a "continuous" prediction but wants to have a tool that will help him to opt for a specific therapeutic choice. Up to now, most of the studies done on risk stratification for FN in adults and children have focused on the identification of low-risk patients with the subsequent goal of simplifying therapy for these patients.

8.3 Risk Stratification Methods

8.3.1 Clinical Approach

This method relies on empirically combining a set of predictive factors published in the literature and/or chosen on the basis of clinical expertise, without formally analyzing the interaction between them. This was the most frequently adopted methodology for the clinical trials which tested oral antibiotic regimens in hospitalized patients considered to be at low-risk [12, 21, 51]. The University of Texas, MD Anderson Cancer Center, has played a pioneering role in delineating the clinical criteria for identifying patients at low-risk for the development of complications and therefore eligible for simplified therapy. Investigators at this institution were among the first to show that low-risk patients could be safely managed as outpatients [38, 41]. This "clinical" approach has the advantage that the definition of low-risk is flexible and may be changed depending on the context of use and on the results of new studies. It is probably more applicable in busy clinical practices but is considered less scientifically stringent when one is trying to conduct multicenter clinical trials (due to transportability and generalizability issues). Because of the flexible nature of clinical criteria, it is very difficult to accurately determine the sensitivity, specificity, and positive and negative predictive values of this approach. The clinical factors considered to delineate low-risk include hemodynamic stability/absence of hypotension, no altered mental status, no respiratory failure, no renal failure, no hepatic dysfunction, good clinical condition, short expected duration of neutropenia, no acute leukemia, no marrow/stem cell transplant, absence of chills, no abnormal chest X-ray, no cellulitis or signs of focal infection, no catheter-related infection, and no need for intravenous supportive therapy [12, 19, 21, 28, 33, 51]. Of note, the first models excluded most patients with hematologic malignancy (direct exclusion of patients with acute leukemia or indirect exclusion through the criterion requiring the expected duration of neutropenia to be short).

8.3.2 Modeling Approach

The second approach has been used to derive risk prediction models by integrating several factors in a unique way and taking into account their independent value and their interactions. This is a more systematic way of constructing prediction models, and their diagnostic characteristics can be studied and optimized depending on the future use of the model. Before being suitable for clinical practice, they need to be tested in distinct patients populations in order to ensure that they are well calibrated (predicted outcomes have to match observed outcomes) and transportable to other settings (other institutions, other underlying tumors, or other antineoplastic therapy). Their discriminant ability needs to be monitored regularly. The advantages of this approach are numerous: the assessment of low-risk as well as the definition of the outcome to be predicted is standardized and more objective; the classifications have known properties; the models can be constructed in a parsimonious way with the use of independent predictive factors making them robust when used in other settings. However, the development process may take years, and the need for validation should not be underestimated since the context of use has to be considered before introducing them in clinical practice.

8.3.3 Validated Models

To date, two scoring systems have been developed and validated in adult patients, both using a similarly defined endpoint, i.e., the occurrence of serious medical complications (Table 8.1). The definition may appear somewhat arbitrary but has the

Table 8.1 Serious medical complications as defined in Talcott et al. [44]

Hypotension (defined as systolic blood pressure <90 mmHg or the need for pressor support to maintain blood pressure)
Respiratory failure (defined as arterial oxygen pressure less than 60 mmHg while breathing room air or need for mechanical ventilation)
Intensive care unit admission
Disseminated intravascular coagulation
Confusion or altered mental state
Congestive cardiac failure seen on chest X-ray and requiring treatment
Bleeding severe enough to require transfusion
Arrhythmia or ECG changes requiring treatment
Renal failure requiring investigation and/or treatment with intravenous fluids, dialysis, or any other intervention
Other complications judged serious and clinically significant by the investigator

Table 8.2 The Talcott classification [44]

Group I	Inpatients (at the time of fever onset)
Group II	Outpatients with acute comorbidity requiring hospitalization
Group III	Outpatients without comorbidity but with uncontrolled cancer
Group IV	Outpatients with controlled cancer and without comorbidity

Group IV is considered to be the low-risk group

merit of having been clearly formulated. Deviations from this definition have been observed in validation series especially when the risk models were used for selecting patients for outpatient treatment. In that setting, it is logical to consider that hospitalization is an event to be avoided although hospitalization is not necessarily a serious medical complication. These adaptations have been used in the studies conducted by Kern et al. [23] and Klastersky et al. [26].

8.3.3.1 The Talcott Model

Talcott and colleagues were the first to propose risk-based subsets in patients with chemotherapy-induced FN. Patients were classified into four groups (Table 8.2). Groups 1, 2, and 3 (all hospitalized patients) were not considered to be low-risk. However, patients in group IV (with controlled cancer and without medical comorbidity, who developed their febrile episode outside the hospital) were considered to be at low-risk [44]. The construction of the groups was done using clinical arguments and expertise and was initially tested in a retrospective series of 261 patients from a single institution. It was then validated in a prospective series of 444 episodes of FN at two institutions [45]. The model was constructed without distinguishing patients with solid tumors or hematologic malignancy although the definition of controlled cancer was different for patients with leukemia (complete response on the last examination) than for patients with solid tumor (initiation of treatment or absence of documentation of progression). The validation series included 24 % of patients with non-Hodgkin's lymphoma and 17 % of patients with

Table. 8.3 The MASCC risk index [24]

Characteristic	Weight
Burden of illness (i.e., febrile neutropenia)	
No or mild symptoms	5
Moderate symptoms	3
No hypotension	5
No chronic obstructive pulmonary disease	4
Solid tumor or no previous fungal infection	4
No dehydration	3
Outpatient status	3
Age <60 years	2

The score is obtained by summing up the different weights (the weights for burden of illness are not cumulative) and ranges from 0 to 26. Patients with a score ≥21 are considered at low-risk

acute myeloid leukemia. The diagnostic characteristics of the model were not stratified by underlying disease. The ultimate goal of the model was to identify low-risk patients, and groups I to III were never defined in order to further refine risk stratification. The model was further applied in a randomized trial [46] that aimed to assess whether outpatient management of predicted low-risk patients increases the risk of medical event. Patients with fever and neutropenia persisting after 24 h inpatient observation were randomized between continued inpatient care and early discharge without changing the antibiotic regimen unless medically required. The study was initially designed to detect an increase from 4 to 8 % in medical complication rate and then revised to detect an increase from 4 to 10 % with a planned sample size of 448 episodes. Stopped early due to poor accrual in 2000, the study was published with 66 episodes randomized in the hospital care arm and 47 episodes in the early discharge arm [46]. Although the study is underpowered, the authors concluded to no evidence of adverse medical consequences of the home arm (9 % complications rate versus 8 % and a 95 % confidence interval for the difference from −10 to 13 %). Having included only predicted low-risk patients, the study cannot be viewed as a full validation one, and we also can wonder why the study hypothesis was the inferiority of the experimental arm.

8.3.3.2 The MASCC Risk Index

The second model was developed as the result of an international prospective study conducted by the Multinational Association for Supportive Care in Cancer (MASCC) [24]. The original design of the study included a validation part. Before carrying out any data analysis, study subjects were split into a derivation set ($n=756$ episodes) and a validation set ($n=383$). The score derived from the first set was obtained after multivariate logistic regression. A numeric risk index score, the so-called MASCC score, was constructed by attributing weights to seven independent factors shown to be associated with a high probability of favorable outcome. This score is presented in Table 8.3. It ranges from 0 to 26, with a score of 21 or more

Table. 8.4 Characteristics of the clinical prediction rules derived from the Talcott and MASCC classifications: validation set from Klastersky et al. [24] ($n=383$ patients)

Group	Sensitivity	Specificity	PPV	NPV	Miscellaneous
Talcott's group IV	0.30	0.90	0.93	0.23	0.59
MASCC ≥21	0.71	0.68	0.91	0.36	0.30

The characteristics were calculated for a test aiming to identify low-risk patients
PPV positive predictive value, *NPV* negative predictive value

defined as being predictive of low-risk for the development of complications. This threshold was chosen from the derivation set, using a complication rate of 5 %, as a compromise between positive predictive value and sensitivity of the prediction rule. Similar to the Talcott model, the intended purpose of this model was to identify patients at sufficiently low-risk for the development of serious complications. The targeted positive predictive value of the score (i.e., the rate of patients without serious medical complication predicted by the rule) decreased, as expected, from 95 to 93 %, on the validation set. The characteristics of both models, based on the validation set are shown in Table 8.4. The MASCC study provides further validation of the Talcott classification in a multicentric setting. Comparing the characteristics of the prediction rules, the MASCC score did improve upon the sensitivity and the overall misclassification rate of the Talcott scheme. On the other hand, the positive predictive value might be considered suboptimal, at least when the threshold of 21 is used. Increasing the threshold might increase the positive predictive value but will also reduce the sensitivity of the model. In the Talcott model, the underlying disease particularly the presence of a solid tumor or hematologic malignancy impacted on the degree of risk only in the form of an interaction with the existence of a previous fungal infection or suspected fungal infection. The underlying disease was a predictive factor on univariate analysis, but was not subsequently identified as an independent risk predictive factor.

8.3.3.3 Independent Validation of the MASCC Score

Due to its immediate validation as planned in the study protocol, its increased sensitivity compared to the Talcott scheme, and its acceptable positive predictive value, the MASCC score has been proposed as a useful tool for predicting low-risk febrile neutropenia in the IDSA guidelines since 2002 [13, 18].

It has also been the subject of several independent validation studies. The primary objective of one of these studies was to attempt to improve the MASCC score through the estimation of the further duration of neutropenia. Indeed, expected further neutropenia duration, if correlated with the underlying tumor, could be the true factor underlying a higher risk for patients with hematologic malignancies than for patients with solid tumors. However, it is difficult to assess at presentation. A multicentric study was therefore conducted with detailed data collection about chemotherapy. This study [35] included 1,003 febrile episodes selected in 1,003 patients from 10 participating institutions. Among them, 546 had hematologic malignancy including 246 with acute leukemia. A model predicting further neutropenia duration as a binary status (long versus short duration) was developed. Almost all leukemic patients were predicted to have a long duration, and all patients with solid tumors were predicted to have a short duration of neutropenia, but the model was unable to split the patients with hematologic malignancies other than leukemia into subgroups with short or long predicted duration. Unfortunately, the addition of this covariate did not result in a risk prediction model more satisfactory than the one obtained with the MASCC risk index.

Table 8.5 summarizes the results of the independent series attempting to validate the MASCC score for identifying low-risk patients. Although some of the series are small, they all show positive predictive values that are above 85 %, except one study [8] not reported in the table. This study used a very different definition of complications which included a change in the empiric antibiotic regimen. Consequently, the reported rate of complications is huge (62 %), and this paper cannot be considered to be a true validation of the MASCC score. Looking at the data summarized in Table 8.5, one can observe that when the proportion of patients with hematologic malignancies increases, the positive predictive value decreases, suggesting that the score should be used with greater caution in patients with hematologic malignancies. One could also consider increasing the threshold for defining low-risk in order to increase the positive predictive value, albeit at the price of decreased sensitivity. Table 8.6 shows how the diagnostic characteristics may evolve with changes in threshold Table 8.7.

Numerous studies [4, 5, 20, 23, 26, 39, 40, 42] have used the MASCC score for selecting low-risk patients in order to simplify therapy, with suggested benefits such as improved quality of life for patients and their families. Some recently published studies confirm as it was hypothesized that costs are decreased [9, 16, 47]. The various therapeutic options for low-risk patients are beyond the scope of this chapter. Nevertheless, it needs to be stressed that prediction of low-risk and the suitability for either oral treatment (one of the approaches for simplifying treatment) or outpatient

Table 8.5 Characteristics of the MASCC clinical prediction rule in independent series

Reference	*N* episodes	Hematologic patients	Predicted at low-risk	Se	Sp	PPV	NPV
Paesmans [35]	1,003	55 %	72 %	79 %	56 %	88 %	40 %
Stratum of hematologic tumors	549	100 %	70 %	77 %	51 %	84 %	40 %
Stratum of solid tumor patients	454	0 %	74 %	81 %	64 %	93 %	38 %
Uys et al. [48]	80	30 %	73 %	95 %	95 %	98 %	86 %
Cherif et al. [5]	279	100 %	38 %	59 %	87 %	85 %	64 %
Klastersky et al. [26]	611	43 %	72 %	78 %	54 %	88 %	36 %
Innes et al. [20]	100	6 %	90 %	92 %	40 %	97 %	20 %
Baskaran et al. [3]	116	100 %	71 %	93 %	67 %	83 %	85 %
Hui et al. [17]	227	20 %	70 %	81 %	60 %	86 %	52 %

The characteristics were calculated for a test aiming to identify low-risk patients and may then differ from the original publications

Table 8.6 MASCC score: characteristics of the clinical prediction rule by threshold and stratified by underlying tumor validation study [35]

Threshold	Se	Sp	PPV	NPV	Misclassified
Hematologic patients (n=549)					
21	77 %	51 %	84 %	40 %	29 %
22	51 %	81 %	90 %	34 %	42 %
24	15 %	97 %	94 %	26 %	65 %
Solid tumor patients (n=454)					
21	81 %	64 %	93 %	38 %	21 %
22	70 %	76 %	94 %	32 %	29 %
24	58 %	81 %	94 %	26 %	38 %

treatment (the other approach for simplifying treatment) are different issues. Prediction of low-risk is a necessary but not exclusive condition for simplified, risk-based therapy. This should be kept in mind [10, 11, 22, 26, 39] when designing studies for low-risk patients. Despite this, there are numerous recent reports showing that outpatient treatment can be as successful as in-hospital treatment, even for some patients with hematologic malignancies [5, 15, 42].

8.3.3.4 Predicting Intermediate or High-Risk Using the Validated Models

The Talcott model was designed to identify low-risk patients, and the classification of high-risk patients into groups I to III had no preplanned purpose. Consequently, this model is unlikely to be helpful in a setting other than the identification of low-risk patients. In the MASCC study, the probability of development of serious complications has been modeled with a “continuous” range of predicted values. This information, however, may not be relevant to the clinician who needs to get a binary answer to help in therapeutic decision making. Initially, the identification of low-risk was considered most relevant in order to facilitate research on oral antibiotic therapy and/or outpatient management. The threshold was set to achieve a positive predictive value of 95 %. A broader use of the score could be envisaged to select patients at intermediate or high-risk of complications. Data collected on validation series show that, indeed, the higher the score, the higher the probability of resolution without the development of serious medical complications, as depicted in Fig. 8.1 [34]. So, intermediate values of the score or even the lowest values of the score may help further categorize patients. However, in each of the categories, the rate of complications never approaches 1. Therefore, a rule trying to identify patients who will develop complications using the available model will lack sensitivity and be unsatisfactory. Furthermore, the number of patients at the lowest values of the score is small, and studies focusing on patients at high-risk of the development of complications might be very difficult to conduct due to low accrual potential. Nevertheless, a study comparing a very “aggressive” therapeutic approach including the administration of growth factors and/or immediate treatment in an intensive care unit, versus standard hospital-based empiric therapy, might be very interesting.

Table 8.7 Bacteremia versus final outcome stratified by the MASCC score and the type of cancer

	MASCC <21					MASCC ≥21					≥21 versus <21		
	Total	Complications (nonlethal)		Death		Total	Complications (nonlethal)		Death		OR[a]	95 % CI	*P*-value
Hematologic													
No bacteremia	262	68	26 %	21	8 %	597	43	7 %	11	2 %	5.17	3.54–7.56	<0.001
Single gram positive	89	26	29 %	8	9 %	133	20	15 %	3	2 %	2.96	1.59–5.50	<0.001
Single gram negative	48	12	25 %	14	29 %	56	8	14 %	3	5 %	4.83	2.03–11.54	<0.001
Polymicrobial	9	3		2		29	7	24 %	2	7 %			
Solid													
No bacteremia	183	33	18 %	20	11 %	601	27	4 %	5	1 %	7.25	4.49–11.70	<0.001
Single gram positive	18	6	33 %	2	11 %	43	5	12 %	–	–	6.08	1.63–22.69	0.01
Single gram negative	39	15	38 %	11	28 %	25	3	12 %	2	8 %	8.00	2.45–26.16	<0.001
Polymicrobial	6	1		2		4	–		–		–	–	
Total													
No bacteremia	445	101	23 %	41	9 %	1,198	70	6 %	16	1 %	6.06	4.51–8.15	<0.001
Single gram positive	107	32	30 %	10	9 %	176	25	14 %	3	2 %	3.42	1.95–5.98	<0.001
Single gram negative	87	27	31 %	25	29 %	81	11	14 %	5	6 %	6.04	3.01–12.09	<0.001
Polymicrobial	15	4	27 %	4	27 %	33	7	21 %	2	6 %			

From Klastersky et al. [27]

[a]Odds ratio of no serious complications (including death) (the complications rate and death rate were only calculated in subgroups of more than ten cases)

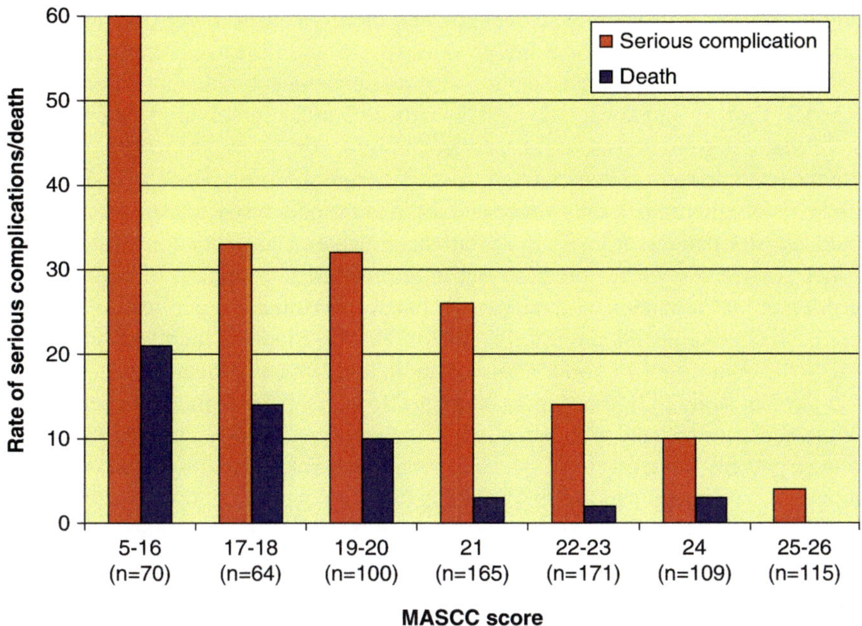

Fig. 8.1 Rate of serious complication or death according to MASCC score values [34]

8.3.3.5 How to Improve Risk Prediction Models?

Although the MASCC score has been satisfactorily validated and reported to be useful for predicting low-risk in different patients populations and settings, it is far from optimal, with a misclassification rate of 30 % and low specificity and negative predictive values. Several attempts to improve the MASCC score have been made. As already mentioned, a multinational study [35] looked in detail at the characteristics of the chemotherapeutic regimen that induced the febrile neutropenic episode and attempted to associate it with further duration of neutropenia. The next step which was to incorporate this information in risk prediction failed.

Utilizing the databases of the original MASCC study and the subsequent study that looked at duration of neutropenia, the issue of the significance of bacteremic status was reviewed [36]. This review found that (1) after stratification for the type of underlying cancer (hematologic malignancy versus solid tumor) and for bacteremic status (no bacteremia, single organism gram-negative bacteremia, single organism gram-positive bacteremia, polymicrobial bacteremia), the MASCC score had a predictive value in all the strata without any detectable interaction term; and (2) prior or early knowledge of bacteremic status, although predictive of outcome, would not be helpful in improving the accuracy of a clinical rule characterizing patients as low and high-risk.

Uys et al. [49] analyzed the predictive role of circulating markers of infection (C-reactive protein, procalcitonin, serum amyloid A, and interleukins IL-1β, IL-6, IL-8, IL-10) in a monocentric series of 78 febrile neutropenic episodes. Although this study is limited by its sample size and power, their conclusion was that none of the markers had an independent predictive value that would improve risk prediction.

De Souza Viana [8] proposed adding information about complex infection status to the MASCC score and to exclude patients with a complex infection (defined as infection of major organs, sepsis, soft tissue wound infection, or oral mucositis grade >2) from the predicted low-risk patients. In a small series of 53 episodes (64 % of patients with hematologic tumor), they suggested that their model restricted the group of predicted low-risk patients from 21 to 15, but that the rate of complications was 0 instead of 4/21 (19 %). However, this proposal used a different definition of complication, considering that a patient with antibiotic change presented a complication although there is no clinical justification of this definition. This model is therefore not comparable to the other proposals and, in our opinion, less clinically meaningful.

In a recent study [37], the authors attempted to develop a risk model targeting high-risk prediction in patients with hematologic malignancies. They suggested that, in this group of patients, progression of infection might be quicker than in patients with solid tumors and that a specific model for predicting high-risk of complications in such patients would be very valuable. In a monocentric study of 259 febrile neutropenic episodes (137 patients), they constructed a score with values 0, 1, 2, or 3. One point is attributed to each of the following factors (measured before the administration of chemotherapy): low albumin level (<3.3 g/dl), low bicarbonate level (<21 mmol/l), and high CRP (≥20 mg/dl). The rates of complications were 7/117 (6 %), 21/71 (30 %), 24/43 (56 %), and 18/18 (100 %) with increasing values of the score. Park and coauthors suggested that patients with a score ≥2 should be considered as high-risk patients. The model needs validation, and the characteristics of the proposed clinical prediction rule should be studied further before being used. It is attractive due to the fact that it is specific to patients with hematologic malignancies and is based on very objective factors (contrary to the MASCC score which needs assessment of burden of FN) which are assessable even before the development of FN (i.e., at the time chemotherapy is initiated). It can however be hypothesized that a high CRP level at initiation of chemotherapy is just reflecting a nondiagnosed infectious disease rather than being predictive of the outcome of a future FN episode.

Conclusions

It is clear that febrile neutropenia occurs in a heterogeneous group of patients and that any accurate risk stratification system is valuable for guiding the management of selected subgroups of patients. Furthermore, evidence-based data and systematic reviews show that oral antibiotic therapy is a safe and feasible alternative to conventional intravenous therapy. The published scoring systems for predicting risk have been validated enough to guide the selection of patients for the administration of an oral regimen. At present, the MASCC risk index is probably the preferred method. However, there is room for improvement, specially in the prediction of low-risk in patients with hematologic malignancies. Further areas of research include the utility of rapid laboratory tests [22] and pattern recognition molecules able to activate the lectin pathway, such as mannose-binding lectin protein or ficolins [2]. One should also look at variables collected in the short-term follow-up. Indeed, the usefulness of reassessment of currently available scoring systems has not been studied much but is probably of limited value as most of the variables included in them are not susceptible to change. The use of risk prediction models for selecting patients for ambulatory treatment is more complex, as factors other than risk have to be taken into account as well as local epidemiology. The recognition of intermediate or high-risk and the provision of aggressive therapy to these patients are a new area for research and need to be formally studied.

References

1. Aapro MS, Cameron DA, Pettengell R, Bohlius J, Crawford J, Ellis M, et al. EORTC guidelines for the use of colony-stimulating factor to reduce the incidence of chemotherapy-induced febrile neutropenia in adult patients with lymphomas and solid tumours. Eur J Cancer. 2006;42:2433–53.
2. Ameye L, Paesmans M, Aoun M, Thiel S, Jensenius JC. Severe infection is associated with lower M-ficolin concentration in patients with hematologic cancer undergoing chemotherapy. Abstract presented at the 12th International Symposium on Febrile Neutropenia, Luxemburg, Luxemburg, Mar 2010.
3. Baskaran ND, Gan GG, Adeeba K. Applying the multinational association for supportive care in cancer risk scoring in predicting outcome of febrile neutropenia patients in a cohort of patients. Ann Hematol. 2008;87:563–9.
4. Chamilos G, Bamias A, Efstathiou E, Zorzou PM, Kastritis E, Kostis E, et al. Outpatient treatment of low-risk neutropenic fever in cancer patients using oral moxifloxacin. Cancer. 2005;103:2629–35.
5. Cherif H, Johansson E, Björkholm M, Kalin M. The feasibility of early hospital discharge with oral antimicrobial therapy in low-risk patients with febrile neutropenia following chemotherapy for hematologic malignancies. Haematologica. 2006;91(2):215–22.
6. Cometta A, Calandra T, Gaya H, et al. Monotherapy with meropenem versus combination therapy with ceftazidime plus amikacin as empiric therapy for fever in granulocytopenic patients with cancer. The International Antimicrobial Therapy Cooperative Group of the European Organization for Research and Treatment of Cancer and the Gruppo Italiano Malattie Ematologiche Maligne dell'Adulto Infection Program. Antimicrob Agents Chemother. 1996;40:1108–15.
7. Cooper KL, Madan J, Whyte S, Stevenson MD, Akehurst RL. Granulocyte-colony stimulating factors for febrile neutropenia prophylaxis following chemotherapy : systematic review and meta-analysis. BMC Cancer. 2011;11:404.
8. de Souza VL, Serufo JC, da Costa Rocha MO, Costa RN, Duarte RC. Performance of a modified MASCC index score for identifying low-risk febrile neutropenia cancer patients. Support Care Cancer. 2008;16:841–6.
9. Elting LS, Lu C, Escalante CP, Giordano SH, Trent JC, Cooksley C, Avritscher BC, Tina Shih YC, Ensor J, Nebiyou Bekele B, Gralla RJ, Talcott JA, Rolston K. Outcomes and cost of outpatient or inpatient management of 712 patients with febrile neutropenia. J Clin Oncol. 2008;26:606–11.
10. Feld R, Paesmans M, Freifeld AG, Klastersky J, Pizzo PA, Rolston KV, Rubenstein E, Talcott JA, Walsh TJ. Methodology for clinical trials involving patients with cancer who have febrile neutropenia : updated guidelines of the Immunocompromised Host Society/Multinational Association for Supportive Care in Cancer, with emphasis on outpatient studies. Clin Infect Dis. 2002;35:1463–8.
11. Finberg RW, Talcott JA. Fever and neutropenia : how to use a new treatment strategy. N Engl J Med. 1999;341:362–62.
12. Freifeld A, Marchigiani D, Walsh T, Chanock S, Lewis L, Hiemenz J, et al. A double-blind comparison of empirical oral and intravenous antibiotic therapy for low-risk febrile patients with neutropenia during chemotherapy. New Engl J Med. 1999;341:305–11.

13. Freifeld AG, Bow EJ, Sepkowitz KA, Boeckh MJ, Ito JI, Mullen CA, Raad II, Rolston KV, Young JA, Wingard JR. Clinical practice guideline for the use of antimicrobial agents in neutropenic patients with cancer: 2010 update by the Infectious Diseases Society of America. Clin Infect Dis. 2011;52:427–31.
14. Gafter-Gvili A, Frase A, Paul M, Vidal L, Lawrie TA, van de Wetering MD, Kremer LCM, Leibovici L. Antibiotic prophylaxis for bacterial infections in afebrile neutropenic patients following chemotherapy. Cochrane Database Syst Rev. 2012;(1):CD004386.
15. Girmenia C, Russo E, Carmosino I, Breccia M, Dragoni F, Latagliata R, Mecarocci S, Morano SG, Stefanizzi C, Alimena G. Early hospital discharge with oral antimicrobial therapy in patients with hematologic malignancies and low-risk febrile neutropenia. Ann Hematol. 2007;86:263–70.
16. Hendriks AM, Trice Loggers E, Talcott JA. Costs of home versus inpatient treatment for fever and neutropenia: analysis of a multicenter randomized trial. J Clin Oncol. 2011;29:3984–9.
17. Hui EP, Leung LKS, Poon TCW, Mo F, Chan VTC, Ma ATW, Poon A, Hui EK, Mak S-s, Kenny ML, Lei KIK, Ma BBY, Mok TSK, Yeo W, Zee BCY, Chan ATC. Prediction of outcome in cancer patients with febrile neutropenia: a prospective validation of the Multinational Association for Supportive Care in Cancer risk index in a Chinese population and comparison with the Talcott model and artificial neural network. Support Care Cancer. 2011;19:1625–35.
18. Hughes WT, Amstrong D, Bodey GP, Bow EJ, Brown AE, Calandra T, et al. 2002 guidelines for the use of antimicrobial agents in neutropenic patients with cancer. Clin Infect Dis. 2002;34:730–51.
19. Innes HE, Smith DB, O'Reilly SM, Clark PI, Kelly V, Marshall E. Oral antibiotics with early hospital discharge compared with in-patient intravenous antibiotics for low-risk febrile neutropenia in patients with cancer: a prospective randomised controlled single centre study. Br J Cancer. 2003;89:43–9.
20. Innes HE, Lim SL, Hall A, Chan SY, Bhalla N, Marshall E. Management of febrile neutropenia in solid tumors and lymphomas using the Multinational Association for Supportive Care in Cancer (MASCC) risk index: feasibility and safety in routine clinical practice. Support Care Cancer. 2008;16:485–91.
21. Kern WV, Cometta A, De Bock R, Langenaeken J, Paesmans M, Gaya H. Oral versus intravenous empirical antimicrobial therapy for fever in patients with granulocytopenia who are receiving cancer chemotherapy. New Engl J Med. 1999;341:312–8.
22. Kern WV. Risk assessment and treatment of low-risk patients with febrile neutropenia. Clin Infect Dis. 2006;42:533–40.
23. Kern WV, Marchetti O, Drgona L, Akan H, Aoun M, Akova M, de Bock R, Paesmans M, Maertens J, Viscoli C, Calandra T. Oral moxifloxacin versus ciprofloxacin plus amoxicillin/clavulanic acid for low-risk febrile neutropenia – a prospective, double-blind, randomised, multicentre EORTC-Infectious Diseases Group (IDG) Trial (protocol 46001, IDG trial XV). 18th European Congress of Clinical Microbiology and Infectious Diseases, Barcelona, 2008.
24. Klastersky J, Paesmans M, Rubenstein EB, Boyer M, Elting L, Feld R, et al. The Multinational Association for Supportive Care in Cancer risk index: a multinational scoring system for identifying low-risk febrile neutropenic cancer patients. J Clin Oncol. 2000;18:3038–51.
25. Klastersky J. Management of patients with different risks of complication. Clin Infect Dis. 2004;39:S32–7.
26. Klastersky J, Paesmans M, Georgala A, Muanza F, Plehiers B, Dubreucq L, et al. Management with oral antibiotics in an outpatient setting of febrile neutropenic cancer patients selected on the basis of a score predictive for complications. J Clin Oncol. 2006;24:4129–34.
27. Klastersky J, Ameye L, Maertens J, Georgala A, Muanza F, Aoun M, Ferrant A, Rapoport B, Rolston K, Paesmans M. Bacteremia in febrile neutropenic cancer patients. Int J Antimicrob Agents. 2007;30:51–9.
28. Klastersky J, Paesmans M. Risk-adapted strategy for the management of febrile neutropenia in cancer patients. Support Care Cancer. 2007;15:477–82.
29. Kuderer NM, Dale DC, Crawford J, Cosler LE, Lyman GH. Mortality, morbidity and cost associated with febrile neutropenia in adult cancer patients. Cancer. 2006;106:2258–66.
30. Leibovici D, Paul M, Cullen M, Bucaneve G, Gafter-Gvili A, Fraser A, Kern WV. Antibiotic prophylaxis in neutropenic patients: new evidence, practical decisions. Cancer. 2006;107:1743–51.

31. Levenga TH, Timmer-Bonte JNH. Review of the value of colony stimulating factors for prophylaxis of febrile neutropenic episodes in adult patients treated for hematologic malignancies. Br J Haematol. 2007;138:146–52.
32. Moreau M, Klastersky J, Schwarzbold A, Muanza F, Georgala A, Aoun M, Loizidou A, Barette M, Costantini S, Delmelle M, Dubreucq L, Vekemans M, Ferrant A, Bron D, Paesmans M. A general chemotherapy myelotoxicity score to predict febrile neutropenia in hematologic malignancies. Ann Oncol. 2009;20:513–9.
33. Paesmans M. Risk factors assessment in febrile neutropenia. Int J Antimicrob Agents. 2000;16:107–11.
34. Paesmans M. Factors predictive for low and high risk of complications during febrile neutropenia and their implications for the choice of empirical therapy: experience of the MASCC Study Group on Infectious Diseases Abstract presented at the 6th International Symposium on Febrile Neutropenia – Brussels, Dec 2003.
35. Paesmans M for the MASCC study section on infectious diseases; the duration of febrile neutropenia. Abstract presented at the 8th International Symposium on Febrile Neutropenia, Athens, Jan 2006.
36. Paesmans M, Klastersky J, Maertens J, Georgala A, Muanza F, Aoun M, Ferrant A, Rapoport B, Rolston K, Ameye L. Predicting febrile neutropenia at low-risk using the MASCC score: does bacteremia matter? Support Care Cancer. 2011;19:1001–8
37. Park Y, Kim DS, Park SJ, Seo HY, Lee SR, Sung HJ, Park KH, Choi IK, Kim SJ, Oh SC, Seo JH, Choi CW, Kim BS, Shin SW, Kim YH, Kim JS. The suggestion of a risk stratification system for febrile neutropenia patients with hematologic disease. Leuk Res. 2010;34:294–300.
38. Rolston K, Rubenstein E, Elting L, Escalante C, Manzullo E, Bodey GP. Ambulatory management of febrile episodes in low-risk neutropenic patients (abstract LM 81). In: Program and Abstracts of the 35th Interscience Conference on Antimicrobial Agents and Chemotherapy, American Society for Microbiology, Washington DC, 2005.
39. Rolston KVI, Manzullo EF, Elting LS, Frisbee-Hume SE, McMahon L, Theriault RL, et al. Once daily, oral, outpatient quinolone monotherapy for low-risk cancer patients with fever and neutropenia. A pilot study for low-risk cancer patients with fever and neutropenia. Cancer. 2006;106:2489–94.
40. Rolston KV, Frisbee-Hume SE, Patel S, et al. Oral moxifloxacin for outpatient treatment of low-risk, febrile neutropenic patients. Support Care Cancer. 2010;18:89–94.
41. Rubenstein EB, Rolston K, Benjamin RS, Loewy J, Escalante C, Manzullo E, et al. Outpatient treatment of febrile episodes in low-risk neutropenic patients with cancer. Cancer. 1993;71:3640–6.
42. Sebban C, Dussart S, Fuhrmann C, Ghesquières H, Rodrigues I, Geoffrois L, Devaux Y, Lancry L, Chvetzoff G, Bachelot T, Chelghoum M, Biron P. Oral moxifloxacin or intravenous ceftriaxone for the treatment of low-risk neutropenic fever in cancer patients suitable for early hospital discharge. Support Care Cancer. 2008;16:1017–23.
43. Smith TJ, Khatcheressian J, Lyman GH, Ozer H, Armitage JO, Balducci L, et al. Update of Recommendations for the use of white blood cell growth factors: an evidence-based clinical practice guideline. J Clin Oncol. 2006;24:3187–205.
44. Talcott JA, Finberg R, Mayer RJ, Goldman L. The medical course of patients with fever and neutropenia: clinical identification of a low-risk subgroup at presentation. Arch Intern Med. 1988;148:2561–8.
45. Talcott JA, Siegel RD, Finberg R, Goldman L. Risk assessment in cancer patients with fever and neutropenia: a prospective, two-center validation of a prediction rule. J Clin Oncol. 1992;10:316–22.
46. Talcott JA, Yeap BY, Clark JA, Siegel RD, Trice Loggers E, Lu C, Godley PA. Safety of early discharge for low-risk patients with febrile neutropenia: a multicenter randomized controlled trial. J Clin Oncol. 2011;29:3977–83.
47. Teuffel O, Amir E, Alibhai S, Beyene J, Shung L. Cost effectiveness of outpatient treatment for febrile neutropenia in adult cancer patients. Br J Cancer. 2011;104:1377–83.
48. Uys A, Rapoport BL, Anderson R. Febrile neutropenia: a prospective study to validate the Multnational Association for Supportive Care in Cancer (MASCC) risk-index score. Support Care Cancer. 2004;12:555–60.

49. Uys A, Rapoport BL, Fickl H, Meyer PWA, Anderson R. Prediction of outcome in cancer patients with febrile neutropenia: comparison of the Multinational Association of Supportive Care in Cancer risk-index score with procalcitonin, C-reactive protein, serum amyloid A, and interleukins-1β, -6, -8 and -10. Eur J Cancer. 2007;16:475–83.
50. Vento S, Cainelli F. Infections in patients with cancer undergoing chemotherapy: aetiology, prevention and treatment. Lancet Oncol. 2003;4:595–604.
51. Vidal L, Paul M, Ben dor I, Soares-Weiser K, Leibovici L. Oral versus intravenous antibiotic treatment for febrile neutropenia in cancer patients: a systematic review and meta-analysis of randomized trials. JAC. 2004;54:29–37.
52. Weycker D, Malin J, Edelsberg J, Glass A, Gokhale M, Oster G. Cost of neutropenic complications of chemotherapy. Ann Oncol. 2008;19:454–60.

Part III

Therapeutic Strategies

Fever of Unknown Origin: Treatment According to Risk Assessment

9

Georg Maschmeyer

Contents

9.1 Infections in Patients with Neutropenia

Although the risk of developing fever and infection is already increased when a patient's neutrophil granulocyte counts fall below 1,000 per mm^3, counts of less than 500 per mm^3 have been demonstrated to be the most critical risk factor for the development of serious infectious complications. Expert groups of the Infectious Diseases Society of America (IDSA) [9], the European Conference on Infections in Leukaemia (ECIL), the Multinational Association for Supportive Care in Cancer [15], the American Society of Clinical Oncology [7], and the German Society of

G. Maschmeyer
Department of Hematology, Oncology and Palliative Care, Klinikum Ernst von Bergmann, Charlottenstrasse 72, Potsdam 14467, Germany
e-mail: gmaschmeyer@klinikumevb.de

G. Maschmeyer, K.V.I. Rolston (eds.), *Infections in Hematology*,
DOI 10.1007/978-3-662-44000-1_9

Hematology and Oncology [18] have categorized neutropenic patients into distinct subgroups with different risk profiles depending upon their duration of neutropenia (see also the chapter by Paesmans). While a strict prospective allocation of all patients to distinct risk groups is not possible in clinical practice, patients with neutropenia lasting for up to 7 days, who have no additional risk factors such as open wounds and tumor-associated obstruction of airways or bile ducts, e.g., patients with malignant lymphoma on standard chemotherapy, are regarded as low-risk patients. In contrast, patients with aggressive hematologic malignancies such as acute leukemias undergoing intensive chemotherapy, who have an expected duration of profound neutropenia of more than 7 days, represent a high-risk group. Sometimes, patients with an expected neutropenia of 7–10 days, e.g., those with lymphomas receiving dose-intensified treatment regimens, are regarded as a separate, so-called intermediate or standard risk group.

Approximately 30–40 % of all febrile episodes in neutropenic patients occur in patients of the low-risk group. It has been shown that oral administration of broad-spectrum antibiotics, i.e., a combination of ciprofloxacin with amoxicillin-clavulanate or with clindamycin, as well as moxifloxacin monotherapy [13], may be a valid option in these patients [3, 8, 12, 14]. However, it is essential to identify patients with a significant risk of treatment failure, i.e., those with bacteremia, pneumonia, sepsis, or other types of serious infection, for whom such a low-risk treatment regimen is not appropriate.

9.2 Diagnostic Procedures in Febrile Neutropenic Patients

Clinical evaluation at first onset of fever in a neutropenic patient is essential for identifying a potential source or focus of infection and thereby discriminating fever of unknown origin from a clinically and/or microbiologically documented infection. A thorough physical examination includes inspection of the oropharyngeal mucosa, the skin (particularly venous access sites, bone marrow puncture sites, and the perianal region), pulmonary auscultation and percussion, abdominal palpation, percussion of paranasal sinuses and renal beds, as well as the assessment of consciousness. Table 9.2 shows typical associations of findings at specific physical sites and the most predominant microbial pathogens involved. If one or more of these findings are made in a febrile neutropenic patient, preemptive modification of antimicrobial therapy targeting at the typically involved pathogens is recommended (see other chapters of this textbook).

9.3 Laboratory Tests for Evaluation of Fever in Neutropenic Patients

Clinical chemistry tests should include a complete blood cell count with a differential leukocyte count, serum creatinine, blood urea nitrogen, electrolytes, hepatic transaminase enzymes, bilirubin, lactate dehydrogenase, clotting tests, C-reactive protein, and in septic patients also lactate. For early assessment of the severity of infection, measurement of interleukin-6 may be helpful [26], while for procalcitonin, clinical experience and published data on its usefulness in febrile neutropenic patients are conflicting [2, 23].

For routine microbiological work-up, a minimum of two separate pairs (aerobic/anaerobic) of blood cultures is recommended. In patients with a central venous catheter, one of the cultures should be taken from the catheter. Culture specimens from other sites should not be obtained routinely, but only if clinically indicated.

9.4 Imaging Procedures at Onset of Febrile Neutropenia

A chest radiograph is recommended routinely but appears to be useful only for patients with respiratory signs or symptoms. Supplemental imaging procedures such as a computed tomography (CT) scan of the paranasal sinuses in patients with clinical signs pointing to sinusitis such as painful orbit, orbitonasal skin alterations, and gingival or hard palate ulcers [21], and abdominal ultrasound or CT scan (with contrast medium) in patients with abdominal complaints [25] may be required in individual patients.

9.5 Empirical First-Line Antimicrobial Therapy in Patients with Fever of Unknown Origin (FUO)

Criteria for the institution of antimicrobial therapy in neutropenic patients are summarized in Table 9.1. The standard of care in patients with granulocytopenia and fever is the prompt institution of broad-spectrum antibiotics active against streptococci, *Staphylococcus aureus*, and gram-negative aerobes including *Pseudomonas aeruginosa*. In more than 50 % of the febrile episodes, the source of infection cannot be identified, so that the selection of antimicrobials must be made empirically (fever of unknown origin, FUO). In order to avoid unselected administration of highly potent intravenous antimicrobial agents to all febrile neutropenic patients, criteria for the differentiation of patients into low-risk and high-risk categories have been elaborated (see above). The stratification is based primarily on the duration of profound neutropenia and the feasibility of outpatient care. In low-risk patients, an ambulatory treatment using oral antibiotics is desirable. In classical clinical studies, Freifeld et al. [8] have demonstrated in a double-blind study that an oral regimen of ciprofloxacin plus amoxicillin-clavulanate was equally effective as a standard intravenous monotherapy with ceftazidime for initial empirical therapy in 116 febrile episodes with low risk for

Table 9.1 Indication for empirical antimicrobial intervention in cancer patients

Granulocyte count <500/μl or <1,000/μl with predicted decline to ≤500/μl
Single oral temperature of >38.3 °C
or ≥38.0 °C × 2 within 12 h
or ≥38.0 °C over ≥1 h
No obvious noninfectious origin
Adverse reaction to blood products, cytokines, other drugs

complications. Similar results have been achieved in a prospective EORTC trial [12], comparing the efficacy of oral ciprofloxacin plus amoxicillin-clavulanate with that of intravenous ceftriaxone plus amikacin. Thus, current guidelines recommend the administration of oral empirical antimicrobial therapy with ciprofloxacin (or levofloxacin) plus amoxicillin-clavulanate (or with clindamycin in case of penicillin allergy) in low-risk patients [7, 9, 24]. Oral antimicrobial monotherapy with once-daily moxifloxacin has been shown to be equivalent to oral ciprofloxacin plus amoxicillin-clavulanate in this setting [13], so that this regimen is feasible as well in low-risk febrile neutropenic patients, provided they did not previously receive fluoroquinolones for systemic antimicrobial prophylaxis and the local prevalence of resistance to fluoroquinolones among gram-negative bacilli is below 20 % [7]. If primary outpatient management is expected to be complicated, short-term hospital admission and initial therapy with intravenous antibiotics followed by a switch to oral antibiotics and early discharge in patients with controlled infection (defervescence, absence of pneumonia, negative blood cultures) may be an alternative [7], as has been well adapted in guidelines for pediatric cancer patients [16].

Patients with a higher risk of a more complicated clinical course of infection should initially be treated with intravenous antimicrobial therapy. Current IDSA guidelines recommend monotherapy with an antipseudomonal beta-lactam such as cefepime, piperacillin-tazobactam, or a carbapenem (meropenem, imipenem-cilastatin) in complicated situations (sepsis, pneumonia) or a duotherapy with an antipseudomonal beta-lactam antibiotic plus an aminoglycoside as appropriate choices for initial empirical therapy in this setting [9]. In general, the combination of the beta-lactam with an aminoglycoside is not required [5, 22]. Fluoroquinolones such as ciprofloxacin are not recommended for initial empirical intravenous monotherapy with respect to inferior efficacy [20] and the considerable emergence of resistance among gram-negative bacilli against quinolones in the past decade [1].

It is not recommended to include an antibacterial agent with specific activity against gram-positive cocci such as vancomycin in the empiric first-line regimen in patients with fever of unknown origin. This combination may be considered in patients with clinical signs of a gram-positive infection (see below) or those with hemodynamic instability in a setting with high prevalence of methicillin-resistant *Staphylococcus aureus* (MRSA).

The initial empiric addition of a broad-spectrum antifungal agent such as voriconazole is not justified in FUO patients, because it does not increase response rates and does not prevent fungal breakthrough infections [19].

9.6 Modification of Antimicrobial Treatment in Patients with Persisting Fever After 4 Days of Initial Therapy

A daily clinical reassessment of neutropenic patients with fever of unknown origin receiving empiric antibacterial therapy is essential. Clinical or radiological findings indicating a specific spectrum of microorganisms have been summarized in Table 9.2.

Table 9.2 Typical clinical findings at specific physical sites and predominant microbial pathogens involved

Clinical symptoms	Typical pathogens
Erythema/pain at venous access	Coagulase-negative staphylococci
Mucosal ulcers	Alpha-hemolytic streptococci, *Candida* spp.
Single point-like erythemas	Gram-positive cocci, *Candida* spp.
Necrotizing skin lesions	*Pseudomonas aeruginosa, Aspergillus* spp.
Retinal infiltrates	*Candida* spp.
Diarrhea, meteorism	*Clostridium difficile,* norovirus
Enterocolitis, perianal lesion	Polymicrobial incl. anaerobes
Lung infiltrates ± sinusitis	*Aspergillus* spp., zygomycetes, *P. jirovecii*

In general, a decision on maintaining or modifying the initial antimicrobial regimen is made after 96 h, after all cultures have tested negative and no clinical or imaging finding enables a more targeted anti-infective treatment. At this point, three options have to be considered: (1) leaving the antimicrobial treatment regimen unchanged, (2) switching to another antibacterial agent, or (3) adding a broad-spectrum antifungal.

Before this decision is made, all potential sites of infection (see Table 9.2) must be reexamined, blood cultured be taken once more (including those drawn from the venous catheter), and the patient be sent to a thoracic CT scan. In individual low-risk patients who are clinically stable and expect the recovery of their neutrophil counts, this procedure might be suspended, but for all other patients, it is strongly recommended. Approximately 50 % of patients without any clinical finding indicative of pneumonia will show pulmonary infiltrates on CT scans [10], which are frequently missed on plain chest radiographs. It can be considered to include paranasal sinuses in CT studies; however, their benefit for treatment decisions in asymptomatic, persistently febrile neutropenic patients has not been conclusively shown as yet. This is different in patients who show pulmonary infiltrates at this time, because pathological findings on CT scans of paranasal sinuses may facilitate the diagnosis of invasive fungal infection [11].

In patients with persistent fever of unknown origin, i.e., with unremarkable results of the abovementioned diagnostic procedures, who are clinically stable, and in whom laboratory parameters such as C-reactive protein and interleukin-6 have not significantly increased in comparison to baseline diagnostics, the antibacterial treatment regimen should be continued without modification [9], irrespective of their risk group allocation. In *low-risk* patients in whom a treatment modification is regarded necessary, because clinical or laboratory findings indicate an uncontrolled febrile complication (clinical instability, increasing proinflammatory laboratory parameters), a change of antibacterial treatment should be prompted. In patients initially treated with ciprofloxacin and amoxicillin-clavulanate, piperacillin-tazobactam may be a suitable second-line regimen. In patients treated with piperacillin-tazobactam or cefepime, a switch to imipenem or meropenem should be considered.

In *high-risk* patients in whom treatment modification is clinically indicated, the antimicrobial regimen should be escalated by the addition of a broad-spectrum antifungal agent, i.e., liposomal amphotericin B or caspofungin (both licensed for this indication). The modification of antibacterial therapy is debatable. It appears justified to switch from piperacillin-tazobactam or cefepime to imipenem or meropenem, because these carbapenems may be effective against pathogens non-susceptible to the former agents. In contrast, in patients already given imipenem or meropenem for first-line therapy, a modification of antibacterial therapy is more speculative. Although apparently logical, the addition of a glycopeptide (vancomycin or teicoplanin) has not been shown to be superior to the addition of placebo [4, 6]. In institutions with a high prevalence of multiresistance among gram-negative microorganisms, the addition of an aminoglycoside might be considered.

Empiric antiviral treatment or the administration of macrolide antibiotics or trimethoprim-sulfamethoxazole should be omitted.

9.7 Approach to Patients with Clinically Documented Infections

A primary ("preemptive") modification of antimicrobial therapy may be beneficial in patients with distinct clinical symptoms, particularly in those with pulmonary infiltrates, a venous catheter-associated infection, and central nervous system or abdominal/perianal infection (Table 9.2). Those scenarios are addressed in separate chapters of this textbook.

9.8 Targeted Treatment in Microbiologically Documented Infections

Microbiological findings can be extremely helpful in order to target antimicrobial treatment; however, they should always be critically interpreted with respect to their causal relationship to the clinical picture of infection. Irrespective of their potentially pathogenic character, some microorganisms may represent nothing but residual flora after antibiotic therapy, e.g., enterococci isolated from oropharyngeal samples. Other findings may point at a separate relevant infection but are irrelevant for the infection that gave reason for taking the sample, e.g., coagulase-negative staphylococci repeatedly isolated from blood cultures in a patient with pneumonia. Moreover, two infections may be present concomitantly or sequentially, e.g., invasive pulmonary aspergillosis in a patient with pneumonia caused by *Klebsiella* spp. not responding to appropriate antibacterial treatment.

9.8.1 Bacteremia

In most cases of bacteremia, the antibiotic regimen selected empirically for febrile neutropenia will be effective, so that no modification after identification of the pathogen is required. In case of coagulase-negative staphylococci, 80–90 % of which being resistant to beta-lactam antibiotics including flucloxacillin, isolated from at least two separate blood cultures, a glycopeptide antibiotic should be supplemented. Although not studied appropriately in prospective clinical trials, linezolid can be recommended as an effective and well-tolerated treatment alternative for staphylococcal and enterococcal bacteremia. It has the favorable property that it can be given orally as well.

9.9 Duration of Antimicrobial Treatment

A prospective randomized study of the appropriate duration of antimicrobial therapy after defervescence and clinical response in febrile neutropenic patients has not yet been conducted. While in most cases treatment may be terminated 7 days after stable defervescence and resolution of clinical symptoms also in persistently neutropenic patients [17, 18], at least 14 days of effective antibiotic treatment are recommended in patients with documented *Staphylococcus aureus* or *Pseudomonas aeruginosa* bacteremia [9].

References

1. Bhusal Y, Mihu CN, Tarrand JJ, Rolston KV. Incidence of fluoroquinolone-resistant and extended-spectrum β-lactamase-producing Escherichia coli at a comprehensive cancer center in the United States. Chemotherapy. 2011;57:335–8.
2. Blijlevens NM, Donnelly JP, Meis JF, De Keizer MH, De Pauw BE. Procalcitonin does not discriminate infection from inflammation after allogeneic bone marrow transplantation. Clin Diagn Lab Immunol. 2000;7:889–92.
3. Cherif H, Johansson E, Björkholm M, Kalin M. The feasibility of early hospital discharge with oral antimicrobial therapy in low risk patients with febrile neutropenia following chemotherapy for hematologic malignancies. Haematologica. 2006;91:215–22.
4. Cometta A, Kern WV, De Bock R, Paesmans M, Vandenbergh M, Crokaert F, Engelhard D, Marchetti O, Akan H, Skoutelis A, Korten V, Vandercam M, Gaya H, Padmos A, Klastersky J, Zinner S, Glauser MP, Calandra T, Viscoli C, International Antimicrobial Therapy Group of the European Organization for Research Treatment of Cancer. Vancomycin versus placebo for treating persistent fever in patients with neutropenic cancer receiving piperacillin-tazobactam monotherapy. Clin Infect Dis. 2003;37:382–9.
5. Del Favero A, Menichetti F, Martino P, Bucaneve G, Micozzi A, Gentile G, Furno P, Russo D, D'Antonio D, Ricci P, Martino B, Mandelli F. A multicenter, double-blind, placebo-controlled trial comparing piperacillin-tazobactam with and without amikacin as empiric therapy for febrile neutropenia. Clin Infect Dis. 2001;33:1295–301.
6. Erjavec Z, de Vries-Hospers HG, Laseur M, Halie RM, Daenen S. A prospective, randomized, double-blinded, placebo-controlled trial of empirical teicoplanin in febrile neutropenia with persistent fever after imipenem monotherapy. J Antimicrob Chemother. 2000;45:843–9.
7. Flowers CR, Seidenfeld J, Bow EJ, Karten C, Gleason C, Hawley DK, Kuderer NM, Langston AA, Marr KA, Rolston KV, Ramsey SD. Antimicrobial prophylaxis and outpatient management of fever and neutropenia in adults treated for malignancy: American Society of Clinical Oncology clinical practice guideline. J Clin Oncol. 2013;31:794–810.
8. Freifeld A, Marchigiani D, Walsh T, Chanock S, Lewis L, Hiemenz J, Hiemenz S, Hicks JE, Gill V, Steinberg SM, Pizzo PA. A double-blind comparison of empirical oral and intravenous

antibiotic therapy for low-risk febrile patients with neutropenia during cancer chemotherapy. N Engl J Med. 1999;341:305–11.

9. Freifeld AG, Bow EJ, Sepkowitz KA, Boeckh MJ, Ito JI, Mullen CA, Raad II, Rolston KV, Young JA, Wingard JR. Infectious Diseases Society of America. Clinical practice guideline for the use of antimicrobial agents in neutropenic patients with cancer: 2010 update by the Infectious Diseases Society of America. Clin Infect Dis. 2011;52:e56–93.
10. Heussel CP, Kauczor HU, Heussel GE, Fischer B, Begrich M, Mildenberger P, Thelen M. Pneumonia in febrile neutropenic patients and in bone marrow and stem cell transplant recipients: use of high-resolution computed tomography. J Clin Oncol. 1999;17:796–805.
11. Ho DY, Lin M, Schaenman J, Rosso F, Leung AN, Coutre SE, Sista RR, Montoya JG. Yield of diagnostic procedures for invasive fungal infections in neutropenic febrile patients with chest computed tomography abnormalities. Mycoses. 2011;54:59–70.
12. Kern WV, Cometta A, DeBock R, Langenaeken J, Paesmans M, Gaya H. Oral versus intravenous empirical antimicrobial therapy for fever in patients with granulocytopenia who are receiving cancer chemotherapy. N Engl J Med. 1999;341:312–8.
13. Kern WV, Marchetti O, Drgona L, Akan H, Aoun M, Akova M, de Bock R, Paesmans M, Viscoli C, Calandra T. Oral antibiotics for fever in low-risk neutropenic patients with cancer: a double-blind, randomized, multicenter trial comparing single daily moxifloxacin with twice daily ciprofloxacin plus amoxicillin/clavulanic acid combination therapy – EORTC infectious diseases group trial X. J Clin Oncol. 2013;31:1149–56.
14. Klastersky J, Paesmans M, Georgala A, Muanza F, Plehiers B, Dubreucq L, Lalami Y, Aoun M, Barette M. Outpatient oral antibiotics for febrile neutropenic cancer patients using a score predictive for complications. J Clin Oncol. 2006;24:4129–34.
15. Klastersky J, Paesmans M. The Multinational Association for Supportive Care in Cancer (MASCC) risk index score: 10 years of use for identifying low-risk febrile neutropenic cancer patients. Support Care Cancer. 2013;21:1487–95.
16. Lehrnbecher T, Phillips R, Alexander S, Alvaro F, Carlesse F, Fisher B, Hakim H, Santolaya M, Castagnola E, Davis BL, Dupuis LL, Gibson F, Groll AH, Gaur A, Gupta A, Kebudi R, Petrilli S, Steinbach WJ, Villarroel M, Zaoutis T, Sung L. Guideline for the management of fever and neutropenia in children with cancer and/or undergoing hematopoietic stem-cell transplantation. J Clin Oncol. 2012;30:4427–38.
17. Link H, Maschmeyer G, Meyer P, Hiddemann W, Stille W, Helmerking M, Adam D. Interventional antimicrobial therapy in febrile neutropenic patients. Study group of the Paul Ehrlich society for chemotherapy. Ann Hematol. 1994;69:231–43.
18. Link H, Böhme A, Cornely OA, Höffken K, Kellner O, Kern WV, Mahlberg R, Maschmeyer G, Nowrousian MR, Ostermann H, Ruhnke M, Sezer O, Schiel X, Wilhelm M, Auner HW. Antimicrobial therapy of unexplained fever in neutropenic patients. Ann Hematol. 2003;82 Suppl 2:S105–17.
19. Maschmeyer G, Heinz WJ, Hertenstein B, Horst HA, Requadt C, Wagner T, Cornely OA, Löffler J, Ruhnke M, On Behalf of the IDEA Study Investigators. Immediate versus deferred empirical antifungal (IDEA) therapy in high-risk patients with febrile neutropenia: a randomized, double-blind, placebo-controlled, multicenter study. Eur J Clin Microbiol Infect Dis. 2013;32:679–89.
20. Meunier F, Zinner SH, Gaya H, Calandra T, Viscoli C, Klastersky J, Glauser M. Prospective randomized evaluation of ciprofloxacin versus piperacillin plus amikacin for empiric antibiotic therapy of febrile granulocytopenic cancer patients with lymphomas and solid tumors. The European Organization for Research on Treatment of Cancer International Antimicrobial Therapy Cooperative Group. Antimicrob Agents Chemother. 1991;35:873–8.
21. Pagano L, Girmenia C, Mele L, Ricci P, Tosti ME, Nosari A, Buelli M, Picardi M, Allione B, Corvatta L, D'Antonio D, Montillo M, Melillo L, Chierichini A, Cenacchi A, Tonso A, Cudillo L, Candoni A, Savignano C, Bonini A, Martino P, Del Favero A, GIMEMA Infection Program, Gruppo Italiano Malattie Ematologiche dell'Adulto. Infections caused by filamentous fungi in patients with hematologic malignancies. A report of 391 cases by GIMEMA Infection Program. Haematologica. 2001;86:862–70.

22. Paul M, Yahav D, Fraser A, Leibovici L. Empirical antibiotic monotherapy for febrile neutropenia: systematic review and meta-analysis of randomized controlled trials. J Antimicrob Chemother. 2006;57:176–89.
23. Robinson JO, Lamoth F, Bally F, Knaup M, Calandra T, Marchetti O. Monitoring procalcitonin in febrile neutropenia: what is its utility for initial diagnosis of infection and reassessment in persistent fever? PLoS One. 2011;6:e18886.
24. Rubenstein EB, Rolston K, Benjamin RS, Loewy J, Escalante C, Manzullo E, Hughes P, Moreland B, Fender A, Kennedy K, Holmes F, Elting L, Bodey GP. Outpatient treatment of febrile episodes in low-risk neutropenic patients with cancer. Cancer. 1993;71:3640–6.
25. Vehreschild MJ, Vehreschild JJ, Hübel K, Hentrich M, Schmidt-Hieber M, Christopeit M, Maschmeyer G, Schalk E, Cornely OA, Neumann S. Diagnosis and management of gastrointestinal complications in adult cancer patients: evidence-based guidelines of the Infectious Diseases Working Party (AGIHO) of the German Society of Hematology and Oncology (DGHO). Ann Oncol. 2013;24:1189–202.
26. von Lilienfeld-Toal M, Dietrich MP, Glasmacher A, Lehmann L, Breig P, Hahn C, Schmidt-Wolf IG, Marklein G, Schroeder S, Stuber F. Markers of bacteremia in febrile neutropenic patients with hematologic malignancies: procalcitonin and IL-6 are more reliable than C-reactive protein. Eur J Clin Microbiol Infect Dis. 2004;23:539–44.

Pulmonary Complications 10

Georg Maschmeyer

Contents

10.1 Introduction

Cancer patients with febrile complications and high-risk neutropenia, i.e., those with granulocytes <0.5 Gpt/l for >10 days, develop lung infiltrates (LI) with a likelihood of 20–25 % [85, 125]. These patients carry a higher risk of treatment

G. Maschmeyer
Department of Hematology, Oncology and Palliative Care, Klinikum Ernst von Bergmann, Charlottenstrasse 72, D-14467 Potsdam, Germany
e-mail: gmaschmeyer@klinikumevb.de

G. Maschmeyer, K.V.I. Rolston (eds.), *Infections in Hematology*,
DOI 10.1007/978-3-662-44000-1_10

failure and fatal outcome as compared to those with fever of unknown origin or most clinically documented infections at other body sites [4, 12, 50, 98], and antimicrobial treatment is often complicated and expensive [79]. In many cases, microbial etiology remains undetermined; in microbiologically documented cases, multiresistant bacteria [63, 128] and pathogens resistant to beta-lactam antibiotics (e.g., filamentous fungi, *Pneumocystis jirovecii*, multiresistant gram-negative aerobes or viruses) are predominant. Important differential diagnoses include alveolar hemorrhage, lung involvement by the underlying malignancy, cryptogenic organizing pneumonia, immune reconstitution syndrome, and lesions caused by chemotherapy or radiation [9, 14, 31, 39, 40, 94, 136, 143, 147, 150].

As yet, it has not been clearly shown that diagnostic procedures such as bronchoscopy and bronchoalveolar lavage, performed in order to identify the etiology of LI in febrile neutropenic patients, improve clinical outcome [10, 48, 98, 126, 136]. However, antimicrobial treatment regimens are modified in a large number of patients based upon the results of these procedures [117]. It has been observed that response to broad-spectrum antibacterial treatment in febrile neutropenic high-risk patients with LI is less than 30 % [98, 119], whereas mold-active systemic antifungals added to the first-line antimicrobial treatment in all febrile, severely neutropenic patients with LI increase the response rate to up to 78 % [130]. In a small prospective study, the incidence of LI in acute leukemia patients could be reduced to 0 % by voriconazole prophylaxis as compared with 33 % under placebo [149]. These observations as well as autopsy studies [14, 32, 45, 61] indicate that the majority of LI in febrile neutropenic patients are caused by filamentous fungi, primarily by *Aspergillus* spp. [3, 111].

In patients with invasive pulmonary aspergillosis (IPA), cultural or histologic proof at an early stage is very rare; however, far advanced, proven IA in neutropenic patients has a very dismal outcome [38, 84]. As a consequence, early ("preemptive") antifungal treatment is frequently started in febrile patients with severe neutropenia and LI presenting with radiological and laboratory findings not indicating a typical non-fungal disease [24, 95].

Successful or ineffective management of IPA will have a substantial impact on further treatment of the patients' underlying malignancy [107], and early initiation of mold-active antifungal treatment has been shown to improve overall survival of febrile neutropenic patients with IPA [37, 60]. At the same time, inadequate overuse of broad-spectrum antifungal agents must be avoided. Early treatment decision may be facilitated by serial *Aspergillus* galactomannan (GM) or beta-D-glucan testing in blood samples of high-risk patients [80, 89]. If LI suspicious of fungal origin emerge in patients receiving posaconazole or voriconazole prophylaxis, diagnostic intervention including fine-needle or open-lung biopsy must be discussed in order to identify rare pathogens such as *Nocardia* and non-fungal causes of LI [28, 132]. In contrast, patients who have been treated with nucleoside analogs such as fludarabine or cladribine or with long-term T-cell-depleting agents such as alemtuzumab or antithymocyte globulin may be affected by microorganisms typical for severe T-cell immunosuppression such as cytomegalovirus, mycobacteria, or yeasts [129], in addition to *Staphylococcus aureus, Pseudomonas aeruginosa*, *Aspergillus* spp., and pneumococci [1], which are very relevant in this context as well.

In febrile neutropenic patients, respiratory viruses such as *influenza*, *parainfluenza*, *human metapneumovirus*, or *respiratory syncytial virus* may be relevant pathogens for respiratory tract infections particularly during cold and wet seasons [68, 92], but typically, allogeneic hematopoietic stem cell transplant recipients are affected [16]. It has been reported that these viral infections are not more frequent in immunocompromised than in non-immunocompromised patients [52, 88]. In immunosuppressed patients affected by these viruses, neutropenia, poor APACHE II score, age over 65 years, and severe lymphocytopenia have been reported prognostic factors resulting in a higher risk of fatal outcome [33, 34]. In many cases, it remains undetermined if respiratory viruses documented in respiratory secretions represent the cause of pneumonia or rather "innocent bystanders." As there are almost no effective antiviral drugs for the treatment of these infections available, no prospective, randomized studies, which could elucidate the relevance of these viruses, have been conducted.

10.2 Diagnostic Procedures

With respect to the critical prognosis of LI in febrile neutropenic patients, diagnostic procedures are of major importance, but should not cause a substantial delay in the start of adequate antimicrobial therapy.

10.2.1 Imaging

Conventional chest radiographs show abnormalities in less than 2 % of febrile neutropenic patients without clinical findings indicating lower respiratory tract infection [78, 106, 109]. It is not exactly known how many of these patients would have abnormalities on computed tomography (CT) scans, because no randomized head-to-head comparisons have been published so far. In patients persistently febrile after more than 48 h of broad-spectrum antibacterial therapy, about 10 % of chest radiographs are abnormal, whereas CT scans at this time reveal pathological findings in approximately 50 % of patients [65, 66]. Early detection of lesions indicating invasive fungal infection, *Pneumocystis* pneumonia (PcP), or cytomegalovirus (CMV) pneumonia is of utmost importance, facilitating targeted bronchoscopy and bronchoalveolar lavage and a prompt institution of preemptive antimicrobial treatment [27, 58, 120], enabling improved survival of these patients. CT findings such as consolidation, "halo sign," and "air crescent" may be important signs of filamentous fungal disease [41, 58]. While the "halo sign" has been described typically in neutropenic patients, in general CT findings indicative of IPA are comparable in neutropenic and in non-neutropenic patients [38]. A "reversed halo sign," showing a focal rounded area of ground-glass opacity surrounded by a crescent or complete ring of consolidation, has been described as relatively specific for fungal pneumonia due to *Mucorales* [58]. Beyond early identification of LI, CT findings may allow for distinguishing fungal from non-fungal LI [26, 49, 55, 62, 67, 143]. Nodular or cavitary lesions are suggestive of invasive filamentous fungal infection. Differential diagnoses include pneumonia due to other microorganisms including mycobacteria [56] (which may be different in regions with specific epidemiology) as well as by underlying malignancies [133], so that comparison to previous CT scans in an individual patient is essential. Combination of CT scan with angiography has been found to increase the diagnostic specificity in patients with pulmonary mold infections [138, 142]; however, this more labor-intensive method has not yet become widely applied and is therefore not included into current clinical practice guidelines. In selected patients where pulmonary CT scan is not wanted or feasible, magnetic resonance tomography (MRI) is a valid alternative [46]. As yet, consensus definitions of invasive fungal diseases have not included thoracic MRI findings. Of note, on follow-up CT scans in patients with IPA, the volume of pulmonary infiltrates frequently increases during the first week despite effective antifungal therapy [25], which should not give reason to assess the treatment course as refractory. The reduction of the "halo" and the development of an "air-crescent" sign, however, typically indicate favorable response [20].

10.2.2 Microbiology and Histopathology

In the majority of febrile neutropenic patients with LI, no indicatory microbiological finding is available, so that the therapeutic management is based upon clinical and imaging findings. In microbiologically documented cases, pathogens are isolated from blood cultures, bronchial secretions, or bronchoalveolar lavage (BAL) fluid. It often means a challenge to assess the diagnostic relevance of culture results [11, 48, 73, 124], because unselected bronchial samples from these patients grow colonizing and contaminating microorganisms with no etiological significance [44], or blood cultures may show isolates not etiologically related to pneumonias. At the same time, if autopsies show invasive fungal infections, 75 % of them have not been detected ante mortem [32]. Therefore, in contrast to the majority of other microbiological findings, isolation of *Aspergillus* spp. or other filamentous fungi from upper respiratory tract specimens of severely immunocompromised patients typically indicates a respiratory tract mycosis [72].

The diagnostic yield of BAL has been described to be 25 % to >50 % [17, 38, 76, 159], depending on the risk profile of patients included. The diagnostic yield and the outcome of clinical management in critically ill, febrile cancer patients with severe pulmonary infiltrates have not been improved by invasive diagnostic procedures [10]. In contrast, one retrospective analysis of microbiological findings from BAL samples in cancer patients with LI showed 34 % bacteria, 22 % CMV, 15 % *Pneumocystis jirovecii*, and 2 % *Aspergillus* spp. [103], and another report of 246 bronchoscopies in 199 febrile patients with hematologic malignancies noted pathogens with possible etiological significance in 48 % of samples, of whom 70 grew only bacteria and 13 samples showed both fungi and bacteria, 15 samples *Aspergillus* spp., 16 samples *Candida* species, and 2 samples both *Aspergillus* and *Candida* spp. [73]. Many LI in severely immunocompromised patients may also have polymicrobial etiology [124], with molds (predominantly *Aspergillus* spp.) plus bacteria in 12 % and multiple fungal species in 22 % of the samples. Although the etiological relevance of BAL findings may be questionable in many cases, the results trigger the change of antimicrobial treatment in up to 50 % of patients [73, 117]. As a diagnostic "gold standard" is lacking, the number of false-positive and false-negative findings is unknown, and the rates of success or failure of "pathogen-directed" antimicrobial treatment there remain undetermined. A proposal for the assessment of the etiological significance of microbiological findings in febrile neutropenic patients with LI is given further below.

While for the proven diagnosis of IPA, cultural isolation of fungi and histological proof from lung tissue are regarded as diagnostic "gold standard" [41], quality standards for diagnostic procedures are not available and patients undergoing biopsy are highly selected. Transbronchial biopsy is not recommended in severely thrombocytopenic patients with lung infiltrates [117], whereas open-lung biopsy (OLB), mini-thoracotomy, or video-assisted thoracoscopic surgery may be safely performed in patients with treatment-refractory LI not cleared up by other diagnostic approaches, primarily in order to rule out noninfectious origin [6, 28, 40, 159]. OLB is a relatively safe procedure, but may cause complications in approximately 6 % of patients [57] including the risk of hemorrhage [6, 155] even in patients with sufficient platelet counts [69, 115]. Histologically, no infection or malignancy, but nonspecific inflammation is detected in the majority of patients [48, 57, 155]. Notably, findings from OLB and BAL obtained simultaneously may show different microbiological results [48].

CT-guided percutaneous fine-needle biopsy (FNB) may provide informative results in approximately 80 % of cases, allowing for species identification using molecular methods for tissue workup [29, 36, 74, 77, 82, 122]. FNB requires platelet counts >50,000/μl and should be limited to patients without an obvious risk of respiratory failure in case of complications such as pneumothorax. As yet, there are no reports from prospective studies comparing different methods for invasive approaches to identify the causes of LI in febrile neutropenic patients.

10.2.3 Non-Culture-Based Diagnostic Methods

While the reference method for detecting *Pneumocystis jirovecii* is microscopic identification, polymerase chain reaction (PCR) has been introduced in the 1990s for early detection of this pathogen with high sensitivity [135]. To distinguish between infection and colonization, which may be present in up to 20 % of individuals without signs or symptoms of PcP, more recently developed real-time PCR assays may be helpful [5]. Beyond that, a negative PCR result from BAL samples allows for discontinuing anti-*Pneumocystis* therapy [8].

CMV may be a relevant cause of LI in immunocompromised hosts, particularly those with cellular immunosuppression secondary to immunosuppressive agents, radiotherapy, or malignant T-cell lymphoma. Primarily, patients who underwent allogeneic hematopoietic stem cell transplantation are affected. In febrile neutropenic patients with LI, CMV PCR applied on BAL samples has a high negative, but low positive predictive value [70], while positive rapid culture, immediate early antigen, direct fluorescent antibody tests, DNA hybridization, and cytology from BAL cultures are required to confirm the diagnosis of CMV pneumonia [15, 86].

Numerous methods have been developed for detecting fungal cell antigens such as *Aspergillus* galactomannan (GM), 1,3-beta-D-glucan, or nuclear amplification assays to identify small amounts of fungal DNA for early noninvasive detection of filamentous fungi in febrile neutropenic patients with LI of undetermined etiology [23, 47, 90, 91, 141]. More recently, a positive GM test not only from blood but also from BAL samples has been accepted as a significant finding indicating a probable invasive fungal infection in severely immunocompromised patients [13, 21]. It is debatable if *Aspergillus* GM assay in blood will become positive earlier than CT scans [154]. Notably, the GM test may give false-positive results in patients treated with semisynthetic beta-lactam antibiotics such as amoxicillin-clavulanate, piperacillin-tazobactam, carbapenems, ceftriaxone, and cefepime [7, 19] as well as in those given enteral nutrition [59], in those with other fungal infections such as fusariosis [148], and in BAL samples obtained using specific lavage solutions such as Plasmalyte™ [64]. Details on antigen testing for fungal infection, including those other than aspergillosis [108], have been reviewed in evidence-based guidelines [127].

Studies on panfungal or *Aspergillus*-specific PCR assays indicate that the use of these techniques on BAL samples seems superior as compared to blood samples, particularly in patients undergoing systemic antifungal therapy [21, 81, 87, 104, 141]. On lung biopsy specimens, PCR added to histopathology and culture may improve specification of pathogens [122]. Since there is no international standardization of these assays available as yet, PCR results have not become part of definition criteria for invasive fungal infections by now [99]. PCR presumably will become part of a diagnostic program for LI, including thoracic CT scans, serology, and conventional microbiology from blood and BAL samples [156].

10.2.4 Biomarkers

Nonspecific pro-inflammatory laboratory parameters like C-reactive protein, interleukin-6 [151], interleukin-8, tumor necrosis factor-alpha, and procalcitonin plasma levels [101] are frequently used to assess the severity of infections and the response to antimicrobial therapy. In febrile neutropenic patients with LI, the predictive value of these parameters has not been investigated in prospective studies as yet. In clinical practice, the repeated measurement of these parameters typically parallels clinical observation and should be used for therapeutic decisions only in the context of these clinical and with imaging findings. Persistent fever, progressive or new emerged LI, and rising pro-inflammatory parameters indicate the need for a change in the antimicrobial treatment regimen [123].

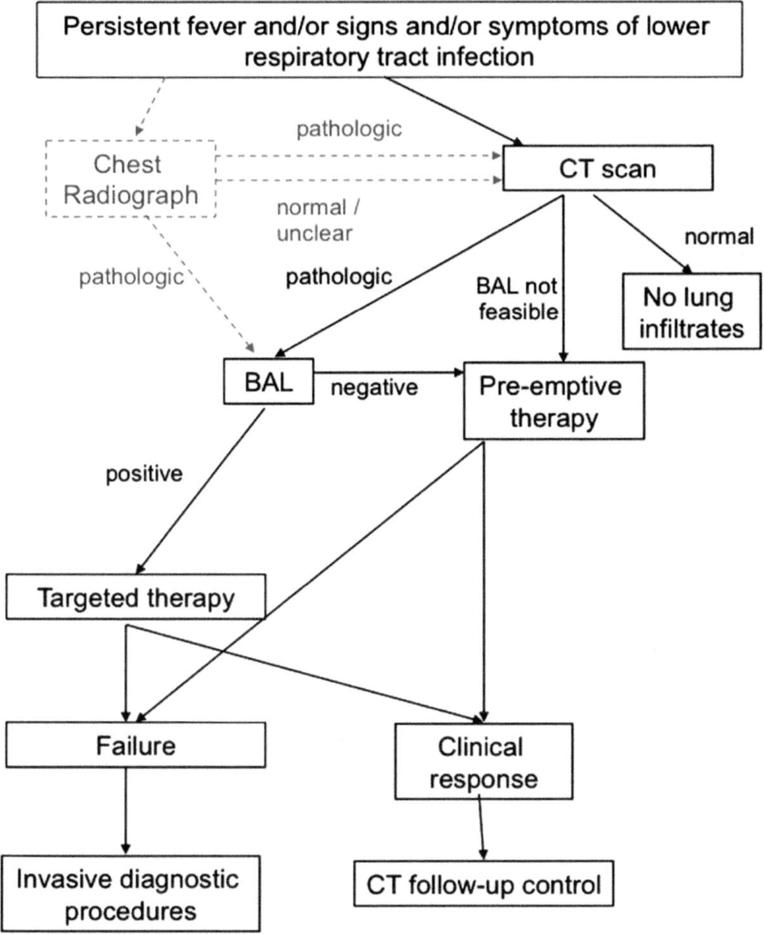

Fig. 10.1 Diagnostic procedures and treatment of neutropenic patients with fever and suspected or proven lung infiltrates. *CT* computed tomography, *BAL* bronchoalveolar lavage. *Dotted lines* indicate exceptions from recommended procedure

10.3 Algorithm for the Diagnostic Management of Febrile Neutropenic Patients with LI

An algorithm for the clinical management of febrile neutropenic patients with LI has been proposed by an expert panel [95] (Fig. 10.1). In patients with acute myeloid leukemia or myelodysplastic syndrome undergoing aggressive myelosuppressive chemotherapy expecting severe neutropenia lasting ≥10 days, serial monitoring of *Aspergillus* galactomannan from blood samples is recommended. The place for 1,3-beta-D-glucan is not yet clearly defined and PCR should be studied in the frame of clinical trials only. Importantly, diagnostic procedures aim at obtaining microbiological results that confirm or help to modify the antimicrobial therapy, which should be initiated preemptively without awaiting results from diagnostic procedures.

Patients with fever of unknown origin not responding to an appropriate first-line therapy after 72–96 h should undergo thorough physical reexamination, imaging, and microbiological diagnostics including thoracic CT scan (see chapter on FUO). When LI are documented, bronchoscopy and BAL should promptly be arranged. BAL samples must be sent immediately to the microbiological laboratory for workup, to be started within 4 h after sampling. Recommended microbiological procedures are listed in Table 10.1.

Table 10.1 Workup of bronchoalveolar lavage samples from febrile neutropenic patients with lung infiltrates [95]

Recommended diagnostic program
Cytospin preparations for distinguishing intracellular from extracellular pathogens and identifying infiltration by underlying malignancy
Gram stain
Giemsa/May-Grünwald-Giemsa stain (assessment of macrophages, ciliated epithelium, leukocytes)
Calcofluor white or equivalent (assessment of fungi and *Pneumocystis jirovecii*)
Direct immunofluorescence test for *Pneumocystis jirovecii* (confirmatory)
Direct immunofluorescence test for *Legionella* spp.
Ziehl-Neelsen/auramine staining
Aspergillus antigen (galactomannan sandwich ELISA)
Quantitative cultures: dilutions of 10^{-2} and 10^{-4}; culture media: blood, McConkey/Endo, Levinthal/blood (bacterial culture), *Legionella* BCYE-α or equivalent (*Legionella* spp.), Löwenstein-Jensen or equivalent (mycobacteria), Sabouraud/Kimmig or equivalent (fungal culture)
Optional program
Enrichment culture (brain-heart infusion, dextrose broth)
Direct immunofluorescence test for *Chlamydia pneumoniae*
Culture for *Chlamydia pneumoniae*
Legionella PCR
Shell vial technique and PCR for influenza, parainfluenza, and adenovirus
Culturing or antigen detection of herpes simplex and varicella zoster virus
Cytomegalovirus early antigen
CMV antibody (ELISA, IgG/IgM)
HSV antibody (ELISA, IgG/IgM)
VZV antibody (ELISA, IgG/IgM/IgA)
Respiratory syncytial virus (PCR, ELISA)
Panfungal/*Aspergillus* PCR
Peripheral blood cultures 1 h after bronchoscopy to detect transient bacteremia
Throat swab to assess oral flora in comparison with BAL
Pneumocystis jirovecii PCR

Invasive procedures such as open-lung or fine-needle biopsy should be considered in patients with undetermined LI who urgently require histological identification.

10.4 Antimicrobial Therapy

Considering the dismal prognosis of febrile neutropenic patients with LI not treated promptly with an appropriate antimicrobial regimen, it is recommended to start therapy preemptively on the basis of clinical, imaging, and/or laboratory findings indicative of a particular infection in patients at risk for, but without proof of, this infection (Table 10.2). The type of underlying malignancy or immunosuppression has an instrumental impact on the selection of antimicrobial agents suitable for preemptive therapy.

10.4.1 Patients with Severe Neutropenia Due to Chemotherapy for Acute Leukemia or Other Aggressive Hematologic Malignancies

In this subgroup of neutropenic patients with LI, broad-spectrum beta-lactam therapy with antipseudomonal activity, as used for empirical treatment of unexplained fever (FUO => see separate chapter), should primarily be combined with a mold-active systemic antifungal, i.e., voriconazole (6 mg/kg every 12 h day 1, 4 mg/kg every 12 h thereafter) or liposomal amphotericin B (3 mg/kg daily) [153]. In patients in whom zygomycosis (mucormycosis) is suspected or who have been pretreated with voriconazole or posaconazole, liposomal amphotericin B is preferred. This high-risk subgroup of patients has a significant benefit from prompt as compared to delayed mold-active antifungal therapy [130]; it has been shown that patients with invasive aspergillosis treated with voriconazole or liposomal amphotericin B had superior response and survival rates when treated early vs. later in the course of the disease [37, 60]. Systemic antifungal treatment should be continued until hematopoietic recovery and regression of clinical and radiological signs of infection.

Table 10.2 Preemptive antimicrobial treatment in febrile neutropenic patients with lung infiltrates [37]

(1) For patients with acute leukaemia and other aggressive haematological malignancies

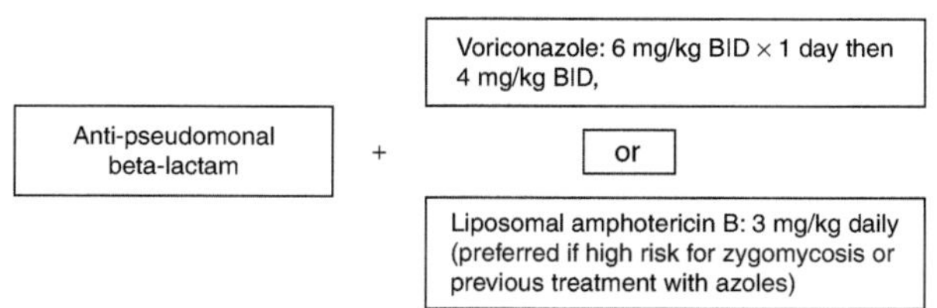

(2) For patients undergoing high-dose chemotherapy and autologous haematopoietic stem cell transplantation (AHSCT)
– No prompt systemic antifungal required
– After CD34-selected AHSCT: Ganciclovir 5 mg/kg BID if positive rapid culture for CMV

The empirical addition of an aminoglycoside or 5-flucytosine is not recommended due to a lack of benefit [116]. In patients who had not taken routine anti-*Pneumocystis* prophylaxis, who have a thoracic CT scan suggesting PcP, and who have a rapid and otherwise unexplained rise of serum lactate dehydrogenase, prompt start of high-dose co-trimoxazole therapy should be considered before bronchoscopy and BAL. In case of PcP, BAL will remain positive for this pathogen over several days despite appropriate antimicrobial therapy.

Except from patients with severe cellular immunosuppression, antiviral agents such as ganciclovir are not recommended for early preemptive therapy in febrile neutropenic patients with LI. In general, glycopeptides or macrolide antibiotics without a specific pathogen isolated from clinically significant samples should not be used as well.

10.4.2 Other Subgroups of Febrile Patients with Hematologic Malignancies

In patients undergoing high-dose chemotherapy and autologous hematopoietic stem cell transplantation (AHSCT) with febrile neutropenia and LI of unknown origin, whose conditioning regimen included total body irradiation or who have received a CD34-selected autograft [71], bronchoscopy with BAL should be performed to check for CMV disease [53]. A positive rapid culture or "immediate early antigen" should prompt ganciclovir treatment (5 mg/kg every 12 h). Foscarnet has not been investigated in this setting, as has not been the serial blood PCR or pp65 antigen monitoring. Since patients after AHSCT have a very low risk of fungal pneumonia [112, 118, 121], antifungal therapy should not be given preemptively.

In patients with profound cellular immunosuppression, respiratory viruses may be the cause of LI, so that diagnostic programs used for workup of BAL or oro-/nasopharyngeal swabs should include CMV as well as influenza, parainfluenza, respiratory syncytial virus, and human metapneumovirus [42, 157].

10.5 Antimicrobial Treatment in Patients with Documented Pathogens

The interpretation of microbiological findings in neutropenic patients with LI is difficult. Isolates typically origin from blood cultures or BAL samples. They may represent nonpathogenic contaminants, colonizers, co-pathogens, or microorganisms causing a separate infection. If etiologically significant pathogens are detected, particularly multiresistant bacteria, immediate modification of antimicrobial treatment to avoid fatal outcome due to delayed effective therapy is recommended [75].

The following findings indicate pathogens causative for lung infiltrates:

- *Pneumocystis jirovecii*, gram-negative aerobic pathogens, pneumococci, *Mycobacterium tuberculosis*, or *Aspergillus* spp. or *Aspergillus* galactomannan or zygomycetes obtained from bronchoalveolar lavage or sputum samples; positive rapid culture for CMV and detection of CMV "immediate early antigen"
- Isolation of pneumococci, alpha-hemolytic streptococci, or gram-negative aerobic pathogens from blood culture
- Any detection of pathogens in biopsy material
- Positive *Legionella* antigen in urine
- Positive (threshold 0.5) *Aspergillus* galactomannan in blood samples or BAL

The following findings do not represent pathogens causative for lung infiltrates:

- Isolation of enterococci from blood culture, swabs, sputum, or BAL
- Coagulase-negative staphylococci or *Corynebacterium* spp. obtained from any sample
- Isolation of *Candida* spp. from swabs, saliva, sputum, or tracheal aspirates
- Findings from surveillance cultures, feces, and urine cultures

Potentially relevant findings are common respiratory viruses; isolation of *Staphylococcus aureus*, *Legionella* spp., or atypical mycobacteria in respiratory secretions; and positive CMV- or *Pneumocystis*-PCR from BAL.

In patients with a documented *P. aeruginosa* pneumonia, the primary combination antibacterial therapy including an antipseudomonal beta-lactam plus preferably an aminoglycoside or (if an aminoglycoside is contraindicated) ciprofloxacin is recommended [54, 114]. Depending on their in vitro susceptibility pattern, multiresistant gram-negative aerobes such as extended-spectrum beta-lactamase (ESBL)-producing *E. coli*, *Enterobacter* spp. or *Klebsiella* spp., as well as *Acinetobacter* spp. or *P. aeruginosa* require antimicrobial treatment combinations selected appropriately according to this pattern. Pharmacokinetic aspects (penetration to lung tissue, possible inactivation by surfactant) must always be included in this selection. In individual patients with pneumonia caused by multiresistant gram-negative pathogens, aerosolized colistin has been successfully used as a part of the antimicrobial strategy [100]. *Stenotrophomonas maltophilia* rarely causes pneumonia, while it is more frequently isolated from respiratory secretions representing selection of opportunistic microorganisms under broad-spectrum antibacterial treatment. In patients with suspected or documented *S. maltophilia* pneumonia, early antimicrobial intervention with high-dose trimethoprim-sulfamethoxazole (15–20 mg/kg/day of trimethoprim) is mandatory [2, 145]. It should be kept in mind that in vitro susceptibility may not predict clinical efficacy of antimicrobial agents in *S. maltophilia* infections [30].

Pneumonias caused by methicillin-resistant *Staphylococcus aureus* (MRSA) should preferably be treated with vancomycin, if no serious renal insufficiency is present. Linezolid is a valid alternative for first-line treatment [158]; however, the risk of severe thrombocytopenia or even pancytopenia associated with linezolid must be taken into consideration [51]. Daptomycin should not be used for treatment of pneumonia, because it is inactivated by surfactant [134].

CMV pneumonia typically affects patients who have undergone allogeneic stem cell transplantation. First-choice antiviral treatment options are foscarnet and ganciclovir. Foscarnet may be preferred because of its lack of myelosuppression, the latter being a serious adverse effect of ganciclovir [102]. On the other hand, reversible nephrotoxicity is one of the typical side effects of foscarnet [152].

10.6 Treatment of Documented Fungal Pneumonia

Detailed recommendations for treatment of documented fungal pneumonia are provided in evidence-based guidelines [18, 83, 153]. Intravenous voriconazole and liposomal amphotericin B are recommended first-line choices for treatment of IPA. For zygomycosis (mucormycosis), liposomal amphotericin B is preferred. In patients with worsening LI and gas exchange within the first week of treatment, failure of antifungal therapy should only be considered if new LI emerge on control CT scans. At the same time, other causes such as a second infection, immune reconstitution syndrome, infiltrates caused by the underlying malignancy, toxicity from cancer treatment, and yet insufficient duration of antifungal treatment should be ruled out [97]. Combination antifungal first-line treatment in patients with invasive mold infections is controversial. A prospective clinical study comparing voriconazole alone with the combination of voriconazole with anidulafungin has not convincingly shown benefit from the combination in patients with proven and probable aspergillosis [93]. For treatment of zygomycosis (mucormycosis), a combination of liposomal amphotericin B and an echinocandin may be promising [139]; however, randomized studies on this subject have not been conducted. A combination of liposomal amphotericin B and the iron chelator deferasirox for the treatment of mucormycoses has shown inferior clinical results for the combination as compared to the antifungal agent alone [140].

10.7 Treatment of Documented *Pneumocystis* Pneumonia (PcP)

Patients with proven PcP should be treated with trimethoprim-sulfamethoxazole (TMP/SMX; co-trimoxazole) at a dosage of TMP 15–20 mg/kg plus SMX 75–100 mg/kg daily, divided into three to four doses and continued for 2–3 weeks. Nonresponders after 14 days of treatment should be evaluated for a secondary infection by repeated bronchoscopy. In individual patients with persistent PcP, dihydropteroate synthase gene mutation may be taken into consideration [105]. In case of confirmed sulfa resistance or TMP/SMX intolerance, atovaquone oral suspension (750 mg three times daily), pentamidine inhalation (600 mg daily), intravenous pentamidine (4 mg/kg daily), and clindamycin (600 mg three times daily) *plus* primaquine (30 mg daily) may represent treatment alternatives [146], with clindamycin + primaquine presumably being the most effective option [137]. Subsequently, patients should be given secondary prophylaxis using oral TMP/SMX at a daily dosage of 160/800 mg given on 2–3 days per week or with monthly pentamidine inhalation at a dose of 300 mg. In patients with respiratory failure due to PcP, systemic corticosteroids may be beneficial, but clinical data from this setting are rare [43, 113].

10.8 Intensive Care Medicine

Analysis of European data on the outcome of cancer patients requiring intensive care has shown an overall mortality rate of 27 %, which is not significantly different from non-cancer patients treated in the intensive care unit [144]. Neutropenic patients with respiratory failure due to LI may have a favorable outcome under appropriate intensive care including mechanical ventilation [35, 96, 110]. Even if respiratory failure is due to invasive pulmonary aspergillosis, survival can be achieved in 33 % of patients [22]. It is therefore not justified to reject cancer patients from intensive care because of their underlying malignancy [131].

References

1. Ahmed S, Siddiqui AK, Rossoff L, Sison CP, Rai KR. Pulmonary complications in chronic lymphocytic leukemia. Cancer. 2003;98:1912–7.
2. Aisenberg G, Rolston KV, Dickey BF, Kontoyiannis DP, Raad II, Safdar A. Stenotrophomonas maltophilia pneumonia in cancer patients without traditional risk factors for infection, 1997–2004. Eur J Clin Microbiol Infect Dis. 2007;26:13–20.
3. Akova M, Paesmans M, Calandra T, Viscoli C. A European Organization for Research and Treatment of Cancer-International Antimicrobial Therapy Group study of secondary infections in febrile, neutropenic patients with cancer. Clin Infect Dis. 2005;40:239–45.
4. Al Ameri A, Koller C, Kantarjian H, et al. Acute pulmonary failure during remission induction chemotherapy in adults with acute myeloid leukemia or high-risk myelodysplastic syndrome. Cancer. 2010;116:93–7.
5. Alanio A, Desoubeaux G, Sarfati C, et al. Real-time PCR assay-based strategy for differentiation between active Pneumocystis jirovecii pneumonia and colonization in immunocompromised patients. Clin Microbiol Infect. 2011;17:1531–7.
6. Armenian SH, La Via WV, Siegel SE, Mascarenhas L. Evaluation of persistent pulmonary infiltrates in pediatric oncology patients. Pediatr Blood Cancer. 2007;48:165–72.
7. Aubry A, Porcher R, Bottero J, et al. Occurrence and kinetics of false-positive Aspergillus galactomannan test results following treatment with beta-lactam antibiotics in patients with hematological disorders. J Clin Microbiol. 2006;44:389–94.
8. Azoulay E, Bergeron A, Chevret S, Bele N, Schlemmer B, Menotti J. Polymerase chain reaction for diagnosing pneumocystis pneumonia in non-HIV immunocompromised patients with pulmonary infiltrates. Chest. 2009;135:655–61.
9. Azoulay E, Darmon M, Delclaux C, et al. Deterioration of previous acute lung injury during neutropenia recovery. Crit Care Med. 2002;30:781–6.
10. Azoulay E, Mokart D, Lambert J, et al. Diagnostic strategy for hematology and oncology patients with acute respiratory failure: randomized controlled trial. Am J Respir Crit Care Med. 2010;182:1038–46.

11. Azoulay E, Mokart D, Rabbat A, et al. Diagnostic bronchoscopy in hematology and oncology patients with acute respiratory failure. Crit Care Med. 2008;36:100–7.
12. Azoulay E, Thiery G, Chevret S, et al. The prognosis of acute respiratory failure in critically ill cancer patients. Medicine. 2004;83:360–70.
13. Becker MJ, Lugtenburg EJ, Cornelissen JJ, et al. Galactomannan detection in computerized tomography-based broncho-alveolar lavage fluid and serum in haematological patients at risk for invasive pulmonary aspergillosis. Br J Haematol. 2003;121:448–57.
14. Bodey G, Bueltmann B, Duguid W, et al. Fungal infections in cancer patients: an international autopsy survey. Eur J Clin Microbiol Infect Dis. 1992;11:99–109.
15. Boeckh M. Complications, diagnosis, management, and prevention of CMV infections: current and future. Hematol Am Soc Hematol Educ Program. 2011;2011:305–9.
16. Boeckh M. The challenge of respiratory virus infections in hematopoietic cell transplant recipients. Br J Haematol. 2008;143:455–67.
17. Boersma WG, Erjavec Z, van der Werf TS, et al. Bronchoscopic diagnosis of pulmonary infiltrates in granulocytopenic patients with hematologic malignancies: BAL versus PSB and PBAL. Respir Med. 2007;101:317–25.
18. Böhme A, Ruhnke M, Buchheidt D, et al. Treatment of invasive fungal infections in cancer patients. Ann Hematol. 2009;88:97–110.
19. Boonsarngsuk V, Niyompattama A, Teosirimongkol C, Sriwanichrak K. False-positive serum and bronchoalveolar lavage Aspergillus galactomannan assays caused by different antibiotics. Scand J Infect Dis. 2010;42:461–8.
20. Brodoefel H, Vogel M, Hebart H, et al. Long-term CT follow-up in 40 non-HIV immunocompromised patients with invasive pulmonary aspergillosis. Am J Roentgenol. 2006;187: 404–13.
21. Buchheidt D, Baust C, Skladny H, et al. Detection of aspergillus species in blood and bronchoalveolar lavage samples from immunocompromised patients by means of 2-step polymerase chain reaction: clinical results. Clin Infect Dis. 2001;33:428–35.
22. Burghi G, Lemiale V, Seguin A, et al. Outcomes of mechanically ventilated hematology patients with invasive pulmonary aspergillosis. Intensive Care Med. 2011;37:1605–12.
23. Busca A, Locatelli F, Barbui A, et al. Usefulness of sequential Aspergillus galactomannan antigen detection combined with early radiologic evaluation for diagnosis of invasive pulmonary aspergillosis in patients undergoing allogeneic stem cell transplantation. Transplant Proc. 2006;38:1610–3.
24. Caillot D, Casasnovas O, Bernard A, et al. Improved management of invasive pulmonary aspergillosis in neutropenic patients using early thoracic computed tomographic scan and surgery. J Clin Oncol. 1997;15:139–47.
25. Caillot D, Couaillier JF, Bernard A, et al. Increasing volume and changing characteristics of invasive pulmonary aspergillosis on sequential thoracic computed tomography scans in patients with neutropenia. J Clin Oncol. 2001;19:253–9.
26. Caillot D, Latrabe V, Thiébaut A, et al. Computer tomography in pulmonary invasive aspergillosis in hematological patients with neutropenia: a useful tool for diagnosis and assessment of outcome in clinical trials. Eur J Radiol. 2010;74:e172–5.
27. Caillot D, Mannone L, Cuisenier B, Couaillier JF. Role of early diagnosis and aggressive surgery in the management of invasive pulmonary aspergillosis in neutropenic patients. Clin Microbiol Infect. 2001;7 Suppl 2:54–61.
28. Camus P, Costabel U. Drug-induced respiratory disease in patients with hematological diseases. Semin Respir Crit Care Med. 2005;26:458–81.
29. Carrafiello G, Lagana D, Nosari AM, et al. Utility of computed tomography and of fine needle aspiration biopsy in early diagnosis of fungal pulmonary infections. Radiol Med. 2006;111:33–41.
30. Carroll KC, Cohen S, Nelson R, et al. Comparison of various in vitro susceptibility methods for testing *Stenotrophomonas maltophilia*. Diagn Microbiol Infect Dis. 1998;32:229–35.
31. Cazzadori A, di Perri G, Todeschini G, et al. Transbronchial biopsy in the diagnosis of pulmonary infiltrates in immunocompromised patients. Chest. 1995;107:101–6.

32. Chamilos G, Luna M, Lewis RE, et al. Invasive fungal infections in patients with hematologic malignancies in a tertiary care cancer center: an autopsy study over a 15-year period (1989–2003). Haematologica. 2006;91:986–9.
33. Chemaly RF, Hanmod SS, Rathod DB, et al. The characteristics and outcomes of parainfluenza virus infections in 200 patients with leukemia or recipients of hematopoietic stem cell transplantation. Blood. 2012;119:2738–45.
34. Chemaly RF, Torres HA, Aguilera EA, et al. Neuraminidase inhibitors improve outcome of patients with leukemia and influenza: an observational study. Clin Infect Dis. 2007;44:964–7.
35. Cherif H, Martling CR, Hansen J, Kalin M, Björkholm M. Predictors of short and long-term outcome in patients with hematological disorders admitted to the intensive care unit for a life-threatening complication. Support Care Cancer. 2007;15:1393–8.
36. Clark BD, Vezza PR, Copeland C, Wilder AM, Abati A. Diagnostic sensitivity of bronchoalveolar lavage versus fine needle aspirate. Mod Pathol. 2002;15:1259–65.
37. Cornely OA, Maertens J, Bresnik M, et al. Efficacy outcomes in a randomised trial of liposomal amphotericin B based on revised EORTC/MSG 2008 definitions of invasive mould disease. Mycoses. 2011;54:e449–55.
38. Cornillet A, Camus C, Nimubona S, et al. Comparison of epidemiological, clinical, and biological features of invasive aspergillosis in neutropenic and nonneutropenic patients: a 6-year survey. Clin Infect Dis. 2006;43:577–84.
39. Danés C, Gonzalez-Martin J, Pumarola T, et al. Pulmonary infiltrates in immunosuppressed patients: analysis of a diagnostic protocol. J Clin Microbiol. 2002;40:2134–40.
40. Daniels CE, Myers JL, Utz JP, Markovic SN, Ryu JH. Organizing pneumonia in patients with hematologic malignancies: a steroid-responsive lesion. Respir Med. 2007;101:162–8.
41. De Pauw B, Walsh TJ, Donnelly JP, et al. Revised definitions of invasive fungal disease from the European Organization for Research and Treatment of Cancer/Invasive Fungal Infections Cooperative Group and the National Institute of Allergy and Infectious Diseases Mycoses Study Group Consensus Group. Clin Infect Dis. 2008;46:1813–21.
42. Debur MC, Vidal LR, Stroparo E, et al. Human metapneumovirus infection in hematopoietic stem cell transplant recipients. Transpl Infect Dis. 2010;12:173–9.
43. Delclaux C, Zahar JR, Amraoui G, et al. Corticosteroids as adjunctive therapy for severe Pneumocystis carinii pneumonia in non-human immunodeficiency virus-infected patients. Clin Infect Dis. 1999;29:670–2.
44. Dettenkofer M, Wenzler-Rottele S, Babikir R, et al. Surveillance of nosocomial sepsis and pneumonia in patients with a bone marrow or peripheral blood stem cell transplant. Clin Infect Dis. 2005;40:926–31.
45. Donhuijsen K, Pfaffenbach B, Samandari S, Leder LD. Autopsy results of deep mycoses in hematologic neoplasms. Mycoses. 1991;34(Suppl):25–7.
46. Eibel R, Herzog P, Dietrich O, et al. Pulmonary abnormalities in immunocompromised patients: comparative detection with parallel acquisition MR imaging and thin-section helical CT. Radiology. 2006;241:880–91.
47. Einsele H, Hebart H, Roller G, et al. Detection and identification of fungal pathogens in blood by using molecular probes. J Clin Microbiol. 1997;35:1353–60.
48. Ellis ME, Spence D, Bouchama A, et al. Open lung biopsy provides a higher and more specific diagnostic yield compared to bronchoalveolar lavage in immunocompromised patients. Scand J Infect Dis. 1995;27:157–62.
49. Escuissato DL, Gasparetto EL, Marchiori E, et al. Pulmonary infections after bone marrow transplantation: high-resolution CT findings in 111 patients. Am J Roentgenol. 2005;185:608–15.
50. Ewig S, Glasmacher A, Ulrich B, et al. Pulmonary infiltrates in neutropenic patients with acute leukemia during chemotherapy. Chest. 1998;114:444–51.
51. Faguer S, Kamar N, Fillola G, Guitard J, Rostaing L. Linezolid-related pancytopenia in organ-transplant patients: report of two cases. Infection. 2007;35:275–7.
52. Falsey AR, Hennessey PA, Formica MA, Cox C, Walsh EE. Respiratory Syncytial Virus infection in elderly and high-risk adults. N Engl J Med. 2005;352:1749–59.

53. Fassas AB, Bolaños-Meade J, Buddharaju LN, et al. Cytomegalovirus infection and non-neutropenic fever after autologous stem cell transplantation: high rates of reactivation in patients with multiple myeloma and lymphoma. Br J Haematol. 2001;112:237–41.
54. Garnacho-Montero J, Sa-Borges M, Sole-Violan J, Barcenilla F, Escoresca-Ortega A, Ochoa M, Cayuela A, Rello J. Optimal management therapy for Pseudomonas aeruginosa ventilator-associated pneumonia: an observational, multicenter study comparing monotherapy with combination antibiotic therapy. Crit Care Med. 2007;35:1888–95.
55. Gasparetto EL, Escuissato DL, Marchiori E, et al. High-resolution CT findings of respiratory syncytial virus pneumonia after bone marrow transplantation. Am J Roentgenol. 2004;182:1133–7.
56. Georgiadou SP, Kontoyiannis DP. Concurrent lung infections in patients with hematological malignancies and invasive pulmonary aspergillosis: how firm is the Aspergillus diagnosis? J Infect. 2012;65:262–8.
57. Georgiadou SP, Sampsonas FL, Rice D, Granger JM, Swisher S, Kontoyiannis DP. Open-lung biopsy in patients with undiagnosed lung lesions referred at a tertiary cancer center is safe and reveals noncancerous, noninfectious entities as the most common diagnoses. Eur J Clin Microbiol Infect Dis. 2013;32:101–5.
58. Georgiadou SP, Sipsas NV, Marom EM, Kontoyiannis DP. The diagnostic value of halo and reversed halo signs for invasive mold infections in compromised hosts. Clin Infect Dis. 2011;52:1144–55.
59. Girmenia C, Santilli S, Ballarò D, Del Giudice I, Armiento D, Mauro FR. Enteral nutrition may cause false-positive results of Aspergillus galactomannan assay in absence of gastrointestinal diseases. Mycoses. 2011;54:e883–4.
60. Greene RE, Schlamm HT, Oestmann JW, et al. Imaging findings in acute invasive pulmonary aspergillosis: clinical significance of the halo sign. Clin Infect Dis. 2007;44:373–9.
61. Groll AH, Shah PM, Mentzel C, Schneider M, Just-Nuebling G, Huebner K. Trends in the postmortem epidemiology of invasive fungal infections at a university hospital. J Infect. 1996;33:23–32.
62. Hachem R, Sumoza D, Hanna H, Girgawy E, Munsell M, Raad I. Clinical and radiologic predictors of invasive pulmonary aspergillosis in cancer patients: should the European Organization for Research and Treatment of Cancer/Mycosis Study Group criteria be revised? Cancer. 2006;106:1581–6.
63. Hachem RY, Chemaly RF, Ahmar CA, et al. Colistin is effective in treatment of infections caused by multidrug-resistant Pseudomonas aeruginosa in cancer patients. Antimicrob Agents Chemother. 2007;51:1905–11.
64. Hage CA, Reynolds JM, Durkin M, Wheat LJ, Knox KS. Plasmalyte as a cause of false-positive results for Aspergillus galactomannan in bronchoalveolar lavage fluid. J Clin Microbiol. 2007;45:676–7.
65. Heussel CP, Kauczor HU, Heussel G, Fischer B, Mildenberger P, Thelen M. Early detection of pneumonia in febrile neutropenic patients: use of thin-section CT. Am J Roentgenol. 1997;169:1347–53.
66. Heussel CP, Kauczor HU, Heussel GE, et al. Pneumonia in febrile neutropenic patients and in bone marrow and blood stem-cell transplant recipients: use of high-resolution computed tomography. J Clin Oncol. 1999;17:796–805.
67. Heussel CP, Kauczor HU, Ullmann AJ. Pneumonia in neutropenic patients. Eur Radiol. 2004;14:256–71.
68. Hicks KL, Chemaly RF, Kontoyiannis DP. Common community respiratory viruses in patients with cancer: more than just "common colds". Cancer. 2003;97:2576–87.
69. Hoffer FA, Gow K, Flynn PM, Davidoff A. Accuracy of percutaneous lung biopsy for invasive pulmonary aspergillosis. Pediatr Radiol. 2001;31:144–52.
70. Hohenthal U, Itälä M, Salonen J, et al. Bronchoalveolar lavage in immunocompromised patients with haematological malignancy–value of new microbiological methods. Eur J Haematol. 2005;74:203–11.
71. Holmberg LA, Boeckh M, Hooper H, et al. Increased incidence of cytomegalovirus disease after autologous CD34-selected peripheral blood stem cell transplantation. Blood. 1999;94:4029–35.

72. Horvath JA, Dummer S. The use of respiratory-tract cultures in the diagnosis of invasive pulmonary aspergillosis. Am J Med. 1996;100:171–8.
73. Hummel M, Rudert S, Hof H, Hehlmann R, Buchheidt D. Diagnostic yield of bronchoscopy with bronchoalveolar lavage in febrile patients with hematologic malignancies and pulmonary infiltrates. Ann Hematol. 2008;87:291–7.
74. Hwang SS, Kim HH, Park SH, Jung JI, Jang HS. The value of CT-guided percutaneous needle aspiration in immunocompromised patients with suspected pulmonary infection. Am J Roentgenol. 2000;175:235–8.
75. Hyle EP, Lipworth AD, Zaoutis TE, Nachamkin I, Bilker WB, Lautenbach E. Impact of inadequate initial antimicrobial therapy on mortality in infections due to extended-spectrum beta-lactamase-producing enterobacteriaceae: variability by site of infection. Arch Intern Med. 2005;165:1375–80.
76. Jain P, Sandur S, Meli Y, et al. Role of flexible bronchoscopy in immunocompromised patients with lung infiltrates. Chest. 2004;125:712–22.
77. Kim K, Lee MH, Kim J, et al. Importance of open lung biopsy in the diagnosis of invasive pulmonary aspergillosis in patients with hematologic malignancies. Am J Hematol. 2002;71:75–9.
78. Korones DN. Is routine chest radiography necessary for the initial evaluation of fever in neutropenic children with cancer? Pediatr Blood Cancer. 2004;43:715–7.
79. Kuderer NM, Dale DC, Crawford J, Cosler LE, Lyman GH. Mortality, morbidity, and cost associated with febrile neutropenia in adult cancer patients. Cancer. 2006;106:2258–66.
80. Lamoth F, Cruciani M, Mengoli C, Third European Conference on Infections in Leukemia (ECIL-3), et al. β-Glucan antigenemia assay for the diagnosis of invasive fungal infections in patients with hematological malignancies: a systematic review and meta-analysis of cohort studies from the Third European Conference on Infections in Leukemia (ECIL-3). Clin Infect Dis. 2012;54:633–43.
81. Lass-Flörl C, Gunsilius E, Gastl G, et al. Diagnosing invasive aspergillosis during antifungal therapy by PCR analysis of blood samples. J Clin Microbiol. 2004;42:4154–7.
82. Lass-Flörl C, Resch G, Nachbaur D, et al. The value of computed tomography-guided percutaneous lung biopsy for diagnosis of invasive fungal infection in immunocompromised patients. Clin Infect Dis. 2007;45:e101–4.
83. Limper AH, Knox KS, Sarosi GA, American Thoracic Society Fungal Working Group, et al. An official American Thoracic Society statement: treatment of fungal infections in adult pulmonary and critical care patients. Am J Respir Crit Care Med. 2011;183:96–128.
84. Lin SJ, Schranz J, Teutsch SM. Aspergillosis case-fatality rate: systematic review of the literature. Clin Infect Dis. 2001;32:358–66.
85. Link H, Maschmeyer G, Meyer P, et al. Interventional antimicrobial therapy in febrile neutropenic patients. Ann Hematol. 1994;69:231–43.
86. Ljungman P, Griffiths P, Paya C. Definitions of cytomegalovirus infection and disease in transplant recipients. Clin Infect Dis. 2002;34:1094–7.
87. Ljungman P, von Dobeln L, Ringholm L, et al. The value of CMV and fungal PCR for monitoring for acute leukaemia and autologous stem cell transplant patients. Scand J Infect Dis. 2005;37:121–7.
88. Luna LK, Panning M, Grywna K, Pfefferle S, Drosten C. Spectrum of viruses and atypical bacteria in intercontinental air travelers with symptoms of acute respiratory infection. J Infect Dis. 2007;195:675–9.
89. Maertens J, Theunissen K, Verhoef G, et al. Galactomannan and computed tomography-based preemptive antifungal therapy in neutropenic patients at high risk for invasive fungal infection. Clin Infect Dis. 2005;41:1242–50.
90. Maertens J, Verhaegen J, Demuynck H, et al. Autopsy-controlled prospective evaluation of serial screening for circulating galactomannan by a sandwich enzyme-linked immunosorbent assay for hematological patients at risk for invasive aspergillosis. J Clin Microbiol. 1999;37:3223–8.
91. Maertens JA, Klont R, Masson C, et al. Optimization of the cutoff value for the Aspergillus double-sandwich enzyme immunoassay. Clin Infect Dis. 2007;44:1329–36.

92. Marcolini JA, Malik S, Suki D, Whimbey E, Bodey GP. Respiratory disease due to parainfluenza virus in adult leukemia patients. Eur J Clin Microbiol Infect Dis. 2003;22:79–84.
93. Marr KA, Schlamm H, Rottinghaus ST, et al. A randomised, double-blind study of combination antifungal therapy with voriconazole and anidulafungin versus voriconazole monotherapy for primary treatment of invasive aspergillosis. 22nd European congress of Clinical Microbiology and Infectious Diseases, London, 31 Mar–3 Apr 2012, abstr # LB2812.
94. Martino R, Ramila E, Rabella N, et al. Respiratory virus infections in adults with hematologic malignancies: a prospective study. Clin Infect Dis. 2003;36:1–8.
95. Maschmeyer G, Beinert T, Buchheidt D, et al. Diagnosis and antimicrobial therapy of pulmonary infiltrates in febrile neutropenic patients. 2008 updated guidelines of the Infectious Diseases Working Party of the German Society of Hematology and Oncology. Eur J Cancer. 2009;45:2462–72.
96. Maschmeyer G, Bertschat FL, Moesta KT, et al. Outcome analysis of 189 consecutive cancer patients referred to the intensive care unit as emergencies during a 2-year period. Eur J Cancer. 2003;39:783–92.
97. Maschmeyer G, Haas A. Defining clinical failure for salvage studies. Med Mycol. 2006;44:S315–8.
98. Maschmeyer G, Link H, Hiddemann W, et al. Pulmonary infiltrations in febrile neutropenic patients. Risk factors and outcome under empirical antimicrobial therapy in a randomized multicenter trial. Cancer. 1994;73:2296–304.
99. Mengoli C, Cruciani M, Barnes RA, Loeffler J, Donnelly JP. Use of PCR for diagnosis of invasive aspergillosis: systematic review and meta-analysis. Lancet Infect Dis. 2009;9:89–96.
100. Michalopoulos A, Kasiakou SK, Mastora Z, Rellos K, Kapaskelis AM, Falagas ME. Aerosolized colistin for the treatment of nosocomial pneumonia due to multidrug-resistant Gram-negative bacteria in patients without cystic fibrosis. Crit Care. 2005;9:R53–9.
101. Monneret G, Doche C, Durand DV, Lepape A, Bienvenu J. Procalcitonin as a specific marker of bacterial infection in adults. Clin Chem Lab Med. 1998;36:67–8.
102. Mori T, Kato J. Cytomegalovirus infection/disease after hematopoietic stem cell transplantation. Int J Hematol. 2010;91:588–95.
103. Mulabecirovic A, Gaulhofer P, Auner HW, et al. Pulmonary infiltrates in patients with haematologic malignancies: transbronchial lung biopsy increases the diagnostic yield with respect to neoplastic infiltrates and toxic pneumonitis. Ann Hematol. 2004;83:420–2.
104. Musher B, Fredricks D, Leisenring W, Balajee SA, Smith C, Marr KA. Aspergillus galactomannan enzyme immunoassay and quantitative PCR for diagnosis of invasive aspergillosis with bronchoalveolar lavage fluid. J Clin Microbiol. 2004;42:5517–22.
105. Nahimana A, Rabodonirina M, Zanetti G, et al. Association between a specific Pneumocystis jiroveci dihydropteroate synthase mutation and failure of pyrimethamine/sulfadoxine prophylaxis in human immunodeficiency virus-positive and -negative patients. J Infect Dis. 2003;188:1017–23.
106. Navigante AH, Cerchietti LC, Costantini P, et al. Conventional chest radiography in the initial assessment of adult cancer patients with fever and neutropenia. Cancer Control. 2002;9:346–51.
107. Offner F, Cordonnier C, Ljungman P, et al. Impact of previous aspergillosis on the outcome of bone marrow transplantation. Clin Infect Dis. 1998;26:1098–103.
108. Ostrosky-Zeichner L, Alexander BD, Kett DH, et al. Multicenter clinical evaluation of the (1,3) beta-D-glucan assay as an aid to diagnosis of fungal infections in humans. Clin Infect Dis. 2005;41:654–9.
109. Oude Nijhuis CS, Gietema JA, Vellenga E, et al. Routine radiography does not have a role in the diagnostic evaluation of ambulatory adult febrile neutropenic cancer patients. Eur J Cancer. 2003;39:2495–8.
110. Owczuk R, Wujtewicz MA, Sawicka W, Wadrzyk A, Wujtewicz M. Patients with haematological malignancies requiring invasive mechanical ventilation: differences between survivors and non-survivors in intensive care unit. Support Care Cancer. 2005;13:332–8.

111. Pagano L, Caira M, Candoni A, et al. The epidemiology of fungal infections in patients with hematologic malignancies: the SEIFEM-2004 study. Haematologica. 2006;91:1068–75.
112. Pagano L, Caira M, Nosari A, et al. Fungal infections in recipients of hematopoietic stem cell transplants: results of the SEIFEM B-2004 study. Clin Infect Dis. 2007;45:1161–70.
113. Pareja JG, Garland R, Koziel H. Use of adjunctive corticosteroids in severe adult non-HIV Pneumocystis carinii pneumonia. Chest. 1998;113:1215–24.
114. Park SY, Park HJ, Moon SM, et al. Impact of adequate empirical combination therapy on mortality from bacteremic Pseudomonas aeruginosa pneumonia. BMC Infect Dis. 2012;12:308.
115. Patel NR, Lee PS, Kim JH, Weinhouse GL, Koziel H. The influence of diagnostic bronchoscopy on clinical outcomes comparing adult autologous and allogeneic bone marrow transplant patients. Chest. 2005;127:1388–96.
116. Paul M, Soares-Weiser K, Leibovici L. Beta lactam monotherapy versus beta lactam-aminoglycoside combination therapy for fever with neutropenia: systematic review and meta-analysis. BMJ. 2003;326:1111–9.
117. Peikert T, Rana S, Edell ES. Safety, diagnostic yield, and therapeutic implications of flexible bronchoscopy in patients with febrile neutropenia and pulmonary infiltrates. Mayo Clin Proc. 2005;80:1414–20.
118. Post MJ, Lass-Floerl C, Gastl G, Nachbaur D. Invasive fungal infections in allogeneic and autologous stem cell transplant recipients. Transpl Infect Dis. 2007;9:189–95.
119. Raad II, Whimbey EE, Rolston KVI, et al. A comparison of aztreonam plus vancomycin and imipenem plus vancomycin as initial therapy for febrile neutropenic cancer patients. Cancer. 1996;77:1386–94.
120. Rámila E, Sureda A, Martino R, et al. Bronchoscopy guided by high-resolution computed tomography for the diagnosis of pulmonary infections in patients with hematologic malignancies and normal plain chest X-ray. Haematologica. 2000;85:961–6.
121. Reich G, Mapara MY, Reichardt P, Dörken B, Maschmeyer G. Infectious complications after high-dose chemotherapy and autologous stem cell transplantation. Bone Marrow Transplant. 2001;27:525–9.
122. Rickerts V, Mousset S, Lambrecht E, et al. Comparison of histopathological analysis, culture, and polymerase chain reaction assays to detect invasive mold infections from biopsy specimens. Clin Infect Dis. 2007;44:1078–83.
123. Robinson JO, Lamoth F, Bally F, Knaup M, Calandra T, Marchetti O. Monitoring procalcitonin in febrile neutropenia: what is its utility for initial diagnosis of infection and reassessment in persistent fever? PLoS One. 2011;6:e18886.
124. Rolston KV, Bodey GP, Safdar A. Polymicrobial infection in patients with cancer: an underappreciated and underreported entity. Clin Infect Dis. 2007;45:228–33.
125. Rossini F, Verga M, Pioltelli P, et al. Incidence and outcome of pneumonia in patients with acute leukemia receiving first induction therapy with anthracycline-containing regimens. Haematologica. 2000;85:1255–60.
126. Rossiter SJ, Miller DC, Churg AM, Carrington CB, Mark JBD. Open lung biopsy in the immunocompromised patient. Is it really beneficial? J Thorac Cardiovasc Surg. 1979;77:338–45.
127. Ruhnke M, Böhme A, Buchheidt D, et al. Diagnosis of invasive fungal infections in hematology and oncology. Ann Oncol. 2012;23:823–33.
128. Safdar A, Rolston KV. Stenotrophomonas maltophilia: changing spectrum of a serious bacterial pathogen in patients with cancer. Clin Infect Dis. 2007;45:1602–9.
129. Samonis G, Kontoyiannis DP. Infectious complications of purine analog therapy. Curr Opin Infect Dis. 2001;14:409–13.
130. Schiel X, Link H, Maschmeyer G, et al. A prospective, randomized multicenter trial of the empirical addition of antifungal therapy for febrile neutropenic cancer patients. Infection. 2006;34:118–26.
131. Sculier JP. Intensive care and oncology. Support Care Cancer. 1995;3:93–105.
132. Segal BH, Almyroudis NG, Battiwalla M, et al. Prevention and early treatment of invasive fungal infection in patients with cancer and neutropenia and in stem cell transplant recipients

in the era of newer broad-spectrum antifungal agents and diagnostic adjuncts. Clin Infect Dis. 2007;44:402–9.
133. Shorr AF, Susla GM, O'Grady NP. Pulmonary infiltrates in the non-HIV-infected immunocompromised patient: etiologies, diagnostic strategies, and outcomes. Chest. 2004;125:260–71.
134. Silverman JA, Mortin LI, Vanpraagh AD, Li T, Alder J. Inhibition of daptomycin by pulmonary surfactant: in vitro modeling and clinical impact. J Infect Dis. 2005;191:2149–52.
135. Sing A, Trebesius K, Roggenkamp A, et al. Evaluation of diagnostic value and epidemiological implications of PCR for Pneumocystis carinii in different immunosuppressed and immunocompetent patient groups. J Clin Microbiol. 2000;38:1461–7.
136. Singer C, Armstrong D, Rosen PP, Walzer PD, Yu B. Diffuse pulmonary infiltrates in immunosuppressed patients. Prospective study of 80 cases. Am J Med. 1979;66:110–20.
137. Smego Jr RA, Nagar S, Maloba B, Popara M. A meta-analysis of salvage therapy for Pneumocystis carinii pneumonia. Arch Intern Med. 2001;161:1529–33.
138. Sonnet S, Buitrago-Téllez CH, Tamm M, Christen S, Steinbrich W. Direct detection of angioinvasive pulmonary aspergillosis in immunosuppressed patients: preliminary results with high-resolution 16-MDCT angiography. AJR Am J Roentgenol. 2005;184:746–51.
139. Spellberg B, Ibrahim A, Roilides E, Lewis RE, Lortholary O, Petrikkos G, Kontoyiannis DP, Walsh TJ. Combination therapy for mucormycosis: why, what, and how? Clin Infect Dis. 2012;54 Suppl 1:S73–8.
140. Spellberg B, Ibrahim AS, Chin-Hong PV, Kontoyiannis DP, Morris MI, Perfect JR, Fredricks D, Brass EP. The Deferasirox-AmBisome Therapy for Mucormycosis (DEFEAT Mucor) study: a randomized, double-blinded, placebo-controlled trial. J Antimicrob Chemother. 2012;67:715–22.
141. Spiess B, Buchheidt D, Baust C, et al. Development of a LightCycler PCR assay for detection and quantification of Aspergillus fumigatus DNA in clinical samples from neutropenic patients. J Clin Microbiol. 2003;41:1811–8.
142. Stanzani M, Battista G, Sassi C, et al. Computed tomographic pulmonary angiography for diagnosis of invasive mold diseases in patients with hematological malignancies. Clin Infect Dis. 2012;54:610–6.
143. Suzuki HI, Asai T, Tamaki Z, Hangaishi A, Chiba S, Kurokawa M. Drug-induced hypersensitivity syndrome with rapid hematopoietic reconstitution during treatment for acute myeloid leukemia. Haematologica. 2008;93:469–70.
144. Taccone FS, Artigas AA, Sprung CL, Moreno R, Sakr Y, Vincent JL. Characteristics and outcomes of cancer patients in European ICUs. Crit Care. 2009;13:R15.
145. Tada K, Kurosawa S, Hiramoto N, Okinaka K, Ueno N, Asakura Y, Kim SW, Yamashita T, Mori SI, Heike Y, Maeshima AM, Tanosaki R, Tobinai K, Fukuda T. Stenotrophomonas maltophilia infection in hematopoietic SCT recipients: high mortality due to pulmonary hemorrhage. Bone Marrow Transplant. 2013;48:74–9.
146. Thomas Jr CF, Limper AH. Pneumocystis pneumonia. N Engl J Med. 2004;350:2487–98.
147. Torres HA, Aguilera EA, Mattiuzzi GN, et al. Characteristics and outcome of Respiratory Syncytial Virus infection in patients with leukemia. Haematologica. 2007;92:1216–23.
148. Tortorano AM, Esposto MC, Prigitano A, et al. Cross-reactivity of Fusarium spp. in the Aspergillus Galactomannan enzyme-linked immunosorbent assay. J Clin Microbiol. 2012;50:1051–3.
149. Vehreschild JJ, Böhme A, Buchheidt D, et al. A double-blind trial on prophylactic voriconazole or placebo during induction chemotherapy for acute myelogenous leukaemia. J Infect. 2007;55:445–9.
150. Vento S, Cainelli F, Temesgen Z. Lung infections after cancer chemotherapy. Lancet Oncol. 2008;9:982–92.
151. von Lilienfeld-Toal M, Dietrich MP, Glasmacher A, et al. Markers of bacteremia in febrile neutropenic patients with haematological malignancies: procalcitonin and IL-6 are more reliable than C-reactive protein. Eur J Clin Microbiol Infect Dis. 2004;23:539–44.

152. Wagstaff AJ, Bryson HM. Foscarnet. A reappraisal of its antiviral activity, pharmacokinetic properties and therapeutic use in immunocompromised patients with viral infections. Drugs. 1994;48:199–226.
153. Walsh TJ, Anaissie EJ, Denning DW, et al. Treatment of aspergillosis: clinical practice guidelines of the Infectious Diseases Society of America. Clin Infect Dis. 2008;46:327–60.
154. Weisser M, Rausch C, Droll A, et al. Galactomannan does not precede major signs on a pulmonary computerized tomographic scan suggestive of invasive aspergillosis in patients with hematological malignancies. Clin Infect Dis. 2005;41:1143–9.
155. White DA, Wong PW, Downey R. The utility of open lung biopsy in patients with hematologic malignancies. Am J Respir Crit Care Med. 2000;161:723–9.
156. White PL, Linton CJ, Perry MD, Johnson EM, Barnes RA. The evolution and evaluation of a whole blood polymerase chain reaction assay for the detection of invasive aspergillosis in hematology patients in a routine clinical setting. Clin Infect Dis. 2006;42:479–86.
157. Williams JV, Martino R, Rabella N, et al. A prospective study comparing human metapneumovirus with other respiratory viruses in adults with hematologic malignancies and respiratory tract infections. J Infect Dis. 2005;192:1061–5.
158. Wunderink RG, Rello J, Cammarata SK, Croos-Dabrera RV, Kollef MH. Linezolid vs vancomycin: analysis of two double-blind studies of patients with methicillin- resistant Staphylococcus aureus nosocomial pneumonia. Chest. 2003;124:1789–97.
159. Zihlif M, Khanchandani G, Ahmed HP, Soubani AO. Surgical lung biopsy in patients with hematological malignancy or hematopoietic stem cell transplantation and unexplained pulmonary infiltrates: improved outcome with specific diagnosis. Am J Hematol. 2005;78:94–9.

Vascular Catheter-Related Infections 11

Luma Dababneh, William Shomali, and Issam I. Raad

Contents

L. Dababneh
Department of Family Medicine,
Summa Barberton Hospital,
Barberton, Ohio 44203, USA
e-mail: ldababneh85@gmail.com

W. Shomali
Department of Internal Medicine,
Cleveland Clinic,
Cleveland, Ohio 44195, USA
e-mail: shomalw@ccf.org

I.I. Raad (✉)
Department of Infectious Diseases, Infection Control and Employee Health, Unit 1460,
The University of Texas MD Anderson Cancer Center,
1515 Holcombe Blvd, Houston, TX 77030, USA
e-mail: iraad@mdanderson.org

G. Maschmeyer, K.V.I. Rolston (eds.), *Infections in Hematology*,
DOI 10.1007/978-3-662-44000-1_11

11.1 Introduction and Epidemiology

Vascular catheters are commonly used in critically ill patients, those with cancer, or in patients undergoing hemodialysis. In the United States, there are more than 150 million intravascular catheters purchased by clinics and hospitals each year. This includes more than five million central venous and pulmonary artery catheters [22].

Catheter use carries the risk of infection, which could be either localized to the catheter site or systemic as bloodstream infections [23]. It is estimated that at least 80,000 catheter-related bloodstream infections (CRBSI) occur in the United States ICUs each year [14]. These infections increase hospital stay and cost of care significantly [1, 21].

A recent systemic review of 200 prospective studies estimated the point incidence rates expressed as CRBSI per 1,000 catheter days to range from 0.5 with peripheral intravenous catheters, 1.6 for cuffed and tunneled catheters, 1.7 for arterial catheters, 2.4 for peripherally inserted central catheters, and 2.7 for short-term non-cuffed and non-medicated central venous catheters (CVCs) [12].

11.2 Pathogenesis

Catheter colonization with microorganisms is a prerequisite for these infections to occur. There are many sources of colonization such as migration of skin surface organisms and colonization of the external surface of catheters (extraluminal), which is usually associated with short-term catheters. Another route involves the transfer of microorganisms to hubs from patients' skin or health-care workers hands and colonization of the internal surface (intraluminal). This is more commonly seen in long-term catheters (>30 days) [15, 25]. Other sources of catheter infections include contaminated infusate through the catheter or hematogenous seeding from another focus of infection [20], as the gut is a common source of candidemia in neutropenic patients [18].

Catheter colonization is promoted by the catheter's material, its surface irregularity and thrombogenicity. Host factors such as fibrin and fibronectin form a sheath around the catheter encasing it and promoting microbial attachment. Other major factors include intrinsic ones, such as extracellular polymeric substance produced by coagulase-negative staphylococci, *Staphylococcus aureus*, *Pseudomonas aeruginosa*, *Stenotrophomonas maltophilia*, and *Candida* species that promote biofilm formation [7, 20].

Biofilms are cellular agglomerations of microorganisms, embedded in a self-produced matrix composed mainly of polysaccharides, enriched with metallic cations such as calcium, iron, and magnesium. This makes it as a solid wall preventing engulfment and killing by polymorphonuclear leukocytes and preventing contact with antimicrobial agents [7, 36].

Localized catheter infections are seen at the insertion site, along the subcutaneous tract in tunneled catheters, along the body and tip of the catheter within the vein, or as a pocket infection. These localized infections are mostly due to pyogenic organisms, particularly *S. aureus* [7, 28], whereas CRBSI are mostly caused by coagulase-negative staphylococci, *S. aureus*, *Candida species*, and enteric gram-negative bacilli [19, 20].

11.3 Diagnosis

Localized infections present with inflammatory manifestations such as erythema, induration, warmth, and tenderness at or around catheter insertion site or as a palpable venous cord. CRBSI presents with bacteremia or fungemia with signs and symptoms of systemic infection: fever, chills, or hypotension. Local catheter infection can be associated with systemic infection but is unreliable in predicting it with a sensitivity of 3 % [28]. CRBSI should be confirmed microbiologically, and cultures should be obtained before the initiation of antibiotics.

Diagnostic methods of CRBSI can be divided according to catheter removal or salvage. It is recommended to assess the possibility of CRBSI before catheter removal, especially in low-risk patients (immunocompetent, no intravascular devices, no evidence of severe sepsis or septic shock, no evidence of infection at catheter insertion site, and no bacteremia or fungemia). This can be done by the following methods:

Simultaneous quantitative blood cultures: by obtaining quantitative blood cultures simultaneously from a central venous catheter and a peripheral vein percutaneously. A threefold or greater colony count from the CVC than from peripheral blood implicates that the CVC is the source of infection. This method is labor intensive and expensive [4].

Differential time to positivity: is suggestive of CRBSI if blood drawn from the CVC becomes positive for bacterial growth ≥2 h before a simultaneously drawn blood from a peripheral vein. However, this method could be compromised when the patient is receiving antibiotics through the CVC [16, 26].

Quantitative blood cultures drawn through a CVC: this method is used when peripheral blood cultures are not withdrawn at the time of culture. Diagnosis of CRBSI can be made if CVC withdrawn blood grows ≥100 CFU/ml. However, this method is unable to differentiate CRBSI from high-grade bacteremia which is a major limitation [2, 16].

Acridine orange leukocyte cytospin: a rapid diagnostic microscopy method within 30 min. But this method has not been widely used in clinical laboratories in the United States [34].

When catheter is removed due to a suspected CRBSI, the following methods can be used for diagnosis:

Semiquantitative CVC tip culture (roll plate method): the distal segment of the CVC is cut and rolled against a blood agar plate at least four times before the plate is incubated overnight. A colony count of ≥15 CFU/ml from 5 cm segment of catheter tip suggests catheter colonization. If catheter colonization is associated with a positive peripheral blood culture growing the same organism, then CRBSI is diagnosed [24, 28].

Quantitative catheter segment cultures: a fixed length of catheter is immersed in broth, sonicated and vortexed to release organisms into suspension that can be plated out and counted quantitatively. A count of $\geq 10^3$ CFU from 5 cm segment is considered positive for colonization. If catheter colonization is associated with a positive peripheral blood culture growing the same organism, then CRBSI is diagnosed [24]. The sonication method is more sensitive than the semiquantitative roll plate method in long-term catheters as it releases organisms from both the external and internal surfaces of the catheter [28].

Microscopy of stained catheters: by using gram stain or acridine orange stain. This method has not been widely used as it is labor intensive and not practical as it only detects extraluminal colonization [28, 33].

11.4 Management

In long-term central venous catheter or implanted catheter: if there is an insertion site infection without systemic signs of infection, a culture from the drainage should be taken, and it should be managed with topical antimicrobials depending on culture and sensitivity (mupirocin ointment for *S. aureus* and ketoconazole or clotrimazole ointment for *Candida*). If systemic signs of infection or pus or positive blood culture are present, systemic antimicrobial should be initiated, and if it fails, catheter should be removed [13, 16].

If tunnel infection or port abscess is found, catheter removal is indicated, with incision and drainage when needed, and 7–10 days of systemic antibiotic therapy in the absence of concomitant bacteremia or candidemia [16].

Empiric antimicrobial therapy is often initiated for suspected CRBSI, after that treatment is modified according to the culture and sensitivity. The most common pathogens causing CRBSI are gram-positive cocci, so vancomycin should be started empirically since the prevalence of methicillin-resistant organisms is increasing [16]. In centers where methicillin-resistant *S. aureus* (MRSA) have high prevalence of isolates with minimum inhibitory concentration for vancomycin greater than 2 mcg/ml or the patient has a contraindication for vancomycin, then daptomycin is the preferred alternative [8, 17]. Linezolid should be avoided as it was associated with worse outcome [37]. It has been shown that linezolid is less efficacious than daptomycin in eradicating staphylococci embedded in biofilm [27].

For empiric gram-negative coverage, antibiotics should be based on local resistance patterns and antimicrobial susceptibility data. Fourth-generation cephalosporin (*cefepime*), carbapenem (ertapenem, imipenem, meropenem, or doripenem), or combined β-lactam/β-lactamase inhibitors (piperacillin/tazobactam or ampicillin/sulbactam) with or without an aminoglycoside (amikacin or tobramycin) can be used. If the patient has risk factors for fungal infection, such as total parenteral nutrition, prolonged use of broad-spectrum antibiotics, hematologic malignancy, stem cell or solid organ transplantation, severe intestinal mucositis, femoral catheter, or colonization with *Candida* species at multiple sites, then empiric antifungal (echinocandin) treatment is recommended [11, 16].

If catheter salvage is needed (no alternative catheter insertion site, severe thrombocytopenia), then systemic antimicrobial therapy can be administered in conjunction with antimicrobial lock therapy. Antimicrobial lock therapy consists of 2–3 ml of an active antimicrobial agent in supratherapeutic concentrations (>1,000 times higher than the MIC of the organism for vancomycin), often mixed with an anticoagulant and used to fill the lumen of the catheter. This therapeutic modality is contraindicated if insertion site, tunnel, or pocket infection is present [16].

Table 11.1 summarizes management of CRBSI according to the causative organism [16, 28].

11.5 Prevention

Catheter-related infections can be prevented by implementing various measures at the time of catheter insertion and after its insertion. Table 11.2 below summarizes the strategies of CRBSI prevention.

11.5.1 Before Catheter Insertion

Proper hand hygiene should be performed using alcohol or antiseptic soap and water [20]. It is also recommended to use maximal sterile barrier precautions

Table 11.1 Management of CRBSI according to the organism[a]

Microorganism	Management
Coagulase-negative staphylococci	Catheter can be removed or retained
	If removed, systemic antibiotics should be administered for 5–7 days
	If catheter is retained, treat with a systemic antibiotic and antibiotic lock therapy for 10–14 days. If there is clinical deterioration, persisting or relapsing bacteremia then the catheter should be removed
Staphylococcus aureus	Catheter should be removed and systemic antibiotics administered for 14 days
Enterococcus spp.	For short-term catheters, catheter should be removed and patient treated with systemic antibiotics for 7–14 days. For long-term CVC or port-related bacteremia, catheter may be retained and systemic antibiotics with antibiotic lock therapy can be used for 10–14 days. If there is clinical deterioration and persisting or relapsing bacteremia, catheter should be removed
Gram-negative bacilli	Catheter should be removed and systemic antibiotics administered for 7–14 days
Candida spp.	Catheter should be removed and antifungal therapy administered for 14 days after the first negative blood culture

[a]If complicated CRBSI is found (suppurative thrombophlebitis, endocarditis, osteomyelitis, endophthalmitis, sepsis, persistent bacteremia or metastatic infection), then the catheter should be removed and the patient treated with antibiotics for 4–6 weeks and for 6–8 weeks for osteomyelitis in adults

Table 11.2 Preventive strategies of CRBSI

Educating health-care workers regarding the proper insertion and maintenance of catheters
Aseptic technique (central line bundle)
Hand hygiene using antiseptic soap and water or alcohol
Maximal sterile barrier (cap, mask, gown, gloves)
Cleaning skin with chlorhexidine solution before insertion
Avoidance of femoral vein for central venous catheters in adults
Removing unnecessary catheter
Using antimicrobial antiseptic impregnated catheters
Using antimicrobial lock solution[a]

[a]Not routinely recommended by the centers for disease control (*CDC*)

including the use of a cap, mask, sterile gown, sterile gloves, and a sterile full body drape for the insertion of CVCs or guidewire exchange [20, 28]. Femoral veins for central venous access in adults should be avoided, and the subclavian vein is preferred instead (subclavian vein should be avoided in patients undergoing hemodialysis as it associated with higher risk of stenosis), because femoral access is associated with greater risk of infection and deep venous thrombosis [20].

Cleaning the skin with an antiseptic (70 % alcohol, tincture of iodine, an Iodophor, or chlorhexidine gluconate) before peripheral venous catheter insertion is recommended. While for central venous catheter and peripheral arterial catheters, a chlorhexidine-based (>0.5 %) skin antiseptic should be used in patients older than 2 months, and the antiseptic should be allowed to dry according the manufacturer's recommendation before insertion. For children younger than 2 months, povidone-iodine solution can be used [20, 28].

11.5.2 After Catheter Insertion

If there is a nonessential catheter, it should be removed. Peripheral catheters should be replaced every 72–96 h, whereas there is no need for replacing CVCs unless indicated. Administration sets should be replaced every 4–7 days (unless blood, blood products, or fat emulsions are given through it, then the administration set should be replaced within 24 h of initiating the infusion) [20].

Another approach of prevention is the usage of impregnated catheters with either minocycline-rifampin or chlorhexidine-silver sulfadiazine. Using these impregnated CVCs has shown to decrease the rate of CRBSI compared to non-impregnated catheters [3, 10]. These impregnated catheters are highly cost-effective and safe and do not appear to select for resistance [5]. These catheters are recommended in patients whose catheter is expected to remain >5 days and the CRBSI rate is not decreasing with the abovementioned methods [16].

Catheters coated with chlorhexidine-silver sulfadiazine have been extensively studied and demonstrated decrease in catheter colonization. The first generation of these catheters is coated on the external surface only. They decrease the risk of CRBSI, but less effectively than minocycline-rifampin catheters, by 12-fold as has been shown in a prospective randomized trial [6, 31]. The second-generation catheters were coated both internally and externally. They showed significant decrease in colonization when compared to first generation, but did not demonstrate statistically significant decrease in CRBSI when compared to non-coated catheters [10, 31, 32].

Catheters coated with minocycline-rifampin have been shown in several studies to reduce the risk of CRBSI [9]. Data suggest that the efficacy of minocycline-rifampin catheters may be prolonged beyond that of chlorhexidine-silver sulfadiazine catheters [6]. First-generation chlorhexidine-silver sulfadiazine catheters are efficient only when the average insertion time is less than 8 days [35]. Minocycline-rifampin catheters are efficient for a longer period of time (around 50 days) [6].

Minocycline-rifampin-coated catheters inhibit the biofilm adherence of resistant gram-positive and gram-negative pathogens with the exception of *Pseudomonas aeruginosa* and *Candida* spp. [29]. In order to expand the spectrum of antimicrobial activity, a second generation of minocycline-rifampin-impregnated catheters has been developed by adding chlorhexidine. These catheters showed better in vitro activity against methicillin-resistant *S. aureus*, *P. aeruginosa*, and *Candida* [29, 30].

We can achieve a near zero rate of CRBSI using aseptic techniques plus impregnated catheters. A study found that the rate of CRBSI was 1.28 per 1,000 catheter days when using uncoated catheters and aseptic techniques, while it was 0.25 per 1,000 catheter days when using both the aseptic techniques and minocycline-rifampin-impregnated catheters [9]. Another study found the rate of CRBSI using only the aseptic techniques as 1.24 per 1,000 catheter days, while in combination with impregnated catheters, the rate was 0.4 cases per 1,000 catheter days [32].

Another approach to prevent CRBSI is the use of antimicrobial lock solutions, by which an antimicrobial solution is used to fill a catheter lumen and then allowed to dwell for a period of time. Antibiotics used include vancomycin, gentamicin, ciprofloxacin, minocycline, amikacin, cefazolin, cefotaxime, and ceftazidime [20]. Antiseptics could be used such as alcohol and taurolidine. These agents are usually combined with anticoagulant such as heparin or EDTA. Using this technique is recommended in patients with long-term catheters who have a history of multiple CRBSI despite adherence to aseptic techniques [20, 28].

References

1. Blot SI, Depuydt P, Annemans L, Benoit D, Hoste E, De Waele JJ, Decruyenaere J, Vogelaers D, Colardyn F, Vandewoude KH. Clinical and economic outcomes in critically ill patients with nosocomial catheter-related bloodstream infections. Clin Infect Dis. 2005;41(11):1591–8.
2. Capdevila JA, Planes AM, Palomar M, Gasser I, Almirante B, Pahissa A, Crespo E, Martínez-Vázquez JM. Value of differential quantitative blood cultures in the diagnosis of catheter-related sepsis. Eur J Clin Microbiol Infect Dis. 1992;5:403–7.

3. Casey AL, Mermel LA, Nightingale P, Elliott TS. Antimicrobial central venous catheters in adults: a systematic review and meta-analysis. Lancet Infect Dis. 2008;8(12):763–76.
4. Chatzinikolaou I, Hanna H, Hachem R, Alakech B, Tarrand J, Raad I. Differential quantitative blood cultures for the diagnosis of catheter-related bloodstream infections associated with short- and long-term catheters: a prospective study. Diagn Microbiol Infect Dis. 2004;50(3):167–72.
5. Crnich CJ, Maki DG. Are antimicrobial-impregnated catheters effective? Don't throw out the baby with the bathwater. Clin Infect Dis. 2004;38(9):12871292.
6. Darouiche RO, Raad II, Heard SO, Thornby JI, Wenker OC, Gabrielli A, Berg J, Khardori N, Hanna H, Hachem R, Harris RL, Mayhall G. A comparison of two antimicrobial-impregnated central venous catheters. Catheter Study Group. N Engl J Med. 1999;340(1):1–8.
7. Donlan RM. Biofilm elimination on intravascular catheters: important considerations for the infectious disease practitioner. Clin Infect Dis. 2011;52(8):1038–45.
8. Fowler Jr VG, Boucher HW, Corey GR, Abrutyn E, Karchmer AW, Rupp ME, Levine DP, Chambers HF, Tally FP, Vigliani GA, Cabell CH, Link AS, DeMeyer I, Filler SG, Zervos M, Cook P, Parsonnet J, Bernstein JM, Price CS, Forrest GN, Fätkenheuer G, Gareca M, Rehm SJ, Brodt HR, Tice A, Cosgrove SE. *S. aureus* Endocarditis and Bacteremia Study Group. Daptomycin versus standard therapy for bacteremia and endocarditis caused by *Staphylococcus aureus*. N Engl J Med. 2006;355(7):653–65.
9. Hanna H, Benjamin R, Chatzinikolaou I, Alakech B, Richardson D, Mansfield P, Dvorak T, Munsell MF, Darouiche R, Kantarjian H, Raad I. Long-term silicone central venous catheters impregnated with minocycline and rifampin decrease rates of catheter-related bloodstream infection in cancer patients: a prospective randomized clinical trial. J Clin Oncol. 2004;22(15):3163–71.
10. Hockenhull JC, Dwan KM, Smith GW, Gamble CL, Boland A, Walley TJ, Dickson RC. The clinical effectiveness of central venous catheters treated with anti-infective agents in preventing catheter-related bloodstream infections: a systematic review. Crit Care Med. 2009;37(2):702–12.
11. Lorente L, Jiménez A, Santana M, Iribarren JL, Jiménez JJ, Martín MM, Mora ML. Microorganisms responsible for intravascular catheter-related bloodstream infection according to the catheter site. Crit Care Med. 2007;35(10):2424–7.
12. Maki DG, Kluger DM, Crnich CJ. The risk of bloodstream infection in adults with different intravascular devices: a systematic review of 200 published prospective studies. Mayo Clin Proc. 2006;81(9):1159–71.
13. Mayhall CG. Diagnosis and management of infections of implantable devices used for prolonged venous access. Curr Clin Top Infect Dis. 1992;12:83–110.
14. Mermel LA. Prevention of intravascular catheter-related infections. Ann Intern Med. 2000;132:391–402. Erratum: Ann Intern Med 2000;133:395.
15. Mermel LA. What is the predominant source of intravascular catheter infections? Clin Infect Dis. 2011;52(2):211–2.
16. Mermel LA, Allon M, Bouza E, Craven DE, Flynn P, O'Grady NP, Raad II, Rijnders BJ, Sherertz RJ, Warren DK. Clinical practice guidelines for the diagnosis and management of intravascular catheter-related infection: 2009 Update by the Infectious Diseases Society of America. Clin Infect Dis. 2009;49(1):1–45.
17. Moise PA, Sakoulas G, Forrest A, Schentag JJ. Vancomycin in vitro bactericidal activity and its relationship to efficacy in clearance of methicillin-resistant Staphylococcus aureus bacteremia. Antimicrob Agents Chemother. 2007;51(7):2582–6.
18. Nucci M, Anaissie E. Revisiting the source of candidemia: skin or gut? Clin Infect Dis. 2001;33(12):1959–67.
19. O'Grady NP, Chertow DS. Managing bloodstream infections in patients who have short-term central venous catheters. Cleve Clin J Med. 2011;78(1):10–7.
20. O'Grady NP, Alexander M, Burns LA, Dellinger EP, Garland J, Heard SO, Lipsett PA, Masur H, Mermel LA, Pearson ML, Raad II, Randolph AG, Rupp ME, Saint S, Healthcare Infection Control Practices Advisory Committee. Guidelines for the prevention of intravascular catheter-related infections. Am J Infect Control. 2011;39(4 Suppl 1):S1–34.

21. Pittet D, Tarara D, Wenzel RP. Nosocomial bloodstream infection in critically ill patients. Excess length of stay, extra costs, and attributable mortality. JAMA. 1994;271(20):1598–601.
22. Raad I. Intravascular-catheter-related infections. Lancet. 1998;351(9106):893–8. Review.
23. Raad II, Bodey GP. Infectious complications of indwelling vascular catheters. Clin Infect Dis. 1992;15(2):197–208.
24. Raad II, Sabbagh MF, Rand KH, Sherertz RJ. Quantitative tip culture methods and the diagnosis of central venous catheter-related infections. Diagn Microbiol Infect Dis. 1992;15(1):13–20.
25. Raad I, Costerton W, Sabharwal U, Sacilowski M, Anaissie E, Bodey GP. Ultrastructural analysis of indwelling vascular catheters: a quantitative relationship between luminal colonization and duration of placement. J Infect Dis. 1993;168(2):400–7.
26. Raad I, Hanna HA, Alakech B, Chatzinikolaou I, Johnson MM, Tarrand J. Differential time to positivity: a useful method for diagnosing catheter-related bloodstream infections. Ann Intern Med. 2004;140(1):18–25.
27. Raad I, Hanna H, Jiang Y, Dvorak T, Reitzel R, Chaiban G, Sherertz R, Hachem R. Comparative activities of daptomycin, linezolid, and tigecycline against catheter-related methicillin-resistant Staphylococcus bacteremic isolates embedded in biofilm. Antimicrob Agents Chemother. 2007;51(5):1656–60.
28. Raad I, Hanna H, Maki D. Intravascular catheter-related infections: advancesin diagnosis, prevention, and management. Lancet Infect Dis. 2007;7(10):645–57.
29. Raad I, Reitzel R, Jiang Y, Chemaly RF, Dvorak T, Hachem R. Anti-adherence activity and antimicrobial durability of anti-infective-coated catheters against multidrug-resistant bacteria. J Antimicrob Chemother. 2008;62(4):746–50.
30. Raad I, Mohamed JA, Reitzel RA, Jiang Y, Raad S, Al Shuaibi M, Chaftari AM, Hachem RY. Improved antibiotic impregnated catheters with extended spectrum activity against resistant bacteria and fungi. Antimicrob Agents Chemother. 2012;56(2):935–41.
31. Ramritu P, Halton K, Collignon P, Cook D, Fraenkel D, Battistutta D, Whitby M, Graves N. A systematic review comparing the relative effectiveness of antimicrobial-coated catheters in intensive care units. Am J Infect Control. 2008;36(2):104–17.
32. Rupp ME, Lisco SJ, Lipsett PA, Perl TM, Keating K, Civetta JM, Mermel LA, Lee D, Dellinger EP, Donahoe M, Giles D, Pfaller MA, Maki DG, Sherertz R. Effect of a second-generation venous catheter impregnated with chlorhexidine and silver sulfadiazine on central catheter-related infections: a randomized, controlled trial. Ann Intern Med. 2005;143(8):570–80.
33. Safdar N, Fine JP, Maki DG. Meta-analysis: methods for diagnosing intravascular device-related bloodstream infection. Ann Intern Med. 2005;142(6):451–66.
34. Tighe MJ, Kite P, Thomas D, Fawley WN, McMahon MJ. Rapid diagnosis of catheter-related sepsis using the acridine orange leukocyte cytospin test and an endoluminal brush. JPEN J Parenter Enter Nutr. 1996;20(3):215–8.
35. Walder B, Pittet D, Tramèr MR. Prevention of bloodstream infections with central venous catheters treated with anti-infective agents depends on catheter type and insertion time: evidence from a meta-analysis. Infect Control Hosp Epidemiol. 2002;23(12):748–56.
36. Wang R, Khan BA, Cheung GY, Bach TH, Jameson-Lee M, Kong KF, Queck SY, Otto M. Staphylococcus epidermidis surfactant peptides promote biofilm maturation and dissemination of biofilm-associated infection in mice. J Clin Invest. 2011;121(1):238–48.
37. Wilcox MH, Tack KJ, Bouza E, Herr DL, Ruf BR, Ijzerman MM, Croos-Dabrera RV, Kunkel MJ, Knirsch C. Complicated skin and skin-structure infections and catheter-related bloodstream infections: noninferiority of linezolid in a phase 3 study. Clin Infect Dis. 2009;48(2):203–12.

Gastrointestinal Complications 12

Nicole M.A. Blijlevens

Contents

12.1 Introduction

Over the past decade, the number of patients with haematological cancer that are being treated for a variety of chemotherapy, radiation therapy or targeted therapy continues to grow. In order to improve patient care and their survival, better

N.M.A. Blijlevens
Department of Haematology, Radboud University Medical Centre, 9101, NL-6500 HB Nijmegen, The Netherlands
e-mail: Nicole.blijlevens@radboudumc.nl

G. Maschmeyer, K.V.I. Rolston (eds.), *Infections in Hematology*,
DOI 10.1007/978-3-662-44000-1_12

recognition and proper management of gastrointestinal complications including infections are warranted.

The entire gastrointestinal (GI) tract is susceptible to a range of acute and chronic complications associated with the treatment of haematological diseases especially if treatment includes a haematopoietic stem cell transplantation (HSCT). Rarely is the intestinal tract itself infiltrated by leukaemia. In general, acute complications are mainly the result of toxicities associated with cytotoxic drugs, while graft-versus-host disease (GVHD) is the main driver of late or chronic GI events. Both conditions hamper the barrier function of the GI tract, enabling both local and systemic infections to occur when the patient is already immunocompromised either by neutropenia or dysfunctional cellular immunity. High-dose chemotherapy conditioning regimens, with or without total body irradiation (TBI), cause severe GI side effects including nausea, vomiting, as well as mucositis along the entire GI tract that cause pain, ulcerations, bloating, malabsorption and diarrhoea. These GI-related symptoms and signs can easily be mistaken for infections by opportunistic microorganisms. The clinical presentation of each complication is nonspecific, and diagnostic procedure includes physical examination, microbiological cultures, imaging and endoscopy with biopsies. Patients undergoing intensive cytotoxic therapy report oral mucositis-induced pain as the most debilitating complication but not emesis or diarrhoea. Aside from pain, discomfort, poor appetite and decreased quality of life, these GI side effects, especially gut mucositis, are associated with increased risk of infection, sepsis and death. Neutropenic enterocolitis is one of the most extreme toxicity accompanied by life-threatening complications. It is obvious that GI toxicities significantly contribute towards increased resource utilisation and prolonged hospital stays.

Real progress has been achieved in treating nausea and vomiting with better antiemetics, but unfortunately the treatment of mucositis either caused by the cytotoxic regimen itself or related to acute or chronic GVHD has been a failure. It is also becoming increasingly clear that some patients are genetically predisposed to certain toxicities and warrant tailored supportive management. Close monitoring of GI complications and awareness of related infections are the critical aspects of supportive care management to optimise the use of specific drugs that can significantly improve treatment outcomes. Management of the following GI toxicities also in relation to infections will be discussed below: cytotoxic therapy-induced nausea and vomiting, mucositis (including oesophagitis and neutropenic enterocolitis) and gastrointestinal GVHD.

12.2 Cytotoxic Therapy-Induced Nausea and Vomiting

12.2.1 Background

Cytotoxic therapy-induced nausea and vomiting (CINV) is commonly feared by patients before start of treatment and can lead to serious medical problems such as dehydration, electrolyte disturbances and renal insufficiency. CINV results in a rise in health care costs, prolonged hospital stay with impairment of quality of life in patients receiving highly and moderately emetogenic therapy [1]. It is obvious that CINV itself is unlikely to ascribe to infection unless the medical history of the preceding days indicates otherwise, for instance, an intercurrent acquired food-borne infection. Nausea, the perception that emesis might occur, can only be judged by the patient, making it difficult to test the efficacy of new drugs in reducing nausea and vomiting. Emesis is basically a defence mechanism based upon different pathways, including the chemoreceptor trigger zone, vestibular nuclei and central nervous system. Emesis has been described as acute (the first 24 h of chemotherapy administration), delayed (from 24 h onwards unto 5 or 7 days after the cytotoxic insult), breakthrough (CINV during antiemetic therapy), anticipatory (before the insult) and refractory (despite antiemetic therapy). The discovery of the importance of the serotonin receptor in the management of CINV was crucial to controlling CINV [2].

12.2.2 Management of CINV

Aprepitant is the first neurokinin-1 receptor antagonist approved for prevention of CINV. NK_1 receptors are the binding sites of the tachykinin substance P and are located in the brainstem emetic centre and in the GI tract. Patients treated with cisplatin or an anthracycline–cyclophosphamide regimen clearly favoured the use of aprepitant in the prevention of acute and delayed emesis [3]. Aprepitant is known to moderately inhibit cytochrome (CYP) P450 3A4 in normal volunteers, and its use is limited in patients receiving high-dose chemotherapy because of concerns about potential drug interactions with some chemotherapeutic and prophylactic agents used for GVHD prevention. CINV is still a significant problem for HSCT recipients as only 20 % completely responded and antiemetic rescue therapy especially for delayed nausea and emesis failed completely [4]. If patients with anticipatory emesis are scheduled to undergo HSCT, anxiolytic drugs such as lorazepam or olanzapine may be useful additions to the antiemetic protocol. The corticosteroids dexamethasone and methylprednisolone are effective as monotherapy or in combination with other drugs for patients treated for cancer. The reader is referred to the recommendations of the American Society of Clinical Oncology Guideline for Antiemetics in Oncology for details [5].

12.3 Mucositis

12.3.1 Pathogenesis

Chemotherapy and radiotherapy damage the entire alimentary mucosa initiating an inflammatory cascade that culminates in mucosal barrier injury (MBI), which manifests itself clinically as mucositis. The alimentary tract undergoes the same embryological development, but mucosal cells at various regions of the alimentary undergo specific differentiation later on in order to evolve site-specific functions. The pathogenesis of MBI is thought to consist of five phases [6, 7]: (1) the activation of nuclear factor-κB directly by chemo-/radiotherapy and indirectly from ROS formation, DNA and non-DNA damage; (2) production and release of pro-inflammatory cytokines and chemokines (IL-1, IL-6, IL-8, TNFα, IL-23, IFNγ) by macrophages, intestinal epithelial cells and endothelial cells; (3) positive feedback loop of TNFα, epithelial cell apoptosis and increased mucosal permeability; (4) translocation of microbes or their cell wall components such as lipopolysaccharide or peptidoglycan; and finally (5) repair and healing. Although the impact of microbes and their cell wall components on the inflammatory response is secondary, stimulation of pattern recognition receptors (PRRs) by pathogen-associated molecular patterns (PAMPs) translocating across the disrupted mucosal barrier with subsequent bacteraemia and endotoxaemia aggravates inflammation.

12.3.2 Clinical Features

The course of mucositis following conditioning regimens is relatively predictable. Clinical evidence of mucosal injury arises about 5 days of conditioning; it peaks at about 12–14 days and then spontaneously resolves 3 weeks after starting chemotherapy. The average duration of severe mucositis when present is almost a week. The exposure to a specific cytotoxic drug or radiation dose is the most prominent factor determining the character, onset and progression of GI mucositis [8]. Symptoms such as diarrhoea or constipation are the net result of clinical mucositis of the entire GI system. The incidence rate of GI mucositis varies from 10 % in patients with advanced disease to around 40 % of patients receiving standard dose chemotherapy. Symptoms of diarrhoea and abdominal complaints affect almost every patient immediately following high-dose chemotherapy and HSCT. These data are retrieved from toxicity scores not specifically designed in documenting the course of specific symptoms [9].

The importance of this observation is highlighted by the incidence of 44 % of severe oral mucositis [World Health Organization (WHO) grade ≥3] found among patients receiving high-dose melphalan or BEAM (carmustine, etoposide, cytarabine and melphalan) before autologous HSCT in a prospective audit [10]. Ulcerative mucositis (WHO Grade ≥2), the major driver of symptoms and infection risk, was noted in 64 %. Because ulceration is, important as major driver of patient related symptoms and risk factors of infection.

12.3.3 Mucositis and Infectious Complications

ASCT recipients with severe oral mucositis (OM) had a significantly higher incidence of fever (68 % versus 47 % of patients), microbiologically defined infection (27 % versus 12 %) and a longer duration of fever (4.2 versus 3.0 days) [11]. Whereas OM is relatively easy to recognise, detection of gut mucositis is more demanding. It was shown that citrulline appeared to be particularly useful to detect gut mucosal damage since blood concentrations of this amino acid directly reflect functioning small intestinal cell mass [12]. Plasma concentrations of citrulline corresponded to the severity and extent of gut injury after intensive myeloablative therapy. Recent exploratory studies in more than 90 HSCT recipients validated a citrulline-based assessment score making it a suitable first choice for measuring and monitoring intestinal MBI [13]. Impaired integrity of the mucosal barrier is thought to promote translocation of microorganisms from the lumen of the digestive tract to the blood stream resulting in bacteraemia. Plasma concentrations of citrulline reached a nadir within 12 days after initiating HDM in 29 patients. Patients with bacteraemia had significantly lower citrulline concentrations on the first day of fever than did those without bacteraemia [14]. Twenty patients (69 %) developed fever that was accompanied by bacteraemia in ten cases, due to oral viridans streptococci (OVS) with or without coagulase-negative staphylococci (CoNS). The lowest citrulline concentrations coincided with the onset of bacteraemia, but not with neutropenia. Low citrulline rather than the duration of neutropenia is associated with bacteraemia indicating the importance of an intact mucosal barrier in neutropenic patients. This suggests that the severity of gut MBI determines whether bacteraemia occurs or not rather than neutropenia per se. This was confirmed in a larger cohort of 67 ASCT patients after HDM where the onset of bacteraemia due to Gram-positive cocci only occurred after a low citrulline level been reached irrespective of duration of neutropenia [15]. A similar association between the presence of gastrointestinal toxicity and the development of OVS bacteraemia was seen in children treated for AML [16].

In out-patients treated with multiple cycles of chemotherapy for lymphoma, myeloma and solid tumours, severe GI mucositis defined and characterised as oesophagitis, gastritis, colitis and typhlitis by NCI common toxicity criteria resulted in significantly more infections than with OM and was associated with prolonged use of antibiotic therapy [17]. The mean duration of hospitalisation of patients receiving myelosuppressive chemotherapy was extended by 2 days during cycles accompanied with only OM, but when gut mucosal damage was also present the length of stay was increased by an average of 8 days [17]. The risk of infection was significantly higher during chemotherapy cycles complicated by any GI mucositis despite the fact that there was no difference in the depth or duration of neutropenia. The risk of infection was almost 100 % during cycles associated with grades 3 and 4 GI mucositis. CoNS are the most frequent isolates, and though CoNS bacteraemia is assumed to be related to the use of central venous catheters, mucosal sites may be as important as source of these bacteria [18]. Indeed, molecular analysis of CoNS isolated from blood cultures indicated that the mucosa was the origin in most of the cases [19]. Bacteraemia due to OVS mainly *Streptococcus mitis* and *Streptococcus oralis* is related to MBI and can be associated with more serious complications such as sepsis and adult respiratory distress syndrome which carries a high mortality (80 %), though MBI is not the sole predictor of the viridans streptococcal shock syndrome [20].

Severe disruption of the mucosal barrier is clearly not the only risk factor for developing bacteraemia, which affected only a third of our patients with low citrulline concentrations. To identify those patients at risk for bacteraemia, citrulline measurements need to be combined with other tests. For instance, the Multinational Association of Supportive Care of Cancer (MASCC) developed a risk score to predict at the onset of fever during neutropenia which patients are at high risk for development of serious medical complications [21].

12.3.4 Mucositis and Fever During Neutropenia

Neutropenia (granulocytes $<0.5 \times 10^9/l$) has been used for more than 40 years to recognise those patients who are at imminent risk of developing infectious complications following intensive chemotherapy [22]. This formed the foundation for developing a successful strategy for managing these patients, namely, administering broad-spectrum antimicrobial therapy promptly as soon as fever occurs during neutropenia. Indeed, empirical antibacterial therapy is still the backbone of the supportive care given to these patients [23]. However, many studies also reported that a substantial number of patients remained febrile without an infection ever being documented [24]. Hence, such episodes of fever were designated 'unexplained fever'.

Patients with severe OM have not only an increased risk of infections, but the incidence of fever and number of days with fever during neutropenia are also higher [25]. Although, the magnitude of the inflammatory response can be aggravated by infections fever as symptom of a systemic inflammatory response is predominantly driven by the course of MBI in HSCT recipients [26]. Data show a clear pattern of an inflammatory response measured by C-reactive protein or IL8, irrespective of the presence or absence of infection, coinciding with the course of mucositis. Consequently, the term 'febrile mucositis' might be suitable in these cases [15].

12.4 Oesophagitis

Oesophagitis causes burning retrosternal chest pain. The differential diagnosis includes cytotoxic therapy-induced oesophagitis and viral or candida infections. Herpes simplex virus (HSV) reactivates commonly in HSV-positive patients after cytoreductive therapy especially in the presence of mucositis after HSCT. Therefore, anti-HSV prophylaxis is routinely given after HSCT. CMV oesophagitis is actually only seen after allogeneic HSCT with active GVHD.

Candida species are part of the commensal flora of the skin and mucosal surfaces, and in many adults they may become the prevalent opportunistic pathogen under the pressures of antimicrobial agents and changes in adherence sites. Under normal circumstances, the intact epithelial surface repel invasion of yeast cells. However, cytoreductive agents and irradiation inflict serious damage to the mucosal barrier, and colonising microorganisms such as *Candida* can gain easy access to the submucosal tissue and subsequently to the bloodstream. The clinical relevance of culturing *Candida albicans* from saliva or stool is a matter of controversy with respect to the diagnosis of *Candida* oesophagitis. It might help in directing initial antifungal therapy in case of suspected candida oesophagitis. Blood cultures mostly remain negative, and results of endoscopy may be delayed. Fluconazole can still be started if the *Candida* species known from the surveillance cultures was shown to be sensitive. Otherwise, echinocandins or lipid formulations of amphotericin B or voriconazole are alternatives.

Oesophagitis was seen in more than 50 % of the upper GI endoscopy procedures performed after intensive chemotherapy (median of 22 days) in 94 patients with leukaemia. The other complications were gastritis, gastric erosions and hiatus hernia and duodenitis. The most therapeutic consequences were the addition of antacid therapy [27]. There is level I evidence that H_2 receptor blockers and proton pump inhibitors can reduce the pain and haemorrhage from standard dose chemotherapy oesophagitis, but there is a link with OVS sepsis [28].

12.5 Neutropenic Enterocolitis

Typhlitis or neutropenic enterocolitis (NE) is used to describe an inflammatory process involving the colon, mainly caecum with or without involving adjacent areas of the small intestine in the context of chemotherapy-induced neutropenia. NE can potentially result in life-threatening complications such as ischemia, necrosis, haemorrhage, bacteraemia and perforation. Mortality rates vary between 5 and 100 % [29]. A prospective survey reported an overall incidence of abdominal infections of 17.7 % and incidence of NE of 6.5 % among adults treated for acute leukaemia [30]. The common clinical manifestations of NE are fever, abdominal pain and diarrhoea. These symptoms are neither specific nor pathognomonic for NE and must be differentiated from other potential causes of abdominal complications such as appendicitis, pseudomembranous colitis, ischemic colitis, obstruction and intussusceptions, and both viral (CMV, adenovirus or rotavirus) and fungal (candidiasis, *Aspergillus* and *Mucorales*) infection can supervene especially after allogeneic HSCT. Typically, NE occurs between 10 and 30 days after starting cytotoxic treatment.

Ultrasound sonography (US) or computer tomography (CT) appears more valuable in the diagnosis and monitoring of suspected NE. Most reports concerning NE adopt the principle that a bowel wall thickness >3 mm is abnormal, and either matches or supports a diagnosis of NE [31]. CT is able to differentiate NE from other intestinal complications in neutropenic patients. For instance, the highest mean BWT (12 mm) was seen in *Clostridium difficile*-related colitis in an analysis of 76 neutropenic patients with various gastrointestinal disorders. Although, US showing BWT >10 mm was associated with a significantly higher mortality rate (60 %) than a BWT ≤10 mm (4.2 %) [32].

Bacteraemia due to *Staphylococcus aureus*, *Pseudomonas aeruginosa*, *Clostridium* species, and *Candida* species are clearly associated with neutropenic enterocolitis [33]. Indeed bacteraemia due to certain species of *Clostridium*, for example, *Clostridium tertium* and *Clostridium septicum*, is considered pathognomonic in the setting of NE. Presumably, prolonged exposure to antibiotics results in a marked shift in the gut microflora towards toxin-producing bacteria such as *Staphylococcus aureus*, *Pseudomonas aeruginosa* and *Clostridium septicum*. Mucosal or transmural necrosis and haemorrhage of the mucosal surface of the ileocecal region probably provide a favourable environment for the spores of *Clostridium* species to germinate and may be their portal of entry into the bloodstream. The pathogenesis of NE seems to require various elements to be present simultaneously, namely, cytotoxic therapy-induced mucosal damage, a perturbed resident microflora and profound neutropenia. The recovery of neutrophils usually resolves the clinical problem of NE but might be deleterious since tissue infiltration of neutrophils in an inflamed bowel wall containing microorganisms could result in perforation.

Treatment with broad-spectrum antibiotics targeting Gram-negative and anaerobic bacteria is mandatory and antifungals to target *Candida* spp. is beneficial. If the patient is a carrier, plus supportive care measures consisting of bowel rest, nasogastric suction, total parenteral nutrition [34]. Surgery should be avoided unless there is perforation or massive bleeding. Pneumatosis intestinalis due to NE is very worrisome as it suggests imminent bowel perforation. The use of G-CSF to hasten neutrophil count or function is still under debate.

12.6 Management of Mucositis and Infections

Despite its frequency and consequences, the prevention and treatment options for mucositis are sparse. Pain control is a major goal of mucositis management. Palifermin, keratinocyte growth factor-1, has been approved for use in the prevention of OM associated with TBI-containing conditioning regimens for autologous HSCT for the treatment of hematologic malignancies. Data demonstrated that palifermin effectively reduces incidence, severity and duration of severe mucositis. There was a striking reduction of febrile neutropenia episodes in the pivotal study of Spielberger et al., and there were fewer episodes of bacteraemia among HSCT recipients given palifermin, albeit not statistically significant (15 vs. 25 %) [35]. A small study showed that treatment with recombinant human IL-11 resulted in less bacteraemia and improved gut permeability [36]. Hence, agents such as recombinant human IL-11 and palifermin which are designed to protect the mucosa may prove helpful in reducing bacterial infection in neutropenic patients. Clinical trials have demonstrated the role of several antimicrobial prophylactic strategies after intensive chemotherapy or HSCT. Patients who are *herpes simplex* seropositive before the transplant procedure have a 70 % change of reactivation within 8–10 days after transplantation. This can be prevented by prophylaxis with acyclovir or valacyclovir. Fluoroquinolones are effective in not only reducing *Gram-negative* bacterial infections but also related mortality and improved overall survival [37]. Fluconazole is effective in reducing *Candida* infections, including fungaemia. In general, broad-spectrum antimicrobial therapy promptly as soon as fever occurs during neutropenia, and subsequent complementary antimicrobial therapy based upon clinical and laboratory results remains the cornerstone of management.

12.7 Gastrointestinal Graft-Versus-Host Disease

12.7.1 Pathogenesis

Acute GVHD results from the complex interaction of donor T cells and host tissues that involves recognition of major and minor histocompatibility antigens in an inflammatory milieu. The pathophysiology of acute GVHD involves both the innate and adaptive immune systems and is thought to follow a reproducible pattern of (1) tissue damage from the conditioning regimen, for example, gastrointestinal mucositis, (2) donor T-cell activation and (3) an inflammatory effector phase. In the first phase, cytotoxic therapy-induced MBI enables translocation of bacteria and microbial wall products, like LPS and peptidoglycan into the bloodstream, with activation of pro-inflammatory cytokines as described earlier. In the second phase activated host antigen presenting cells (APCs), and less important donor APCs, present host antigens to alloreactive T-lymphocytes. Subsequent activation and proliferation of T-lymphocytes, predominantly Th1-lymphocytes and probably Th17, ensues. The last phase concerns trafficking of alloreactive T- and natural killer (NK) cells to inflamed tissues and the occurrence of damage to these target tissues. Subsequently, translocation of bacterial products in intestinal GVHD leads to amplification of inflammation.

12.7.2 Clinical Features

Acute GVHD is a syndrome mostly involving the skin, liver and intestinal tract. The median time to diagnosis of acute GVHD varies with conditioning, with recipients of high-dose therapy and transplantation being diagnosed at a median of 17 days post-HSCT, as compared with recipients of reduced-intensity conditioning and transplantation being diagnosed at a median of 3 months post-HSCT where it is commonly associated with tapering of immunosuppressive agents. Similar to OM, conditioning regimen-induced lower GI toxicity can persist until the development of acute GVHD thereby complicating the diagnosis. The symptoms of gastrointestinal GVHD are similar as those associated with chemotherapy consisting of nausea, vomiting, anorexia, malabsorption, malnutrition, abdominal complaints and diarrhoea. Even when typical erythematous skin lesions erupt, biopsy is still necessary for definitive diagnosis. Infectious diarrhoea also needs to be considered. However, despite all this, infectious diarrhoea is not that common early post-HSCT, except maybe for *Clostridium difficile*-related pseudomembranous enterocolitis. The intestinal tract is a prevalent site for post-HSCT thrombotic microangiopathy. Although rare the clinical picture mimics gut GVHD, but laboratory findings of intravascular hemolysis are discriminatory.

Chronic GVHD is a multisystem immune-mediated disorder characterised by immunosuppression and immune dysregulation, resulting in increased risk of infection, impaired organ function, and reduced quality of life. Incidence of chronic GVHD is increasing, likely because of increasing age of patients undergoing HSCT, decreased early post-transplant mortality, use of peripheral blood cells as the stem cell source and increased utilisation of unrelated donors.

12.7.3 Management of GVHD and Infections

The recommended initial dose of corticosteroids for moderate to severe acute GVHD is 2 mg/kg/day of methylprednisolone or its equivalent. The response rate to single-agent corticosteroid therapy is approximately 50 %; however, complete durable responses are noted in fewer patients. Patients with steroid-refractory GVHD (either acute or chronic) have a poor survival, and second-line therapy, such as polyclonal (ATG) or monoclonal antibodies (daclizumab, inolimomab, basiliximab, alemtuzumab, rituximab) or TNF-α blockade (infliximab or etanercept) only further diminishes the activity of remaining innate and adoptive immunity. GVHD itself is an immunosuppressive condition, but therapy is extremely immunosuppressive making the patient prone to systemic infections especially viral and fungal diseases. Intestinal GVHD after nonmyeloablative HSCT significantly increased the risk of invasive aspergillosis over time [38]. Sometimes, symptoms of severe abdominal pain and nausea or diarrhoea due to visceral involvement of *varicella zoster*, CMV or H1N1 infection are misdiagnosed as GVHD. *Varicella zoster* is revealed only after eruption of skin vesicles. Intestinal adenovirus infections are associated with significant morbidity and potentially life-threatening primary in paediatric transplant recipients. The intestinal tract maybe the primary site of adenovirus reactivation [39]. Endoscopy with biopsies, CT scanning and extensive microbial culturing are mandatory in these clinically difficult patients to establish the cause(s) of their misery. Often patients with severe GI tract GVHD need intravenous hyperalimentation for prolonged periods exposing them to additional risks of infections related to the use of a central venous catheter.

Many patients with steroid-refractory GVHD will succumb to systemic infections. Therefore, standard infection prophylaxis to prevent *Pneumocystis jiroveci* pneumonia, herpesvirus reactivation and prophylaxis against invasive fungal diseases with an azole antifungal agent is recommended. In case of CMV reactivation prophylactic ganciclovir or valganciclovir is required. Patients with chronic GVHD are at risk for infection particularly by encapsulated organisms. Rare intestinal opportunistic infections with *non-tuberculous Mycobacteria*, *Mucorales species* or *Cryptosporidium species* can occur demanding meticulous diagnostic procedures if the clinical condition of the patient deteriorates.

12.8 Future Options of Management

The role of innate immunity in cancer patients has been brought to attention by the impact of single nucleotide polymorphisms (SNP) of innate immune genes (Toll-like receptors (TLRs), the Nod-like receptors (NLRs) and C-type lectin receptors (CLRs)), which result in enhanced or attenuated expression and/or function, on treatment-related complications including infections. Polymorphisms in PRRs of importance in intestinal host–microbe interactions like NOD2, originally described in Crohn's disease, and TLRs have been implicated in the occurrence of GvHD and infections.

Dectin-1, a C-type lectin that recognises 1,3-b-glucans from fungal pathogens, including *Candida species*, is involved in the initiation of the immune response against fungi. The Y238X polymorphism demonstrated a loss of function in functional assays by decreased cytokine production. Patients undergoing an allogeneic HSCT bearing this polymorphism *DECTIN-1* Y238X polymorphism had an increased oral and gastrointestinal colonisation with *Candida species* necessitating more frequent use of fluconazole in the prevention of systemic *Candida* infection [40]. Furthermore, patients from patient–donor pairs bearing the wild-type allele who where colonised with *Candida species* had a significant increased incidence of acute GVHD compared to non-colonised patients (OR=2.6, P=0.04), but this was not the case in patients from pairs with the Y238X polymorphism (OR=1.2, ns) [41]. This might suggest that *Candida* could have a role in the pathogenesis of acute GvHD. There are also several reports indicating the role of NOD2 polymorphisms on GVHD and infections [42]. Intriguing is the fact that the impact of NOD2 polymorphisms on GVHD disappears with the use of comprehensive antimicrobial prophylaxis suggesting a role of intestinal sensing of a microbial product in such a way that the balance of immunity is influenced.

Conclusions

All these preliminary findings point out that selection of high-risk patients with the use of SNP of innate immune genes in the future might offer another tool in optimising supportive care in an attempt to prevent life-threatening gastrointestinal complications and related infections (Table 12.1).

Table 12.1 Gastrointestinal complications of haematological therapy

	Early onset <28 days	**Management**
GI mucositis	Chemotherapy/irradiation complicated by OVS or CoNS bacteraemia	Pain killers (morphine) and antibiotics
Oesophagitis	Chemotherapy	Antacids
	Herpes simplex	Antiviral prophylaxis
	Candida spp.	Antifungal therapy
Gastritis	Chemotherapy/irradiation	Antacids
Neutropenic enterocolitis	Multifactorial origin	Conservative approach
	High risk of candidaemia and bacteraemia with *Clostridia* spp. and *Staph. aureus*	Broad antimicrobial coverage
	late onset >28 days	**Management**
GI mucositis	GVHD high risk of invasive fungal diseases	Start corticosteroids antifungal therapy
Colitis	*Clostridium difficile*	Metronidazole
	CMV, adenovirus, H1N1	Antiviral treatment
	Other opportunistic pathogens:	Targeted therapy
	Cryptosporidium spp.	
	Mucorales spp.	
	Non-tuberculous mycobacteriae spp.	

References

1. Bloechl-Daum B, Deuson RR, Mavros P, Hansen M, Herrstedt J. Delayed nausea and vomiting continue to reduce patients' quality of life after highly and moderately emetogenic chemotherapy despite antiemetic treatment. J Clin Oncol. 2006;24(27):4472–8.
2. Warr DG, Hesketh PJ, Gralla RJ, Muss HB, Herrstedt J, Eisenberg PD, et al. Efficacy and tolerability of aprepitant for the prevention of chemotherapy-induced nausea and vomiting in patients with breast cancer after moderately emetogenic chemotherapy. J Clin Oncol. 2005;23(12):2822–30.
3. Warr DG, Grunberg SM, Gralla RJ, Hesketh PJ, Roila F, Wit R, et al. The oral NK(1) antagonist aprepitant for the prevention of acute and delayed chemotherapy-induced nausea and vomiting: pooled data from 2 randomised, double-blind, placebo controlled trials. Eur J Cancer. 2005;41(9):1278–85.
4. Lopez-Jimenez J, Martin-Ballesteros E, Sureda A, Uralburu C, Lorenzo I, del Campo R, et al. Chemotherapy-induced nausea and vomiting in acute leukemia and stem cell transplant patients: results of a multicenter, observational study. Haematologica. 2006;91(1):84–91.
5. Kris MG, Hesketh PJ, Somerfield MR, Feyer P, Clark-Snow R, Koeller JM, et al. American Society of Clinical Oncology guideline for antiemetics in oncology: update 2006. J Clin Oncol. 2006;24(18):2932–47.
6. Blijlevens NM, Donnelly JP, de Pauw BE. Mucosal barrier injury: biology, pathology, clinical counterparts and consequences of intensive treatment for haematological malignancy: an overview. Bone Marrow Transplant. 2000;25(12):1269–78.
7. Sonis ST. The pathobiology of mucositis. Nat Rev Cancer. 2004;4(4):277–84.
8. Wardley AM, Jayson GC, Swindell R, Morgenstern GR, Chang J, Bloor R, et al. Prospective evaluation of oral mucositis in patients receiving myeloablative conditioning regimens and haematopoietic progenitor rescue. Br J Haematol. 2000;110(292):299.
9. Jones JA, Avritscher EB, Cooksley CD, Michelet M, Bekele BN, Elting LS. Epidemiology of treatment-associated mucosal injury after treatment with newer regimens for lymphoma, breast, lung, or colorectal cancer. Support Care Cancer. 2006;14(6):505–15.
10. Blijlevens N, Schwenkglenks M, Bacon P, D'Addio A, Einsele H, Maertens J, et al. Prospective oral mucositis audit: oral mucositis in patients receiving high-dose melphalan or BEAM conditioning chemotherapy–European Blood and Marrow Transplantation Mucositis Advisory Group. J Clin Oncol. 2008;26(9):1519–25.
11. McCann S, Schwenkglenks M, Bacon P, Einsele H, D'Addio A, Maertens J, et al. The Prospective Oral Mucositis Audit: relationship of severe oral mucositis with clinical and medical resource use outcomes in patients receiving high-dose melphalan or BEAM-conditioning chemotherapy and autologous SCT. Bone Marrow Transplant. 2008;43:141–7.
12. Crenn P, Vahedi K, Lavergne-Slove A, Cynober L, Matuchansky C, Messing B. Plasma citrulline: a marker of enterocyte mass in villous atrophy-associated small bowel disease. Gastroenterology. 2003;124:1210–9.
13. Herbers AH, Feuth T, Donnelly JP, Blijlevens NM. Citrulline-based assessment score: first choice for measuring and monitoring intestinal failure after high-dose chemotherapy. Ann Oncol. 2010;21(8):1706–11.
14. Herbers AH, Blijlevens NM, Donnelly JP, de Witte TJ. Bacteraemia coincides with low citrulline concentrations after high-dose melphalan in autologous HSCT recipients. Bone Marrow Transplant. 2008;42(5):345–9.
15. van der Velden W, Blijlevens NM, Feuth T, Donnelly JP. Febrile mucositis in haematopoietic SCT recipients. Bone Marrow Transplant. 2008;43:55–60.
16. Gamis AS, Howells WB, Swarte-Wallace J, Feusner JH, Buckley JD, Woods WG. Alpha hemolytic streptococcal infection during intensive treatment for acute myeloid leukemia: a report from the children's cancer group study CCG-2891. J Clin Oncol. 2000;18(9):1845–55.
17. Elting LS, Cooksley C, Chambers M, Cantor SB, Manzullo E, Rubenstein EB. The burdens of cancer therapy: clinical and economic outcomes of chemotherapy-induced mucositis. Cancer. 2003;98:1531–9.

18. Costa SF, Miceli MH, Anaissie EJ. Mucosa or skin as source of coagulase-negative staphylococcal bacteraemia? Lancet Infect Dis. 2004;4(5):278–86.
19. Costa SF, Barone AA, Miceli MH, van der Heijden I, Soares RE, Levin AS, et al. Colonization and molecular epidemiology of coagulase-negative Staphylococcal bacteremia in cancer patients: a pilot study. Am J Infect Control. 2006;34(1):36–40.
20. Gassas A, Grant R, Richardson S, Dupuis LL, Doyle J, Allen U, et al. Predictors of viridans streptococcal shock syndrome in bacteremic children with cancer and stem-cell transplant recipients. J Clin Oncol. 2004;22(7):1222–7.
21. Klastersky J, Paesmans M, Rubenstein EB, Boyer M, Elting L, Feld R, et al. The Multinational Association for Supportive Care in Cancer risk index: a multinational scoring system for identifying low-risk febrile neutropenic cancer patients. J Clin Oncol. 2000;18(16):3038–51.
22. Bodey GP, Buckley M, Sathe YS, Freireich EJ. Quantitative relationships between circulating leukocytes and infection in patients with acute leukemia. Ann Intern Med. 1966;64(2):328–40.
23. Bow EJ. Management of the febrile neutropenic cancer patient: lessons from 40 years of study. Clin Microbiol Infect. 2005;11 Suppl 5:24–9.
24. De Pauw BE, Deresinski SC, Feld R, lane-Allman EF, Donnelly JP. Ceftazidime compared with piperacillin and tobramycin for the empiric treatment of fever in neutropenic patients with cancer – a multicenter randomized trial. Ann Intern Med. 1994;120:834–44.
25. Vera-Llonch M, Oster G, Ford CM, Lu J, Sonis S. Oral mucositis and outcomes of allogeneic hematopoietic stem-cell transplantation in patients with hematologic malignancies. Support Care Cancer. 2006;15:491–6.
26. Blijlevens NM, Donnelly JP, DePauw BE. Inflammatory response to mucosal barrier injury after myeloablative therapy in allogeneic stem cell transplant recipients. Bone Marrow Transplant. 2005;36(8):703–7.
27. Gorschluter M, Schmitz V, Mey U, Hahn-Ast C, Schmidt-Wolf IG, Sauerbruch T. Endoscopy in patients with acute leukaemia after intensive chemotherapy. Leuk Res. 2008;32(10):1510–7.
28. Elting LS, Bodey GP, Keefe BH. Septicemia and shock syndrome due to viridans streptococci: a case-control study of predisposing factors. Clin Infect Dis. 1992;14(6):1201–7.
29. Gomez L, Martino R, Rolston KV. Neutropenic enterocolitis: spectrum of the disease and comparison of definite and possible cases. Clin Infect Dis. 1998;27:695–9.
30. Gorschluter M, Marklein G, Hofling K, Clarenbach R, Baumgartner S, Hah C, et al. Abdominal infections in patients with acute leukaemia: a prospective study applying ultrasonography and microbiology. Br J Haematol. 2002;117:351–8.
31. Dietrich CF, Hermann S, Klein S, Braden B. Sonographic signs of neutropenic enterocolitis. World J Gastroenterol. 2006;12(9):1397–402.
32. Cartoni C, Dragoni F, Micozzi A, Pescarmona E, Mecarocci S, Chirletti P, et al. Neutropenic enterocolitis in patients with acute leukemia: prognostic significance of bowel wall thickening detected by ultrasonography. J Clin Oncol. 2001;19:756–61.
33. Cunningham SC, Fakhry K, Bass BL, Napolitano LM. Neutropenic enterocolitis in adults: case series and review of the literature. Dig Dis Sci. 2005;50(2):215–20.
34. Davila ML. Neutropenic enterocolitis. Curr Treat Options Gastroenterol. 2006;9(3):249–55.
35. Spielberger R, Stiff P, Emmanouilides C. Efficacy of recombinant human keratinocyte growth factor (rHuKGF) in reducing mucositis in patients with hematologic malignancies undergoing autologous peripheral blood progenitor cell transplantation (auto-PBPCT) after radiation-based conditioning: results of a phase 2 trial (abstract no. 25). Proc Am Soc Clin Oncol. 2001;20(Pt 1):7a.
36. Ellis M, Zwaan F, Hedstrom U, Poynton CH, Kristensen J, Jumaa P, et al. Recombinant human interleukin 11 and bacterial infection in patients with haemological malignant disease undergoing chemotherapy: a double-blind placebo-controlled randomised trial. Lancet. 2003;361:275–80.
37. Gafter-Gvili A, Fraser A, Paul M, Leibovici L. Meta-analysis: antibiotic prophylaxis reduces mortality in neutropenic patients. Ann Intern Med. 2005;142(12 Pt 1):979–95.
38. Labbe AC, Su SH, Laverdiere M, Pepin J, Patino C, Cohen S, et al. High incidence of invasive aspergillosis associated with intestinal graft-versus-host disease following nonmyeloablative transplantation. Biol Blood Marrow Transplant. 2007;13(10):1192–200.

39. Lion T, Kosulin K, Landlinger C, Rauch M, Preuner S, Jugovic D, et al. Monitoring of adenovirus load in stool by real-time PCR permits early detection of impending invasive infection in patients after allogeneic stem cell transplantation. Leukemia. 2010;24(4):706–14.
40. Plantinga TS, van der Velden, Ferwerda B, van Spriel AB, Adema G, Feuth T, et al. Early stop polymorphism in human DECTIN-1 is associated with increased candida colonization in hematopoietic stem cell transplant recipients. Clin Infect Dis. 2009;49(5):724–32.
41. van der Velden W, Plantinga TS, Feuth T, Donnelly JP, Netea MG, Blijlevens NM. The incidence of acute graft-versus-host disease increases with Candida colonization depending the dectin-1 gene status. Clin Immunol. 2010;136(2):302–6.
42. van der Velden W, Blijlevens NM, Maas FM, Schaap NP, Jansen JH, van der Reijden BA, et al. NOD2 polymorphisms predict severe acute graft-versus-host and treatment-related mortality in T-cell-depleted haematopoietic stem cell transplantation. Bone Marrow Transplant. 2009;44(4):243–8.

Central Nervous System Infections 13

Martin Schmidt-Hieber

Contents

13.1 General Aspects of CNS Infections in Hematology Patients

13.1.1 Introduction

The first part of this chapter provides an overview that covers general aspects of central nervous system (CNS) infections in hematology patients, while the second part discusses selected causative organisms in detail. Noteworthy is the scarcity of data on CNS infections in hematology patients. Thus, diagnostic and therapeutic

M. Schmidt-Hieber
Clinic for Hematology, Oncology and Tumorimmunology,
Helios Clinic Berlin-Buch, Berlin, Germany
e-mail: Martin.schmidt-hieber@charite.de

G. Maschmeyer, K.V.I. Rolston (eds.), *Infections in Hematology*,
DOI 10.1007/978-3-662-44000-1_13

recommendations may be based on studies performed mainly in non-immunocompromised patients or those with acquired immunodeficiency syndrome (AIDS).

13.1.2 Epidemiology and Causative Organisms

Only limited data are available on the general epidemiology of CNS infections in hematology patients, and most analyses focus on specific patient cohorts such as patients after allogeneic stem cell transplantation (AlloSCT) or selected causative organisms (e.g., fungi or viruses). AlloSCT patients are among those at highest risk for infection and have a 1–15 % incidence of CNS infection [14, 32, 60].

Aspergillus spp. and *Toxoplasma gondii* are among the most frequent causative organisms of CNS infections in hematology patients, though the spectrum of organisms may vary considerably according to the underlying disease (including its treatment), geographical conditions, and other parameters. For example, *Toxoplasma gondii* has been identified as the leading causative agent of CNS infections among AlloSCT patients in Europe, whereas fungal CNS infections seem to prevail in North America [14, 20, 32]. The higher *Toxoplasma gondii* seroprevalence in Europe than in North America might explain this observation [73]. *In vivo* T cell depletion with agents such as alemtuzumab or OKT-3 prior to AlloSCT may enhance the risk of viral CNS infections [54, 69]. Invasive mucormycosis is a rare opportunistic infection that can directly invade the CNS from adjacent regions like the sinuses and should be considered particularly in patients with uncontrolled diabetes mellitus [6, 47]. Bacterial CNS infections are seldom seen in hematology patients but occur more often in conjunction with neurological malignancies or neurosurgical interventions [48, 59]. In addition, parasitic CNS infections (e.g., malaria, microsporidiosis, leishmaniasis, or trypanosomiasis) or CNS infections caused by other rare organisms such as West Nile virus have to be considered in some geographic areas [43, 70].

13.1.3 Clinical Symptoms

Two major types of cerebral infections can be distinguished according to clinical presentation and neuroimaging findings: localized parenchymatous infections such as abscesses or strokes and diffuse (meningo)encephalitis. The former typically presents with focal neurological symptoms like pareses and the latter with headache, nuchal rigidity, and consciousness alterations. However, clinical manifestations are frequently unspecific, particularly in immunocompromised patients, and may include both types of symptoms [48]. Neurological symptoms of CNS infections may initially be attenuated in patients who receive immunosuppressive treatment; they may also be mimicked by other conditions such as side effects of drugs (e.g., cyclosporine), cranial irradiation, metabolic disturbances, or CNS affection by the underlying malignancy.

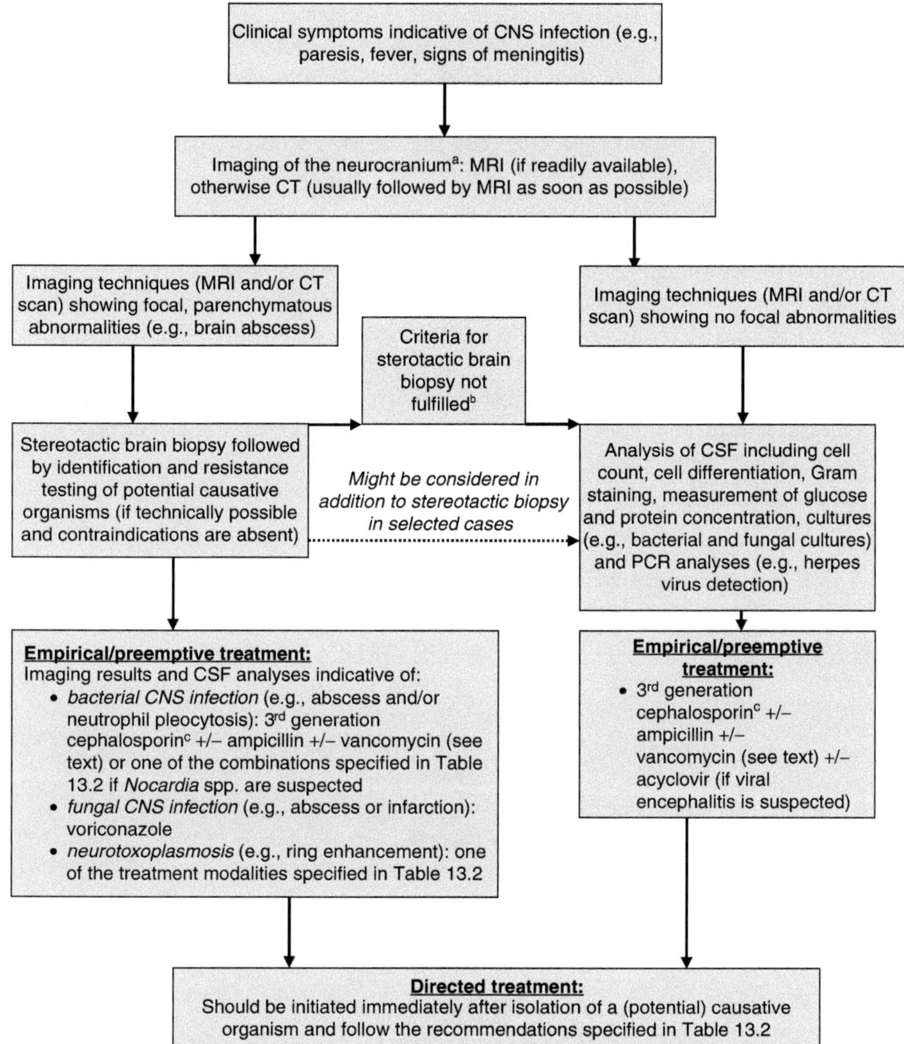

Fig. 13.1 Algorithm to diagnose and to treat empirically/preemptively CNS infections in hematology patients

13.1.4 Diagnostic Procedures

Definitive diagnosis of CNS infections still remains a major challenge in hematology patients and is often achieved only at autopsy. Diagnostic procedures may follow the algorithm depicted in Fig. 13.1. Any patient with suspected CNS infection should undergo neuroimaging as soon as possible. Magnetic resonance imaging (MRI) should be preferred, since studies have shown that a standard computed tomography (CT) scan may fail to demonstrate even severe cerebral involvement in conjunction with several CNS infections like human herpes virus-6 (HHV-6) encephalitis or neurotoxoplasmosis [38, 71]. Several reports have indicated that special MRI sequences such as diffusion-weighted imaging, apparent diffusion coefficient maps, perfusion-weighted imaging, and magnetic resonance spectroscopy may enhance the ability of standard MRI to detect CNS infections and distinguish them from other CNS abnormalities [8, 35].

Lumbar puncture and cerebrospinal fluid (CSF) analysis should follow the algorithm in Fig. 13.1 and are generally performed after neuroimaging in the absence of contraindications such as transfusion-refractory thrombocytopenia or critically increased intracranial pressure. Routine CSF analyses should be performed according to published guidelines and include the differential cell count, determination of the glucose and protein concentration, Gram staining, and bacterial cultures [13]. Additional CSF examinations such as specific PCR assays or India ink smears are useful in some situations (see below, also Table 13.1). The aim is to make an

Table 13.1 Recommended examinations of biopsy material or CSF to diagnose CNS infections caused by fungi, *Toxoplasma gondii*, or viruses in hematology patients

Causative organism		Recommended diagnostic examinations
Fungi	*Aspergillus* spp.	Biopsy material
		Fungal cultures and direct microscopy
		CSF (*Aspergillus meningitis*)
		Detection of *Aspergillus* DNA (PCR) or galactomannan (ELISA) (if feasible)
	Candida spp.	Biopsy material
		Fungal cultures and direct microscopy
		CSF
		Fungal cultures (sensitivity about 40–80 %) and direct microscopy (sensitivity about 40 %)[a]
		Enzyme immunoassay formats for rapid detection of species-specific amplicons and the use of real-time PCR (if feasible)
		Detection of *Candida* antigen mannan (if feasible)
	Cryptococcus neoformans	Biopsy material
		Direct microscopy (e.g., after PAS or H&E staining)
		CSF
		Fungal cultures (sensitivity and specificity up to 90–100 %)
		India ink smear examination (sensitivity 50–94 %), latex antigen test (sensitivity and specificity up to 100 %), and PCR (sensitivity and specificity nearly 100 %)
	Zygomycetes	Biopsy material
		Fungal cultures and direct microscopy
		Molecular-based tests (if feasible)

Table 13.1 (continued)

Causative organism		Recommended diagnostic examinations
Parasites	*Toxoplasma gondii*	Biopsy material or CSF Demonstration of tachyzoites and/or cysts after Wright-Giemsa and/or immunoperoxidase staining (can also be done after mouse inoculation or tissue cultures) CSF PCR (sensitivity about 50–90 %; specificity 90–100 %) Serological investigations (ELISA is more sensitive than latex agglutination test)
Viruses[b]	HHV-6	CSF PCR (sensitivity above 95 %, PCR in CSF can be positive without evidence of HHV-6 encephalitis in brain biopsy or autopsy specimens)
	EBV (virus encephalitis)	CSF PCR (can be combined with serological techniques)
	HSV	CSF PCR (sensitivity and specificity 90–100 % compared to brain biopsy) Immunoassays for intrathecal anti-HSV antibody production
	CMV	CSF PCR (sensitivity 82–100 %; specificity 86–100 %; PCR results may be confirmed by cultures)
	VZV	CSF PCR (sensitivity 80–95 %, specificity >95 %; copy number in real-time PCR may correlate with the clinical severity of encephalitis) Sensitivity of PCR might be enhanced by serological tests (e.g., detection of CSF VZV IgM)
	JC virus (PML)	Biopsy Required for definitive diagnosis: demonstration of the typical histopathologic triad (demyelination, bizarre astrocytes, and enlarged oligodendroglial nuclei), might be combined with tissue JC virus PCR CSF PCR (sensitivity 75–100 %), might be false positive (e.g., due to JC virus viremia in healthy individuals)

Obtical brighteners such as Calcofluor White or Blankophor and silver staining are recommended for staining of tissue samples whenever fungal infection is suspected

CMV cytomegalovirus, *EBV* Epstein-Barr virus, *ELISA* Enzyme-linked Immunosorbent Assay, *H&E* hematoxylin and eosin, *HHV-6* human herpesvirus-6, *HSV* herpes simplex virus, *PAS* periodic acid Schiff, *PML* progressive multifocal leukoencephalopathy, *VZV* varicella-zoster virus

[a]Sensitivity of *Candida* isolation in CSF can be improved by (1) culturing a large CSF volume (at least 5 mL), (2) analyzing ventricular CSF, (3) performing CSF centrifugation or using submicron filters, and (4) inoculating CSF into enriched liquid medium

[b]In some cases stereotactic or open brain biopsy followed by immunohistochemistry studies might be required to achieve the definitive diagnosis

unambiguous diagnosis of CNS infections, but this cannot always be achieved by the combination of clinical symptoms, CSF analyses, and neuroimaging. In patients with focal lesions, biopsy (e.g., stereotactic) and/or neurosurgical interventions (e.g., abscess drainage or resection of lesions) should therefore be considered as modalities for identifying causative organisms and determining their *in vitro* susceptibilities in individual patients [72].

13.1.5 Treatment

Efforts should always be directed towards identifying a causative organism and testing its susceptibility prior to the initiation of anti-infective drug therapy. Empirical or preemptive anti-infective drug therapy should typically be started immediately, as long as the causative pathogen has not yet been identified, since treatment delay may increase the mortality rate [65, 66]. Figure 13.1 specifies empirical or preemptive anti-infective drug regimens for different suspected organisms, while Table 13.2 summarizes recommendations for anti-infective drug therapy of defined CNS infections, including categories of evidence [28, 53].

However, other measures can be applied in addition to anti-infective drug therapy in some situations. For example, a significant increase in survival has been achieved by combined neurosurgical and voriconazole treatment in patients with cerebral aspergillosis [55]. Indwelling CNS devices should always be removed in patients with suspected or proven CNS *Candida* infections [33]. A placebo-controlled trial demonstrated improved outcome in adult bacterial meningitis patients, who received concomitant glucocorticoid therapy, but this could not be confirmed by a more recently published meta-analysis [12, 68]. Concomitant therapy with voriconazole and glucocorticoids has also been successfully used in the treatment of CNS aspergillosis [24]. However, adjunctive glucocorticoid therapy cannot be generally recommended in hematology patients with CNS infections, since data on this approach are still limited and were mainly acquired in immunocompetent hosts.

13.2 CNS Infections Related to Specific Causative Agents

13.2.1 Fungi

Though rarely associated with CNS infections in non-immunocompromised hosts, fungi are among the most common causative agents in hematology patients, particularly after AlloSCT or in conjunction with neutropenia. The predominant fungal pathogens are *Aspergillus* spp., mainly *A. fumigatus* and less frequently other species such as *A. nidulans*, *A. terreus*, and *A. flavus*, whereas *Candida* spp. and *Cryptococcus neoformans* are only occasionally detected in these patients [20, 39, 55]. Patients with CNS aspergillosis typically present with persistent fever, altered mental status, and focal neurological symptoms. MRI may reveal areas consistent

Table 13.2 Anti-infective drug therapy recommended for selected CNS infections in hematology patients

Causative organism		Recommended therapy
Fungi	*Aspergillus* spp.	Voriconazole (6 mg/kg q12h for the first 24 h, then 4 mg/kg q12h) [A II]
		Alternative
		Liposomal amphotericin B (3–5 mg/kg/d) or ABLC (5 mg/kg/d) [B III]
	Candida spp.	Voriconazole (6 mg/kg q12h for the first 24 h, then 4 mg/kg q12h) [BIII]
		Alternative
		Liposomal amphotericin B (3–4 mg/kg/d) or ABLC (5 mg/kg/d) [B III]
	Cryptococcus neoformans	Liposomal amphotericin B (3–4 mg/kg/d) + 5-fluorocytosine (25 mg/kg q6h) [A III][a]
		Alternative
		Liposomal amphotericin B (3–5 mg/kg/d) [B I] or ABLC (5 mg/kg/d) [B III] or
		Amphotericin B deoxycholate (0.7 mg/kg/d) + 5-fluorocytosine (25 mg/kg q6h) [B I] or
		Voriconazole (6 mg/kg q12h for the first 24 h, then 4 mg/kg q12h) [B III]
	Zygomycetes	Liposomal amphotericin B (3–5 mg/kg/d) [A II] or ABLC (5 mg/kg/d) [B III]
		Alternative
		Posaconazole (orally, 400 mg q12h or 200 mg q6h) [C III]
Parasites	*Toxoplasma gondii*	Pyrimethamine (orally, 100 mg load then 50 mg/d)[b] + sulfadiazine (orally, 50 mg/kg/d) [A I][c]
		Alternative
		Pyrimethamine (orally, 100 mg load then 50 mg/d)[b] + clindamycin (600 mg q6h)[d] [B II][c] or
		Trimethoprim/sulfamethoxazole (orally or intravenously, 10 mg/kg/d and 50 mg/kg/d) [B II][c]
Viruses	HHV-6	Ganciclovir (5 mg/kg q12h) [B III] or foscarnet (60 mg/kg q8h) [B III][e]
	EBV (virus encephalitis)	No antiviral treatment [C III] or ganciclovir (5 mg/kg q12h) [C III]
		Acyclovir is not recommended [D III]
	HSV	Acyclovir (10 mg/kg q8h) [A I]
	CMV	Ganciclovir (5 mg/kg q12h) or foscarnet (60 mg/kg q8h) as single agent [A III] or a combination of both [B III]
	VZV	Acyclovir (10 mg/kg q8h) [A III] or ganciclovir (5 mg/kg q12h) [C III]
	JC virus (PML)	Cidofovir is not recommended [D II]

Table 13.2 (continued)

Causative organism		Recommended therapy
Bacteria	*Listeria monocytogenes*	Ampicillin (2 g q4h) +/– aminoglycoside (for at least the first 7–10 days) [B III] or meropenem (2 g q8h) [C III]
	Pseudomonas spp.	Ceftazidime (2 g q8h) +/– aminoglycoside [B III] or
		Meropenem (2 g q8h) +/– aminoglycoside [C III]
	Nocardia spp.	Imipenem (0.5 g q6h) + amikacin (5 mg/kg q8h) [B III][f] or
		Trimethoprim/sulfamethoxazole (5–10 mg/kg q12h)[g] + imipenem (0.5 g q6h) + amikacin (5 mg/kg q8h) [B III][f] or
		Trimethoprim/sulfamethoxazole (5–10 mg/kg q12h)[g] + ceftriaxone (2 g/d) + amikacin (5 mg/kg q8h) [B III][f]
	MSSA	Oxacillin (1.5–2 g q4h) [B III] or nafcillin (1.5–2 g q4h) [B III] or meropenem (2 g q8h) [B III]
	MRSA	Vancomycin (0.5 g q6h or 1.0 g q12h) [B III] or linezolid (0.6 g q12h) [B III]

Evidence level and strength of recommendation are given in parenthesis. Treatment should commonly be started intravenously if not otherwise be specified. Possible contraindications or dosage adjustments, as in the case of renal insufficiency, should follow recommendations specified in the investigator's brochure. Anti-infective treatment should be adjusted according to the results of *in vitro* susceptibility testing. Reversal of immunosuppression (e.g., following AlloSCT) should be aimed whenever possible

ABLC amphotericin B lipid complex, *MSSA* methicillin-sensitive *S. aureus*, *MRSA* methicillin-resistant *S. aureus*

[a]For 2 weeks, followed by fluconazole for at least 6 months

[b]Should be combined with folinic acid

[c]For 4–6 weeks, then half of the original dosage as maintenance therapy for 3 months

[d]Can be given intravenously for 3 weeks and then orally

[e]Or a combination of both agents

[f]Might be adjusted to oral monotherapy (e.g., trimethoprim/sulfamethoxazole) according to *in vitro* susceptibility test results if the patient improves

[g]Referring to the trimethoprim component

with infarction, ring-enhanced lesions due to abscess formation, or dural or vascular infiltration from adjacent regions (Fig. 13.2a) [18]. CSF fungal cultures are typically negative for *Aspergillus* spp. but recent observations indicate that CSF galactomanan or PCR assays might be useful tools to diagnose CNS aspergillosis in selected cases [2, 45, 58]. Definitive diagnosis of CNS aspergillosis frequently requires biopsy of lesions. Typical septate hyphae might be demonstrated after Grocott silver or H&E staining (Fig. 13.3).

Voriconazole should be preferred for CNS aspergillosis, since it has acceptable CSF penetration and a relatively favorable overall response rate of 35 % [55]. Liposomal amphotericin B might be a second treatment option (Table 13.2). Conventional amphotericin B deoxycholate should not be used

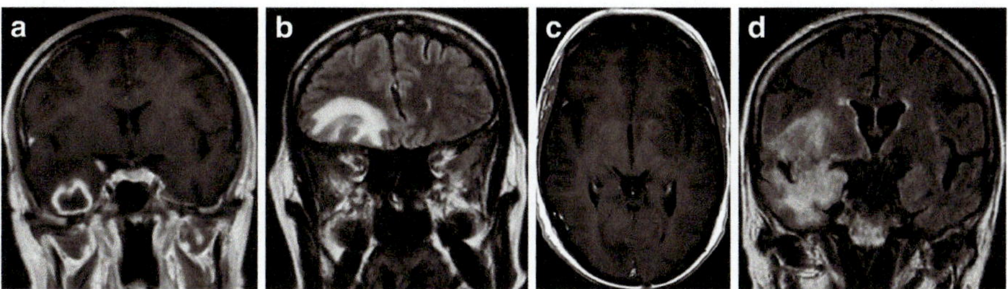

Fig. 13.2 Cranial MRI images illustrating typical abnormalities of different CNS infections in hematology patients. Shown are T1-weighted sequences after intravenous application of contrast medium (**a**, **c**) and dark fluid sequences (**b**, **d**). (**a**) CNS aspergillosis with a partially liquid lesion in the right temporal lobe surrounded by pronounced edema. (**b**) CNS mucormycosis with a large, frontobasal lesion and perifocal edema. (**c**) Neurotoxoplasmosis with multiple punctual and ring-configured hyperintense lesions in the cerebellum, basal ganglia, and cortical, subcortical, and subependymal regions. (**d**) Hyperintense laminar lesions with right frontotemporal preponderance in a patient with herpes encephalitis (The MRI images were kindly provided by W. Grassl, Clinic for Radiology and Nuclear Medicine, Charité Campus Benjamin Franklin, Berlin, Germany)

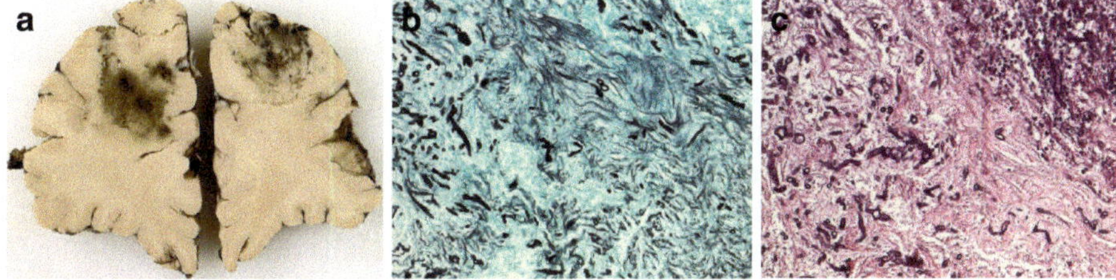

Fig. 13.3 (**a**) Gross photograph of a coronal brain section showing multiple ill-defined lesions in the frontal lobe in a patient with cerebral aspergillosis. (**b**, **c**) Photomicrographs (original magnification: ×200) show septate hyphae diffusely scattered throughout these lesions (Grocott silver stain (**b**) and H&E staining (**c**)) (The photographs were kindly provided by W. Stenzel, Department of Neuropathology, Charité Campus Mitte, Berlin, Germany)

anymore because of its unfavorable toxicity profile and inferior clinical efficacy [23]. The prognosis of CNS aspergillosis is still poor in adults with a mortality of about 70 %, but more favorable in children with a mortality of about 40 % (after 1990) [15, 55].

C. albicans and recently also other *Candida* spp. such as *C. tropicalis* or *C. glabrata* may cause meningitis presenting with subacute onset and with fever and headache [33]. However, *Candida* spp. may also cause cerebral microabscesses and occasionally macroabscesses presenting with focal neurological signs. Since CT and CSF analysis are rarely diagnostic for *Candida* microabscesses, they are often only diagnosed at autopsy [50]. In patients with *Candida* meningitis, CT might show hydrocephalus, and yeasts can be detected in the CSF in about 40 % by direct microscopy and in about 80 % by fungal cultures (Table 13.1) [50, 53]. Despite the lack of systematic data comparing MRI and CT in the diagnosis of *Candida* CNS infections, MRI is considered more sensitive and should thus be preferred. New techniques such as the PCR or detection of the *Candida* antigen mannan in the CSF might also be useful and are currently being further evaluated [3, 53]. *Candida* CNS infection might respond to voriconazole or liposomal amphotericin B, but only limited (mainly preclinical) data are available on their use in the treatment of *Candida* CNS infections [31, 51].

Cryptococcus neoformans typically causes meningitis. In hematology patients, it may present with acute or subacute onset and atypical symptoms, including fever, confusion, headache, or diplopia [39]. MRI may reveal signs of meningitis, dilated Virchow-Robin spaces, cyst-like structures, and granuloma of the choroid plexus [1, 62]. The diagnosis can be made in most cases by CSF fungal cultures, PCR analysis, and India ink smear microscopy (Table 13.1) [49]. Treatment of cryptococcal meningitis can comprise a combination of amphotericin B deoxycholate (preferentially as continuous infusion) and 5-fluorocytosine (Table 13.2) [4, 16, 41]. However, liposomal amphotericin B or voriconazole also seem to be useful treatment options since these two agents may have a better toxicity profile than amphotericin B deoxycholate [5, 9, 22, 25, 30, 41].

Mucormycosis is a rare opportunistic infection caused by *Zygomycetes*. The most frequent species include *Absidia corymbifera*, *Rhizopus* spp. and *Apophysomyces elegans*, but the spectrum shows geographic variations [6, 47]. It affects mainly the lungs and more rarely the soft tissue or the rhino-sinu-orbital region; the brain is involved in about 15 % of cases [47]. The rhinocerebral type typically presents with facial pain and swelling. Though this disease is often suspected initially from clinical appearance and imaging results (Fig. 13.2b), the diagnosis should always be confirmed by biopsy. Liposomal amphotericin B now seems to be the most active anti-infective agent for invasive mucormycosis (Table 13.2) [10, 40, 47, 56, 61]. Preliminary data further suggest that a combination of (liposomal) amphotericin B and caspofungin might be useful to treat invasive [10, 27, 44].

Posaconazole can be used in the case of intolerance, contraindications, or unresponsiveness to liposomal amphotericin B [10, 19]. However, it should be noted that this agent has poor CSF penetration, at least if the blood-CSF barrier is intact, and that breakthrough mucormycosis has been reported under posaconazole prophylaxis [47]. In addition, surgical debridement and correction of uncontrolled diabetes mellitus should always be considered in patients with invasive mucormycosis, since both these measures might improve clinical outcome [6, 10, 40, 61].

13.2.2 Parasites

Only neurotoxoplasmosis, one of the most frequent types of CNS infections in hematology patients, will be presented here in detail. Most data on neurotoxoplasmosis have been acquired in AIDS patients, and there have thus far been few reports on CNS infection by *Toxoplasma gondii* in hematology patients [17, 34, 37, 46, 52, 57]. Common clinical symptoms of neurotoxoplasmosis after AlloSCT include psychiatric abnormalities, seizures, and paresis [46]. MRI typically shows multiple lesions located in basal ganglia and subcortically located in supra- and infratentorial regions (Fig. 13.2c). However, typical nodular or ring enhancement surrounded by edema is observed in only about 60 % of patients after AlloSCT [36]. The diagnosis of neurotoxoplasmosis is also based on the detection of tachyzoites and/or cysts in the CSF or tissue sections, cultures, CSF PCR analysis, and serological CSF studies (Table 13.1) [52]. Detection of IgM antibodies in CSF is of negligible value in the diagnosis of neurotoxoplasmosis [7]. Neurotoxoplasmosis should primarily be treated with a combination of pyrimethamine and sulfadiazine or, alternatively, with a combination of pyrimethamine and clindamycin or the fixed combination trimethoprim-sulfamethoxazole [11, 26, 63]. However, it should be noted that these recommendations are based on trials performed in AIDS patients with neurotoxoplasmosis. AlloSCT recipients have received various combinations of these agents, and treatment was efficient in some of them [21]. The mortality of neurotoxoplasmosis in AlloSCT recipients is still high at 60–90 % [37, 46, 52].

13.2.3 Viruses

Hematology patients develop viral CNS infections mainly after AlloSCT or secondary to intensive T cell immunosuppressive treatment, e.g., with fludarabine or alemtuzumab. Viral encephalitis is observed in up to 12 % of AlloSCT recipients after *in vivo* T cell depletion with agents such as alemtuzumab or OKT-3 [54, 69]. Viral CNS infection after AlloSCT is most often caused by HHV-6 and less frequently by Epstein-Barr virus (EBV), herpes simplex virus (HSV), JC virus (progressive multifocal leukoencephalopathy (PML)), varicella-zoster virus (VZV), cytomegalovirus (CMV), or adenovirus. More than one virus can be detected in the CSF in about 15 % of AlloSCT recipients with viral encephalitis [54]. Viral CNS infections present mainly as (meningo)encephalitis but also as strokes (e.g., VZV infection), leukoencephalopathy (e.g., JC virus infection), or mass lesions (e.g., EBV-associated lymphoma) [42]. Typical clinical symptoms are consciousness disturbances, personality changes, fever, seizures, and pareses. The method of choice for diagnosing viral encephalitis is PCR on CSF samples, which provides 80–100 % sensitivity and specificity for the majority of viral pathogens (Table 13.1). However, a systematic comparison of CSF virus PCR and brain biopsy, the former reference standard of viral encephalitis, has only been conducted for selected viruses such as HSV, while valid data on diagnosis of viral encephalitis in hematology patients are still lacking [29]. CSF analysis frequently reveals lymphocytic pleocytosis and a slightly elevated protein concentration, but the CSF cell count and the protein concentration may both be normal in about 50 % of AlloSCT recipients [54]. Viral encephalitis can often be diagnosed by the combination of clinical symptoms, neuroimaging results (Fig. 13.2d), and CSF PCR, but some cases require stereotactic or even open brain biopsy (e.g., PML or EBV-associated lymphoma) to achieve the definitive diagnosis [64]. Recommendations for antiviral treatment are summarized in Table 13.2. Despite the poor overall prognosis of viral encephalitis with a median survival of 94 days after onset in AlloSCT recipients, it should be noted that a more favorable outcome may be achieved for selected causative viruses such as HSV [54].

13.2.4 Bacteria

Compared to fungal CNS infections and neurotoxoplasmosis, bacterial CNS infections are generally rare in hematology patients, including AlloSCT recipients. However, they occur occasionally in selected subgroups of patients such as those who have undergone neurosurgical interventions or suffer from CNS malignancies [48, 59]. Bacterial meningitis can be caused in immunocompetent as well as immunocompromised patients by bacteria such as *Neisseria meningitidis*, *S. pneumoniae*, *Listeria* spp., *Enterobacteriaceae*, *Pseudomonas* spp., and *Staphylococcus* spp. A shift towards Gram-positive cocci, particularly *S. aureus* and coagulase-negative *Staphylococcus* spp., has recently been reported in cancer patients with bacterial encephalitis [48]. However, bacterial brain abscesses caused by *S. aureus*, *Nocardia* spp., and *Bacteroides* have been reported in these patients as well. Common clinical symptoms of bacterial meningitis in cancer patients are fever, headache (in about 50 % each), an altered mental status (in about 35 %), focal neurological deficits, and nuchal rigidity (in about 15 % each). Noteworthy is the fact that the triad of fever, nuchal rigidity, and altered mental status, characteristic for bacterial meningitis in non-immunocompromised hosts, seems to have a much lower incidence (approximately 5 %) in patients with malignancies [48]. Diagnosis is based on imaging techniques and CSF analysis. Whenever possible, CSF analysis should precede the initiation of antibiotic treatment, since Gram staining and CSF cultures are less frequently positive thereafter [66]. About 75 % of cancer patients with bacterial encephalitis have an elevated CSF cell count with polymorphonuclear preponderance [66]. The abovementioned analysis disclosed a median CSF white blood cell count of only 74 cells/μl in cancer patients, though it is ≥100 cells/μl in more than 90 % of non-immunocompromised patients with bacterial meningitis [48, 67]. The CSF might be only unspecifically altered in the case of bacterial brain abscesses, and definitive diagnosis may require brain biopsy. Empirical or definitive treatment of bacterial meningitis should be initiated immediately and should follow the recommendations specified in Table 13.2 and Fig. 13.1. For empirical therapy of purulent meningitis, the Infectious Disease Society of America (IDSA) recommends a combination of vancomycin, a third-generation cephalosporin, and ampicillin for patients over 50 years and vancomycin combined with a third-generation cephalosporin in patients aged 2–50 years, provided that *Listeria monocytogenes* is not suspected (Fig. 13.1) [65].

Acknowledgment The author would like to thank Dr. J. Weirowski for her editorial support.

References

1. Andreula CF, Burdi N, Carella A. CNS cryptococcosis in AIDS: spectrum of MR findings. J Comput Assist Tomogr. 1993;17:438–41.
2. Antinori S, Corbellino M, Meroni L, Resta F, Sollima S, Tonolini M, et al. Aspergillus meningitis: a rare clinical manifestation of central nervous system aspergillosis. Case report and review of 92 cases. J Infect. 2013;66:218–38.
3. Biesbroek JM, Verduyn Lunel FM, Kragt JJ, Amelink GJ, Frijns CJ. Culture-negative Candida meningitis diagnosed by detection of Candida mannan antigen in CSF. Neurology. 2013;81:1555–6.
4. Brouwer AE, Rajanuwong A, Chierakul W, Griffin GE, Larsen RA, White NJ, et al. Combination antifungal therapies for HIV-associated cryptococcal meningitis: a randomised trial. Lancet. 2004;363:1764–7.
5. Chaaban S, Wheat LJ, Assi M. Cryptococcal meningitis post autologous stem cell transplantation. Transpl Infect Dis. 2014;16:473–6.
6. Chakrabarti A, Chatterjee SS, Das A, Panda N, Shivaprakash MR, Kaur A, et al. Invasive zygomycosis in India: experience in a tertiary care hospital. Postgrad Med J. 2009;85: 573–81.
7. Chandramukhi A. Diagnosis of neurotoxoplasmosis by antibody detection in cerebrospinal (CSF) fluid using Latex Agglutination Test and ELISA. J Commun Dis. 2004;36:153–8.
8. Charlot M, Pialat JB, Obadia N, Boibieux A, Streichenberger N, Meyronnet D, et al. Diffusion-weighted imaging in brain aspergillosis. Eur J Neurol. 2007;14:912–6.
9. Coker RJ, Viviani M, Gazzard BG, Du Pont B, Pohle HD, Murphy SM, et al. Treatment of cryptococcosis with liposomal amphotericin B (AmBisome) in 23 patients with AIDS. AIDS. 1993;7:829–35.
10. Cornely OA, Arikan-Akdagli S, Dannaoui E, Groll AH, Lagrou K, el Chakrabarti A. ESCMID and ECMM joint clinical guidelines for the diagnosis and management of mucormycosis 2013. Clin Microbiol Infect. 2014;20:5–26.
11. Dannemann B, McCutchan JA, Israelski D, Antoniskis D, Leport C, Luft B, et al. Treatment of toxoplasmic encephalitis in patients with AIDS. A randomized trial comparing pyrimethamine plus clindamycin to pyrimethamine plus sulfadiazine. The California Collaborative Treatment Group. Ann Intern Med. 1992;116:33–43.
12. De Gans J, van de Beek D, European Dexamethasone in Adulthood Bacterial Meningitis Study Investigators. Dexamethasone in adults with bacterial meningitis. N Engl J Med. 2002;347: 1549–56.
13. Deisenhammer F, Bartos A, Egg R, Gilhus NE, Giovannoni G, Rauer S, EFNS Task Force, et al. Guidelines on routine cerebrospinal fluid analysis. Report from an EFNS task force. Eur J Neurol. 2006;13:913–22.
14. Denier C, Bourhis JH, Lacroix C, Koscielny S, Bosq J, Sigal R, et al. Spectrum and prognosis of neurologic complications after hematopoietic transplantation. Neurology. 2006;67: 1990–7.
15. Dotis J, Iosifidis E, Roilides E. Central nervous system aspergillosis in children: a systematic review of reported cases. Int J Infect Dis. 2007;11:381–93.
16. Falci DR, Lunardi LW, Ramos CG, Bay MB, Aquino VR, Goldani LZ. Continuous infusion of amphotericin B deoxycholate in the treatment of cryptococcal meningoencephalitis: analysis of safety and fungicidal activity. Clin Infect Dis. 2010;50:e26–9.
17. Fricker-Hidalgo H, Bulabois CE, Brenier-Pinchart MP, Hamidfar R, Garban F, Brion JP, et al. Diagnosis of toxoplasmosis after allogeneic stem cell transplantation: results of DNA detection and serological techniques. Clin Infect Dis. 2009;48:e9–15.
18. Gabelmann A, Klein S, Kern W, Krüger S, Brambs HJ, Rieber-Brambs A, et al. Relevant imaging findings of cerebral aspergillosis on MRI: a retrospective case-based study in immunocompromised patients. Eur J Neurol. 2007;14:548–55.

19. Greenberg RN, Mullane K, van Burik JA, Raad I, Abzug MJ, Anstead G, et al. Posaconazole as salvage therapy for zygomycosis. Antimicrob Agents Chemother. 2006;50:126–33.
20. Hagensee ME, Bauwens JE, Kjos B, Bowden RA. Brain abscess following marrow transplantation: experience at the Fred Hutchinson Cancer Research Center, 1984–1992. Clin Infect Dis. 1994;19:402–8.
21. Hakko E, Ozkan HA, Karaman K, Gulbas Z. Analysis of cerebral toxoplasmosis in a series of 170 allogeneic hematopoietic stem cell transplant patients. Transpl Infect Dis. 2013;15: 575–80.
22. Hamill RJ, Sobel JD, El-Sadr W, Johnson PC, Graybill JR, Javaly K, et al. Comparison of 2 doses of liposomal amphotericin B and conventional amphotericin B deoxycholate for treatment of AIDS-associated acute cryptococcal meningitis: a randomized, double-blind clinical trial of efficacy and safety. Clin Infect Dis. 2010;51:225–32.
23. Herbrecht R, Denning DW, Patterson TF, Bennett JE, Greene RE, Oestmann JW, Invasive Fungal Infections Group of the European Organisation for Research and Treatment of Cancer and the Global Aspergillus Study Group, et al. Voriconazole versus amphotericin B for primary therapy of invasive aspergillosis. N Engl J Med. 2002;347:408–15.
24. Hiraga A, Uzawa A, Shibuya M, Numata T, Sunami S, Kamitsukasa I. Neuroaspergillosis in an immunocompetent patient successfully treated with voriconazole and a corticosteroid. Intern Med. 2009;48:1225–9.
25. Jadhav MP, Bamba A, Shinde VM, Gogtay N, Kshirsagar NA, Bichile LS, et al. Liposomal amphotericin B (Fungisome) for the treatment of cryptococcal meningitis in HIV/AIDS patients in India: a multicentric, randomized controlled trial. J Postgrad Med. 2010;56:71–5.
26. Katlama C, De Wit S, O'Doherty E, Van Glabeke M, Clumeck N. Pyrimethamine-clindamycin vs. pyrimethamine-sulfadiazine as acute and long-term therapy for toxoplasmic encephalitis in patients with AIDS. Clin Infect Dis. 1996;22:268–75.
27. Kazak E, Aslan E, Akalın H, Saraydaroğlu O, Hakyemez B, Erişen L, et al. A mucormycosis case treated with a combination of caspofungin and amphotericin B. J Mycol Med. 2013;23:179–84.
28. Kish MA, Infectious Diseases Society of America. Guide to development of practice guidelines. Clin Infect Dis. 2001;32:851–4.
29. Lakeman FD, Whitley RJ. Diagnosis of herpes simplex encephalitis: application of polymerase chain reaction to cerebrospinal fluid from brain-biopsied patients and correlation with disease. National Institute of Allergy and Infectious Diseases Collaborative Antiviral Study Group. J Infect Dis. 1995;171:857–63.
30. Loyse A, Wilson D, Meintjes G, Jarvis JN, Bicanic T, Bishop L, et al. Comparison of the early fungicidal activity of high-dose fluconazole, voriconazole, and flucytosine as second-line drugs given in combination with amphotericin B for the treatment of HIV-associated cryptococcal meningitis. Clin Infect Dis. 2012;54:121–8.
31. Majithiya J, Sharp A, Parmar A, Denning DW, Warn PA. Efficacy of isavuconazole, voriconazole and fluconazole in temporarily neutropenic murine models of disseminated Candida tropicalis and Candida krusei. J Antimicrob Chemother. 2009;63:161–6.
32. Maschke M, Dietrich U, Prumbaum M, Kastrup O, Turowski B, Schaefer UW, et al. Opportunistic CNS infection after bone marrow transplantation. Bone Marrow Transplant. 1999;23:1167–76.
33. Mattiuzzi G, Giles FJ. Management of intracranial fungal infections in patients with haematological malignancies. Br J Haematol. 2005;131:287–300.
34. Meers S, Lagrou K, Theunissen K, Dierickx D, Delforge M, Devos T, et al. Myeloablative conditioning predisposes patients for Toxoplasma gondii reactivation after allogeneic stem cell transplantation. Clin Infect Dis. 2010;50:1127–34.
35. Muccio CF, Esposito G, Bartolini A, Cerase A. Cerebral abscesses and necrotic cerebral tumours: differential diagnosis by perfusion-weighted magnetic resonance imaging. Radiol Med. 2008;113:747–57.
36. Mueller-Mang C, Mang TG, Kalhs P, Thurnher MM. Imaging characteristics of toxoplasmosis encephalitis after bone marrow transplantation: report of two cases and review of the literature. Neuroradiology. 2006;48:84–9.

37. Mulanovich VE, Ahmed SI, Öztürk T, Khokhar FA, Kontoyiannis DP, de Lima M. Toxoplasmosis in allo-SCT patients: risk factors and outcomes at a transplantation center with a low incidence. Bone Marrow Transplant. 2011;46:273–7.
38. Noguchi T, Yoshiura T, Hiwatashi A, Togao O, Yamashita K, Nagao E, et al. CT and MRI findings of human herpesvirus 6-associated encephalopathy: comparison with findings of herpes simplex virus encephalitis. AJR Am J Roentgenol. 2010;194:754–60.
39. Pagano L, Fianchi L, Caramatti C, D'Antonio D, Melillo L, Caira M, Gruppo Italiano Malattie EMatologiche dell'Adulto Infection Program, et al. Cryptococcosis in patients with hematologic malignancies. A report from GIMEMA-infection. Haematologica. 2004;89:852–6.
40. Pagano L, Valentini CG, Posteraro B, Girmenia C, Ossi C, Pan A, et al. Zygomycosis in Italy: a survey of FIMUA-ECMM (Federazione Italiana di Micopatologia Umana ed Animale and European Confederation of Medical Mycology). J Chemother. 2009;21:322–9.
41. Perfect JR, Dismukes WE, Dromer F, Goldman DL, Graybill JR, Hamill RJ, et al. Clinical practice guidelines for the management of cryptococcal disease: 2010 update by the Infectious Diseases Society of America. Clin Infect Dis. 2010;50:291–322.
42. Pruitt AA. Central nervous system infections in cancer patients. Semin Neurol. 2004;24: 435–52.
43. Reddy P, Davenport R, Ratanatharathorn V, Reynolds C, Silver S, Ayash L, et al. West Nile virus encephalitis causing fatal CNS toxicity after hematopoietic stem cell transplantation. Bone Marrow Transplant. 2004;33:109–12.
44. Reed C, Bryant R, Ibrahim AS, Edwards Jr J, Filler SG, Goldberg R, et al. Combination polyene-caspofungin treatment of rhino-orbital-cerebral mucormycosis. Clin Infect Dis. 2008;47:364–71.
45. Reinwald M, Buchheidt D, Hummel M, Duerken M, Bertz H, Schwerdtfeger R, et al. Diagnostic performance of an Aspergillus-specific nested PCR assay in cerebrospinal fluid samples of immunocompromised patients for detection of central nervous system aspergillosis. PLoS One. 2013;8:e56706.
46. Roemer E, Blau IW, Basara N, Kiehl MG, Bischoff M, Günzelmann S, et al. Toxoplasmosis, a severe complication in allogeneic hematopoietic stem cell transplantation: successful treatment strategies during a 5-year single-center experience. Clin Infect Dis. 2001;32:E1–8.
47. Rüping MJ, Heinz WJ, Kindo AJ, Rickerts V, Lass-Flörl C, Beisel C, et al. Forty-one recent cases of invasive zygomycosis from a global clinical registry. J Antimicrob Chemother. 2010;65:296–302.
48. Safdieh JE, Mead PA, Sepkowitz KA, Kiehn TE, Abrey LE. Bacterial and fungal meningitis in patients with cancer. Neurology. 2008;70:943–7.
49. Saha DC, Xess I, Biswas A, Bhowmik DM, Padma MV. Detection of Cryptococcus by conventional, serological and molecular methods. J Med Microbiol. 2009;58:1098–105.
50. Sánchez-Portocarrero J, Pérez-Cecilia E, Corral O, Romero-Vivas J, Picazo JJ. The central nervous system and infection by Candida species. Diagn Microbiol Infect Dis. 2000;37:169–79.
51. Scarcella A, Pasquariello MB, Giugliano B, Vendemmia M, de Lucia A. Liposomal amphotericin B treatment for neonatal fungal infections. Pediatr Infect Dis J. 1998;17:146–8.
52. Schmidt M, Sonneville R, Schnell D, Bigé N, Hamidfar R, Mongardon N, et al. Clinical features and outcomes in patients with disseminated toxoplasmosis admitted to intensive care: a multicenter study. Clin Infect Dis. 2013;57:1535–41.
53. Schmidt-Hieber M, Zweigner J, Uharek L, Blau IW, Thiel E. Central nervous system infections in immunocompromised patients: update on diagnostics and therapy. Leuk Lymphoma. 2009;50:24–36.
54. Schmidt-Hieber M, Schwender J, Heinz WJ, Zabelina T, Kühl JS, Mousset S, et al. Viral encephalitis after allogeneic stem cell transplantation: a rare complication with distinct characteristics of different causative agents. Haematologica. 2011;96:142–9.
55. Schwartz S, Ruhnke M, Ribaud P, Corey L, Driscoll T, Cornely OA, et al. Improved outcome in central nervous system aspergillosis, using voriconazole treatment. Blood. 2005;106: 2641–5.

56. Skiada A, Pagano L, Groll A, Zimmerli S, Dupont B, Lagrou K, et al. European Confederation of Medical Mycology Working Group on Zygomycosis. Zygomycosis in Europe: analysis of 230 cases accrued by the registry of the European Confederation of Medical Mycology (ECMM) Working Group on Zygomycosis between 2005 and 2007. Clin Microbiol Infect. 2011;17:1859–67.
57. Small TN, Leung L, Stiles J, Kiehn TE, Malak SA, O'Reilly RJ, et al. Disseminated toxoplasmosis following T cell-depleted related and unrelated bone marrow transplantation. Bone Marrow Transplant. 2000;25:969–73.
58. Soeffker G, Wichmann D, Loderstaedt U, Sobottka I, Deuse T, Kluge S. Aspergillus galactomannan antigen for diagnosis and treatment monitoring in cerebral aspergillosis. Prog Transplant. 2013;23:71–4.
59. Sommers LM, Hawkins DS. Meningitis in pediatric cancer patients: a review of forty cases from a single institution. Pediatr Infect Dis J. 1999;18:902–7.
60. Sostak P, Padovan CS, Yousry TA, Ledderose G, Kolb HJ, Straube A. Prospective evaluation of neurological complications after allogeneic bone marrow transplantation. Neurology. 2003;60:842–8.
61. Sun HY, Forrest G, Gupta KL, Aguado JM, Lortholary O, Julia MB, et al. Rhino-orbital-cerebral zygomycosis in solid organ transplant recipients. Transplantation. 2010;90:85–92.
62. Tien RD, Chu PK, Hesselink JR, Duberg A, Wiley C. Intracranial cryptococcosis in immunocompromised patients: CT and MR findings in 29 cases. AJNR Am J Neuroradiol. 1991;12:283–9.
63. Torre D, Casari S, Speranza F, Donisi A, Gregis G, Poggio A, et al. Randomized trial of trimethoprim-sulfamethoxazole versus pyrimethamine-sulfadiazine for therapy of toxoplasmic encephalitis in patients with AIDS. Italian Collaborative Study Group. Antimicrob Agents Chemother. 1998;42:1346–9.
64. Tunkel AR, Glaser CA, Bloch KC, Sejvar JJ, Marra CM, Roos KL, et al. The management of encephalitis: clinical practice guidelines by the Infectious Diseases Society of America. Clin Infect Dis. 2008;47:303–27.
65. Tunkel AR, Hartman BJ, Kaplan SL, Kaufman BA, Roos KL, Scheld WM, et al. Practice guidelines for the management of bacterial meningitis. Clin Infect Dis. 2004;39:1267–84.
66. Tunkel AR, Scheld WM. Acute bacterial meningitis. Lancet. 1995;346:1675–80.
67. Van de Beek D, de Gans J, Spanjaard L, Weisfelt M, Reitsma JB, Vermeulen M. Clinical features and prognostic factors in adults with bacterial meningitis. N Engl J Med. 2004;351:1849–59.
68. Van de Beek D, Farrar JJ, de Gans J, Mai NT, Molyneux EM, Peltola H, et al. Adjunctive dexamethasone in bacterial meningitis: a meta-analysis of individual patient data. Lancet Neurol. 2010;9:254–63.
69. Vu T, Carrum G, Hutton G, Heslop HE, Brenner MK, Kamble R. Human herpesvirus-6 encephalitis following allogeneic hematopoietic stem cell transplantation. Bone Marrow Transplant. 2007;39:705–9.
70. Walker M, Kublin JG, Zunt JR. Parasitic central nervous system infections in immunocompromised hosts: malaria, microsporidiosis, leishmaniasis, and African trypanosomiasis. Clin Infect Dis. 2006;42:115–25.
71. Weenink JJ, Weenink AG, Geerlings SE, van Gool T, Bemelman FJ. Severe cerebral toxoplasma infection cannot be excluded by a normal CT scan. Neth J Med. 2009;67:150–2.
72. Xiao F, Tseng MY, Teng LJ, Tseng HM, Tsai JC. Brain abscess: clinical experience and analysis of prognostic factors. Surg Neurol. 2005;63:442–9.
73. Zuber P, Jacquier P. Epidemiology of toxoplasmosis: worldwide status. Schweiz Med Wochenschr Suppl. 1995;65:19S–22.

Part IV

Antimicrobial Treatment (Including Important Pitfalls, Toxicities and Interactions)

Antibacterial Agents

14

Winfried V. Kern

Contents

Traditionally, antipseudomonal penicillins combined with an aminoglycoside have been the standard choice for the initial therapy of fever and neutropenia [42, 87]. These regimens were covering primarily *Enterobacteriaceae*, *Pseudomonas aeruginosa*, and streptococci. The activity of the former antipseudomonal penicillins (such as carbenicillin, cefsulodin, azlocillin, and ticarcillin) against many Gram-negative rods was, however, rather limited, and the addition of an aminoglycoside was needed to compensate for this limited activity. In the 1980s, ceftazidime was one of the first drugs studied as monotherapy in febrile neutropenia. It was more active

W.V. Kern
Department of Medicine, Center for Infectious Diseases and Travel Medicine,
IFB-Center for Chronic Immunodeficiency, University Hospital,
Hugstetter Strasse 55, D-79106 Freiburg, Germany
e-mail: kern@if-freiburg.de

G. Maschmeyer, K.V.I. Rolston (eds.), *Infections in Hematology*,
DOI 10.1007/978-3-662-44000-1_14

in vitro against *P. aeruginosa* than most of the penicillins and highly active against *Escherichia coli* and *Klebsiella* species.

The development of new effective and well-tolerated drugs such as the carbapenems and the problems of emerging resistance among bacterial pathogens in critically ill patients including patients with neutropenia have broadened the spectrum of antibacterial drugs and drug regimens used and needed in febrile neutropenic patients. Today, piperacillin-tazobactam or meropenem are very (if not the most) common drugs used for initial therapy in patients with infection and cancer [23, 30, 77, 86, 113]. Targeted therapy with narrow-spectrum drugs such as vancomycin or linezolid may still be needed and/or be beneficial in the setting of proven infection, and the prescription of unconventional drugs and drug combinations including older agents may be necessary in patients with infection due to multidrug-resistant organisms that have now become quite common in cancer hospitals throughout the world. The present chapter describes the most important features of the most commonly used and needed antibacterial drugs for the treatment of fever and bacterial infection in patients with neutropenia.

14.1 Betalactam Antibiotics

Betalactam antibiotics exhibit time-dependent antibacterial activity [76]. Drug concentrations need to be maintained for some time above the minimum inhibitory concentration (MIC) of pathogenic bacteria. For bactericidal activity, the fraction of the dosing interval during which the free (unbound) betalactam drug concentration is above (i.e., two to four times greater than) the bacterial MIC (fT > MIC) should be at least 40–50 %. In a clinical study of febrile neutropenic patients treated with meropenem, a calculated T > MIC of 83 % was found in responders, while those with a poor clinical response had a T > MIC of only 60 % [3]. Vice versa, neutropenic patients given broad-spectrum cephalosporins with a T > MIC of 100 % had better clinical and microbiological outcomes than patients with shorter T > MIC [81]. Simulation experiments with betalactams with short half-lives and clinical observations have shown that extended and continuous infusion dosing regimens are superior compared with bolus or short infusion dosing in achieving the recommended pharmacodynamic targets against most Gram-negative pathogens, in particular against less susceptible *P. aeruginosa*, *Acinetobacter* species, and *Klebsiella* species [22, 27, 57–59, 81, 103].

Table 14.1 shows how the probabilities of pharmacodynamic target attainment ratios will depend on the MIC of the causative organism, the infusion times with intermittent dosing versus extended/continuous infusion, and the total daily dose. As a rule, the less susceptible the microorganism is and the more critically ill or immunodeficient the patient is, the more is optimal dosing with higher total daily doses and extended infusion times beneficial and required [72, 103]. Conversely, in a patient with documented infection due to a highly susceptible microorganism, the total daily dose of a betalactam and/or infusion times can often be reduced without losing therapeutic efficacy. These pharmacokinetic/pharmacodynamic properties of

Table 14.1 Comparison of pharmacokinetic-pharmacodynamic target attainment probabilities by dosing regimen, duration of infusion, and MIC

Dosing regimen	Duration of infusion (h)	MIC (μg/mL)	Probability of patients achieving a target T > MIC of			
			30 %	35 %	40 %	45 %
500 mg every 8 h	1/2/3	1	100/100/100	100/100/100	100/100/100	99/100/100
500 mg every 8 h	1/2/3	2	100/100/100	99/100/100	77/100/100	25/90/100
1,000 mg every 12 h	4/5/6	4	100/100/100	100/100/100	92/100/100	23/96/100
1,000 mg every 8 h	1/2/3	4	100/100/100	99/100/100	77/100/100	25/90/100
1 g/2 g/3 g every 24 h	24	4	0/98/100	0/98/100	0/98/100	0/98/100
1,000 mg every 8 h	1/2/3	8	100/100/100	100/100/99	84/99/99	26/90/95
1 g/2 g/3 g every 24 h	24	8	0/0/46	0/0/46	0/0/46	0/0/46

The data are based on a doripenem population pharmacokinetic model with Monte Carlo simulations (Adapted from Bhavnani et al [9]). Short infusions are worse than extended infusions, and continuous infusion (24 h) can be worse than intermittent extended infusion

Table 14.2 Commonly recommended standard and high doses (in adult patients with normal renal function) per day for selected betalactams and their plasma half-life and chemical stability at room temperature which are relevant for extended infusion regimens

	Standard dose per day	High dose per day	Half-life	Chemical stability (at room temperature)	Commonly used extended infusion times
Flucloxacillin	2 g every 8 h	3 g every 6 h	1 h	24 h	4–6 h
Aztreonam	1 g every 12 h	2 g every 6 h	1.5 h	>24 h	4–8 h
Piperacillin-tazobactam	3/0.375 g every 6 h	4/0.5 g every 6 h	1 h	24 h	4–6 h
Ceftazidime	1 g every 12 h	2 g every 8 h	2 h	24 h	4–8 h
Cefepime	1 g every 12 h	2 g every 8 h	2 h	24 h	4–8 h
Imipenem	0.5 g every 8 h	1 g every 6 h	1 h	3–4 h	3–4 h
Meropenem	0.5 g every 8 h	2 g every 8 h	1 h	4–8 h	3–4 h
Doripenem	0.5 g every 8 h	0.5 g every 6 h	1 h	4 h	3–4 h

betalactams are different from those of a number of other antibacterial drug classes and need to be considered in medical practice. Table 14.2 shows commonly used daily doses for selected betalactams and their plasma half-life and chemical stability at room temperature which are relevant for extended infusion regimens.

Most betalactams are hydrophilic antibiotics with small distribution volumes similar to extracellular water. Tissue concentrations are usually not higher than plasma concentrations and largely depend on protein binding. Most studies in the field indicate that the higher the protein binding is, the lower is the tissue concentration. The ability to penetrate into various deep compartments differs for specific betalactams, depending on additional characteristics, notably physicochemical properties in relationship to tissue/cell binding and to drug carriers/active transporters across anatomical barriers.

14.1.1 Piperacillin-Tazobactam

Piperacillin is an ureidopenicillin which, in the absence of a betalactamase inhibitor, is inactivated by most betalactamases which are now very common among various *Enterobacteriaceae*. The distribution of MICs of the drug alone and in combination with tazobactam for *E. coli*, *K. pneumoniae*, and *P. aeruginosa* is shown in Fig. 14.1. As can be seen, piperacillin alone has limited activity against both *E. coli* and *K. pneumoniae*. In the presence of tazobactam, the MICs of both *E. coli* and *Klebsiella* are shifted to the "susceptible" range, while the addition of tazobactam does less alter the distribution of piperacillin MICs against *P. aeruginosa* [35]. The activity of the drug combination is better than that of ticarcillin-clavulanic acid which is still marketed in many countries (Table 14.3). Most *A. baumannii* and *Stenotrophomonas maltophilia*, however, are resistant to piperacillin-tazobactam [35].

Depending on the particular type(s) of extended-spectrum betalactamase (ESBL) enzyme(s), the drug is also quite active in vitro against ESBL-positive *Enterobacteriaceae*, and good clinical responses with the drug have been observed in bacteremic infection due to ESBL-positive *E. coli* if the MIC was <8 μg/mL [96]. Interestingly, in such cases amoxicillin-clavulanic acid (if tested susceptible) may be even more active due to the fact that clavulanic acid binds much more tightly to the ESBL enzyme than tazobactam (and sulbactam) – hence the designation "suicide" betalactamase inhibitor for clavulanic acid [31].

The antibacterial activity of piperacillin includes ampicillin-susceptible *Enterococcus* species, streptococci (including *Streptococcus pneumoniae*), and – if combined with tazobactam or other betalactamase inhibitors – many anaerobes and methicillin-susceptible staphylococci. For targeted therapy of proven staphylococcal infections, however, oxacillin and derivatives (in the case of methicillin-susceptible *S. aureus*) are superior.

Piperacillin-tazobactam is marketed as fixed combination formulation with 2/0.25 g, 3/0.375 g, and 4/0.5 g. In many countries a dose of 4/0.5 g every 6–8 h is the recommended daily dosage in adults with normal renal function. After a single dose of 4 g of piperacillin, peak plasma concentrations are in the range of 300–400 μg/mL. The half-life of piperacillin is approximately 1 h. The plasma concentration 6 h after short (~30 min) infusion is usually <2 μg/mL. The breakpoint for resistance according to EUCAST (*European Committee on Antimicrobial Susceptibility Testing*, www.eucast.org) is >16 μg/mL. The drug is stable for 24 h at room temperature [95, 112]. Extended infusion times including 24 h of continuous infusion are possible and safe. We recommend intermittent administration with extended infusion for 4–6 h.

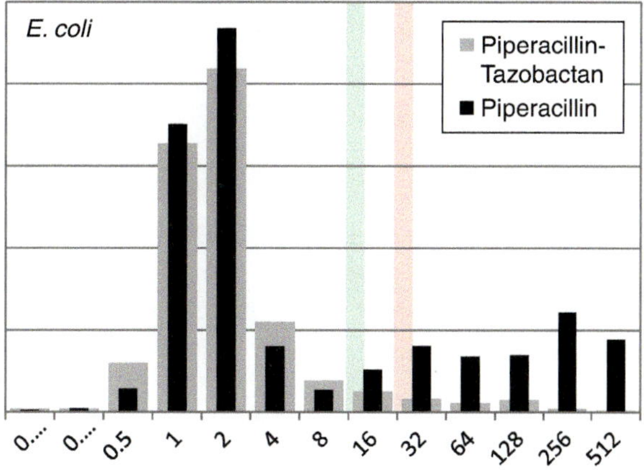

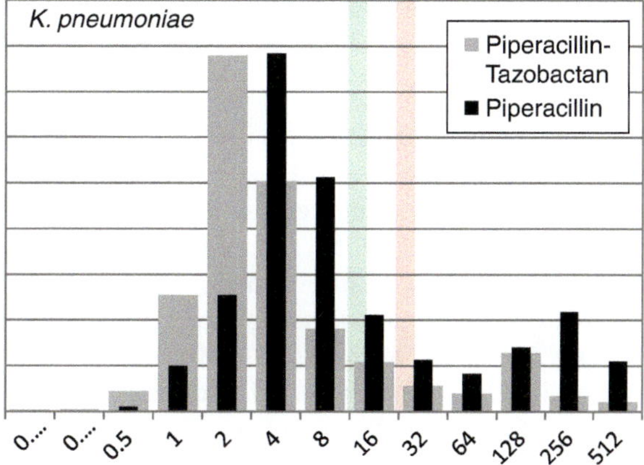

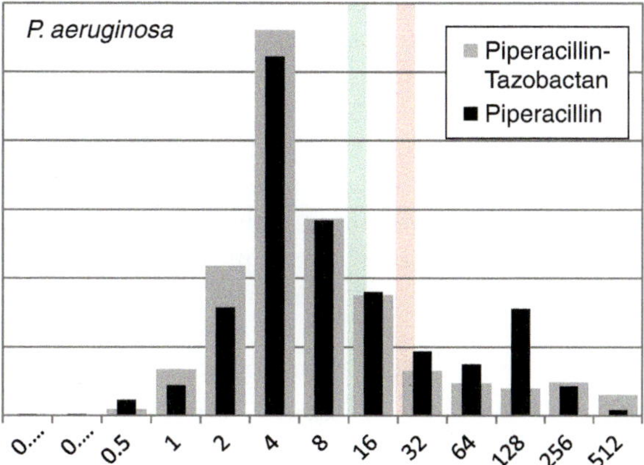

Fig. 14.1 The distribution of MICs of the piperacillin with and without tazobactam for *E. coli*, *K. pneumoniae*, and *P. aeruginosa* (Data are from EUCAST [35]). The *green line* indicates the breakpoint for susceptibility. The *red line* indicates the breakpoint for resistance

Table 14.3 Comparison of rates of resistance (in %) to betalactam versus betalactam/betalactamase inhibitor combinations according to EUCAST [35]

	E. coli	*K. pneumoniae*	*P. aeruginosa*
Ampicillin	43 %	89 %	–
Ampicillin-sulbactam	→34 %	→28 %	–
Ticarcillin	50 %	97 %	73 %
Ticarcillin-clavulanic acid	→23 %	→22 %	→78 %
Piperacillin	30 %	26 %	24 %
Piperacillin-tazobactam	→3 %	→10 %	→14 %

Resistance rates may vary locally

The efficacy of initial monotherapy with piperacillin-tazobactam in patients with fever and neutropenia has been demonstrated in several clinical trials including a large double-blind trial from Italy in which the drug was compared with the initial combination of piperacillin-tazobactam plus amikacin [30].

14.1.2 Ceftazidime

Ceftazidime was the first antipseudomonal cephalosporin with excellent activity also against most *Enterobacteriaceae*. The drug was extensively evaluated in clinical trials in patients with fever and neutropenia [29, 36, 43, 49, 88, 89]. Typically, the MIC for susceptible *P. aeruginosa* is 1–4 µg/mL while the MIC for non-ESBL-positive *E. coli* and *Klebsiella* is in the order of 0.1–0.2 µg/mL [35]. The activity of ceftazidime against streptococci (including pneumococci) is somewhat lower than that of cefotaxime/ceftriaxone and of cefepime (MICs, ~0.25 versus <0.1 µg/mL). Similarly, the drug has more limited activity against methicillin-susceptible staphylococci compared with cefotaxime/ceftriaxone and cefepime (MICs, ~4 versus ~2 µg/mL) and is not recommended as targeted therapy in proven infections due to staphylococci or streptococci.

After intravenous infusion of 1 and 2 g doses of ceftazidime over 20–30 min in volunteers, peak plasma concentrations of ~70–100 and 120–180 µg/mL, respectively, are achieved. The half-life is approximately 2 h, and less than 10 % of the drug is protein bound. Elimination is almost completely by the renal route. Continuous infusion (6 g per day in patients with normal renal function) yields steady-state plasma concentrations of 30–50 µg/mL. Some centers use continuous infusion of 4 g per day (after an initial 2 g loading dose) [34, 88].

Pivotal trials of ceftazidime monotherapy in patients with fever and neutropenia have been published in the early to mid 1980s and established the efficacy and non-inferiority of ceftazidime versus cephalothin plus gentamicin plus carbenicillin, ceftazidime plus flucloxacillin, or piperacillin or azlocillin each plus an aminoglycoside [29, 36, 49, 89], and a large clinical trial reported equal efficacy of ceftazidime monotherapy compared with imipenem [43].

Today, the usefulness of the drug in particular for initial therapy has become limited primarily due to the emergence of ESBL-positive *Enterobacteriacaeae* [4, 74]. Using a breakpoint for resistance in *Enterobacteriaceae* of >4 μg/mL (EUCAST), approximately 60–70 % of ESBL-positive isolates will be resistant to ceftazidime (compared with 20–30 % resistance to piperacillin-tazobactam in such strains). Of note is that the breakpoint for resistance in *P. aeruginosa* was set at >8 μg/mL (dosage, 6 g per day) so that it is quite possible that ceftazidime at high dose and given by extended or continuous infusion will cover some more *Enterobacteriaceae* than EUCAST-defined in vitro resistance rates do suggest. Clinical experience with the drug in infection due to ESBL-positive Gram-negative bacteria is, however, limited.

Ceftazidime is currently developed in combination with a new betalactamase inhibitor, avibactam [116]. The potent in vitro activity of this new ceftazidime plus avibactam combination against *Enterobacteriaceae* producing betalactamases of Ambler class A, and more importantly class C and some class D, has been confirmed in vivo in murine pneumonia, bacteremia, and pyelonephritis models, and it is likely that clinical trials will show the usefulness of this new drug in patients with fever and neutropenia. Ceftazidime plus avibactam is a promising regimen for infections due to *Klebsiella* with carbapenem resistance due to KPC enzymes.

14.1.3 Cefepime

Cefepime was brought to market in the mid 1990s. The antimicrobial activity is similar to that of ceftazidime with somewhat lower MICs of cefepime for staphylococci and streptococci. As with ceftazidime, the MIC for susceptible *P. aeruginosa* is typically 1–4 μg/mL, while the MIC for non-ESBL-positive *E. coli* and *Klebsiella* is in the order of <0.1–0.2 μg/mL [35]. The drug is more stable than ceftazidime to AmpC-type betalactamases which are typically found in *Enterobacter* species.

There still are major discrepancies between the USA and Europe in setting clinical breakpoints for the drug. According to the so-called CLSI (*Clinical and Laboratory Standards Institute*, proposing breakpoints in the USA, www.clsi.org) standards, the breakpoint of cefepime for resistance in *Enterobacteriaceae* had earlier been set at >32 μg/mL, while according to EUCAST criteria, it is now >4 μg/mL. This has implications for estimating and interpreting susceptibility rates, particularly for ESBL-producing *K. pneumoniae* and *E. cloacae*. The rates of cefepime susceptibility for such strains may differ substantially, for example, 61 % (CLSI) versus 12 % (EUCAST) for *K. pneumoniae* or 58 % versus 32 % for *E. cloacae*, respectively [114]. Since the pharmacokinetic characteristics of cefepime are similar to those of ceftazidime and dosing is also similar for the two drugs, it may be more logical to apply breakpoints which are also similar. The most recent CLSI criteria revision (in 2014) consequently changed the breakpoint of cefepime for resistance in *Enterobacteriaceae* to >8 μg/mL (breakpoint for susceptibility, ≤2 μg/mL). In India, cefepime is also available as a fixed combination with sulbactam and with tazobactam – no clinical trials with those combinations have been reported as yet [109].

Cefepime was approved in 1997 for use as empiric monotherapy in febrile neutropenic patients in the USA. In 2007, a meta-analysis noted increased 30-day mortality associated with the use of cefepime versus other betalactams (risk ratio, 1.26) [115]. Among subcategories of patients, the increased mortality with cefepime was statistically significant only among neutropenic patients [87, 115]. The USA Food and Drug Administration reevaluated the data in collaboration with the drug sponsor that provided additional unpublished material and, 2 years later, concluded that the data would not confirm a higher rate of death in cefepime-treated patients [65]. There has still been some concern over cefepime's safety, and there continue to appear reports about possibly dose-related neurotoxicity including nonconvulsive status epilepticus that can be severe and life-threatening [44, 62, 107].

14.1.4 Carbapenems

Imipenem was the first carbapenem introduced into the market [61]. It can be hydrolyzed in the mammalian kidney by an enzyme dubbed dihydropeptidase-I. This brush-border enzyme is inhibited by the co-drug cilastatin. With this imipenem/cilastatin combination, high urinary concentrations and recovery are obtained, and imipenem does not enter into the proximal tubular epithelium of the kidney and cannot be metabolized to a metabolite causing tubular necrosis.

Meropenem was the second carbapenem approved in both the USA and Europe and has been extensively studied in patients with fever and neutropenia. Meropenem is – besides piperacillin-tazobactam – now commonly used for initial empirical monotherapy in cancer patients [23, 39, 40, 43, 45, 77]. The advantage of meropenem is its broad-spectrum activity and excellent tolerability. Other carbapenems in the market include ertapenem, a carbapenem for single daily dosing that has no activity against *P. aeruginosa*; doripenem which is similar to meropenem [45]; and two other compounds only approved in Japan (panipenem and biapenem) [69].

The carbapenems are stable to most betalactamases including AmpC and ESBL enzymes. Resistance develops when bacteria acquire so-called metallobetalactamases or Ambler class A-type KPC enzymes that are capable of degrading carbapenems or when changes in membrane permeability arise usually as a result of loss of specific outer membrane porins. The activity of carbapenems so far remains excellent against wild-type *Enterobacteriaceae* (MIC in *E. coli* and *K. pneumoniae*, 0.01–0.06 μg/mL) with few exceptions. Species of *Proteus*, *Morganella*, and *Providencia* often are marginally susceptible or (low-level) resistant to imipenem and ertapenem [35].

Most isolates of *P. aeruginosa* and of *A. baumannii* show an MIC of meropenem in the range of 0.2–2 μg/mL [35]. Carbapenems are active against most clinically relevant anaerobes. They are poorly active against enterococci (typical MIC of meropenem, 2–16 μg/mL) and inactive at clinically achievable concentrations against *S. maltophilia* (typical MIC of meropenem, >32 μg/mL). *Listeria* are surprisingly susceptible to meropenem and imipenem which also have activity against *Nocardia* species and (extracellular) mycobacteria including multidrug-resistant *M. tuberculosis*.

Table 14.4 The breakpoints of meropenem for susceptibility and resistance (μg/mL) for Gram-negative bacteria according to EUCAST and CLSI

		CLSI		EUCAST	
		S	R	S	R
Meropenem	*Enterobacteriaceae*	≤1	>2	≤2	>8
	Acinetobacter	≤4	>8	≤2	>8
	P. aeruginosa	≤2	>16	≤2	>8
Imipenem	*Enterobacteriaceae*	≤1	>2	≤2	>8
	Acinetobacter	≤4	>8	≤2	>8
	P. aeruginosa	≤2	>16	≤4	>8

S susceptible, *R* resistant

Imipenem, meropenem, and doripenem have in vivo half-lives of approximately 1 h, while ertapenem has a half-life of approximately 4 h. Imipenem reaches higher CSF concentrations than meropenem, but meropenem is usually preferred for the treatment of CNS infections due to its lower incidence of seizures. The carbapenems are chemically less stable at room temperature than ceftazidime and piperacillin-tazobactam, in particular in concentrated (>4 g/100 mL) aqueous solution, and the rate of inactivation within 24 h can exceed 50 % [7, 112]. Although there is some experience with longer infusion times [68], we believe extended infusion regimens >4 h cannot currently be recommended.

Meropenem has extensively been evaluated in patients with fever and neutropenia. In the largest study (already published in 1996 and) involving more than 1,000 subjects [23], meropenem was associated with a slightly higher clinical response than ceftazidime plus amikacin (56 % versus 52 %, respectively). In a second large trial with 411 adult cancer patients, a similar response rate was observed with meropenem (54 % versus 44 % in patients receiving ceftazidime monotherapy, respectively) [39]. In children, a response rate of 56 % was reported (versus 40 % in pediatric patients receiving ceftazidime monotherapy, respectively) [40]. Some trials noted diarrhea with or without *Clostridium difficile* infection as a frequent significant adverse event, but carbapenems were otherwise usually well tolerated. There are very limited data on head-to-head comparisons of carbapenems for empirical therapy in febrile neutropenia.

The breakpoints of meropenem for resistance in Gram-negative bacteria are >8 μg/mL (EUCAST) and between >2 and >8 μg/mL (last CLSI revision, depending on whether *Enterobacteriaceae*, *P. aeruginosa*, or *A. baumannii* is tested) (Table 14.4). Such "more or less" carbapenem-resistant Gram-negative microorganisms show variable MICs ranging from 4 to >64 μg/mL. Importantly, meropenem used at high dosage (3 × 2 g by extended infusion instead of 3 × 1 g) is likely to cover microorganisms with an MIC of 16 and 32 μg/mL with a T>MIC of 50–60 % and 20–30 %, respectively [58]. The safety of such a dosage regimen has recently been shown in a comparative clinical trial [22]. Such a regimen can be considered as important adjunct and combination therapy partner to effectively treat infections due to carbapenemase-producing organisms [4, 25, 74].

14.1.5 Other Betalactams

Among the various other betalactams commonly used and potentially useful in patients with fever and neutropenia are oxacillin and its derivatives, amoxicillin-clavulanic acid, ceftriaxone, and aztreonam. Cefixime has also been evaluated in step-down therapy in a very limited number of children with low-risk febrile neutropenia without documented infection. There is insufficient information to consider this drug as a suitable alternative to amoxicillin-clavulanic acid in patients with fever and neutropenia.

14.1.5.1 Oxacillin

The oxacillin derivatives cloxacillin, dicloxacillin, and flucloxacillin (like nafcillin) are narrow-spectrum penicillins with activity against methicillin-susceptible staphylococci and many streptococci, but no relevant antimicrobial activity against enterococci and *Listeria*. Oxacillin and its derivatives are important drugs in severe staphylococcal infection and are considered to be superior to vancomycin and also to cefazolin and to cefuroxime in patients with bacteremic *S. aureus* infection. The MIC of oxacillin in staphylococci is typically ~0.25–0.5 μg/mL [35]. Based on population pharmacokinetic data, a daily dose of 6 g given as 2 g by 4 h extended infusion every 8 h is likely to provide an fT > MIC of 50 % at an MIC of 0.75–1 μg/mL [71]. Short infusion regimes will require higher daily dosages to maintain high probabilities of response. These data have been the basis for recommendations of 2 g given every 6–8 h daily for serious staphylococcal infection. Higher dosages (Table 14.2) may be required in staphylococcal endocarditis and central nervous system infection.

The most critical adverse event apart from rash associated with oxacillin and its derivatives is cholestatic jaundice and hepatitis. Risk factors appear to be older age, preexisting hepatic impairment, long-term use (>14 days), and probably the daily dose. It is unknown whether continuous or extended infusion regimens can lower the risk of hepatotoxicity. Flucloxacillin is stable at room temperature for at least 24 h.

14.1.5.2 Amoxicillin-Clavulanic Acid

As an oral drug, amoxicillin-clavulanic acid is commonly used together with ciprofloxacin for therapy in low-risk febrile neutropenia patients [42]. Amoxicillin is well absorbed. Its oral bioavailability is approximately 70 %. A dose of 500 mg yields a mean peak plasma concentration of ~7–10 μg/mL [41, 94]. The usual oral dose of 500 mg (together with 125 mg of clavulanic acid) every 8 h provides a ~55 % or greater T > MIC for *Haemophilus* and streptococci incl. pneumococci [6]. Almost similar results (T > MIC [1 μg/mL], 44 %) are obtained with the 875/125 mg tablets given every 12 h [5]. Elimination of amoxicillin is predominantly by the renal route (52 %), and high concentrations are achieved in the urine sufficient to treat urinary tract infection (including those due to Gram-negative bacteria susceptible at the breakpoint of 8 μg/mL) [41, 94]. Parenteral therapy with higher doses is needed to treat systemic infections due to susceptible Gram-negative bacteria. In some countries, organisms with an MIC of 1–8 μg/mL are therefore categorized as intermediate susceptible. Resistance in *E. coli* is not uncommon and is primarily due to enzymatic inactivation by OXA-1- or inhibitor-resistant TEM (IRT) enzymes and chromosomal AmpC hyperproduction [97].

Clavulanic acid is extensively metabolized and eliminated in urine and feces. Adverse effects include rash, gastrointestinal disturbances, and – rarely – cholestatic hepatitis usually associated with clavulanic acid rather than with amoxicillin. Age, preexisting liver disease, therapy duration, and probably genetic factors play a role in the risk for drug-induced hepatitis [106].

14.1.5.3 Ceftriaxone

Ceftriaxone has become a most popular parenteral broad-spectrum cephalosporin because of its long half-life and the ease of the corresponding once daily dosing. It is a third-generation cephalosporin with antimicrobial activity very similar to that of cefotaxime. The usual dose in adults for infections outside the brain is 2 g every 24 h. This dosing regimen yields ~100 % fT > MIC (≤1 μg/mL), thus providing excellent in vivo activity against streptococci, *Haemophilus*, and wild-type *Enterobacteriaceae*. It has no relevant activity against *P. aeruginosa* (MIC typically >8 μg/mL). The breakpoint for resistance has been set at >2 μg/mL (EUCAST). The drug is very well tolerated. Gastrointestinal disturbance may occur, and *Clostridium difficile* infections are more common than with most other broad-spectrum cephalosporins due to its substantial effects on the intestinal microflora.

14.1.5.4 Ceftaroline and Ceftobiprole

Both compounds are broad-spectrum cephalosporins approved for the treatment of skin and soft tissue infection and pneumonia. The two drugs have enhanced activity against MRSA and in the future might become interesting treatment options in febrile neutropenia. There is increasing experience with them in salvage therapy for MRSA infection [18].

14.1.5.5 Aztreonam

Aztreonam is a monobactam available for clinical use since the 1980s. The antimicrobial activity comprises exclusively Gram-negative bacteria. Wild-type *E. coli* and *Klebsiella* species are highly susceptible with MICs typically <0.1 μ/mL [35]. Aztreonam is moderately active against *P. aeruginosa* (MIC, ~4 μg/mL) and has no clinically relevant activity against *Acinetobacter* and *Stenotrophomonas* [35]. The MIC distribution for *E. coli*, *P. aeruginosa*, and *A. baumannii* is shown in Fig. 14.2. Aztreonam is not inactivated by Ambler class B betalactamases (metalloenzymes) and represents an important therapeutic option in infections due to *P. aeruginosa* with metallobetalactamase-associated carbapenem resistance. In some countries, the drug (as aztreonam-lysine with a dose of 75 mg administered every 8 h using an ultrasonic nebulizer) has been approved for inhalation [92].

Recommended doses for an adult patient with normal renal function are 1–2 g every 6–8 h. Monte Carlo simulations with a target of an fT > MIC of 50–60 % at a dose of 1 g (infused over 1 h) every 8 h indicate a clinical breakpoint of 1–4 μg/mL. Thus, infections due to susceptible *E. coli* do not require high-dose therapy.

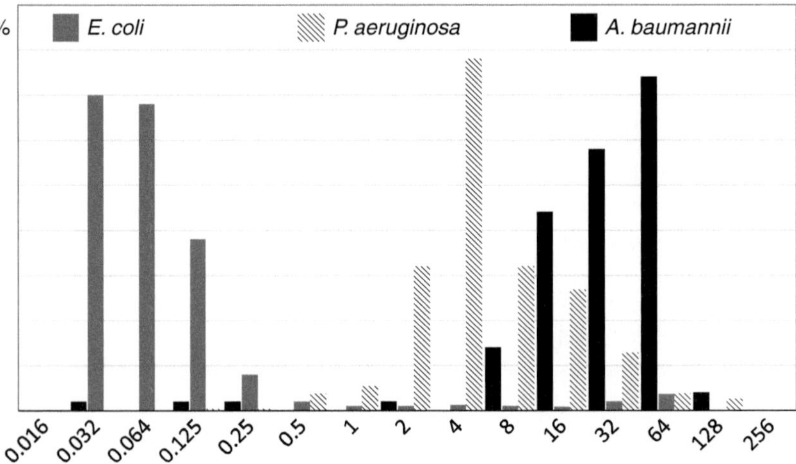

Fig. 14.2 The in vitro activity of aztreonam against *E. coli*, *K. pneumoniae*, and *P. aeruginosa* (Data are from EUCAST [35]). Aztreonam is moderately active against *P. aeruginosa* (MIC, ~4 µg/mL) and has no clinically relevant activity against *Acinetobacter*

The drug can be given as continuous infusion (24 h). Continuous infusion of 6–8 g per day produces plasma concentrations of ~40–50 µg/mL [16]. Such a regimen should be sufficient to treat infection due to low-level resistant *P. aeruginosa*.

The addition of avibactam to aztreonam is currently being evaluated in clinical trials [24]. The advantage of such a drug combination would be the restored activity of aztreonam against ESBL-positive organisms and its intrinsic activity in organisms with metalloenzyme-associated carbapenem resistance.

14.2 Aminoglycosides

In view of many clinical trials establishing the noninferiority of betalactam monotherapy for fever and neutropenia [86], many clinicians now limit the use of aminoglycosides in these and other critically ill patients to an initial, often single-shot therapy in patients with severe sepsis/septic shock or recommend their use only for targeted combination therapy for infection due to otherwise difficult-to-treat or resistant organisms [13, 79, 82]. This strategy may change in the future if betalactam monotherapy becomes unreliable due to emerging resistance, and it is conceivable that there will be an increasing need to reinitiate initial empirical combination therapies with short courses of aminoglycosides.

The most commonly used aminoglycosides for systemic use are gentamicin, tobramycin, and amikacin. Other aminoglycosides such as netilmicin, isepamicin, and arbekacin are uncommonly used and/or not available in many countries [91]. New developments include plazomicin (a "neoglycoside") which is stable against common aminoglycoside-inactivating enzymes [117].

The older aminoglycosides are most active in many Gram-negative bacteria [35]. Wild-type *E. coli* and *Klebsiella* exhibit gentamicin and tobramycin MICs in the range of 0.5–1 μg/mL and amikacin MICs in the range of 2–4 μg/mL. Aminoglycosides show a concentration-dependent bactericidal activity in Gram-negative organisms and an interesting so-called post-antibiotic effect that is also dependent on the ratio of drug concentration versus MIC and can last several hours [9]. Additional doses during this phase do not produce additional bacterial killing and the killing efficacy is reduced for subsequent repeated exposures (so-called adaptive resistance) compared to the initial exposure. Once daily dosing is therefore advantageous despite the relatively short half-life of the aminoglycosides of 2–3 h [9, 54, 79, 80, 83].

Fortunately, extended-interval dosing is also advantageous regarding the typical adverse effects of aminoglycosides, nephrotoxicity, and ototoxicity [9]. The toxic effects require drug uptake and binding to the brush borders of renal cells and to the cochlea and vestibular membranes. Binding to these membranes, however, demonstrates saturable kinetics and is less efficient at high intermittent drug levels. The half-life of aminoglycosides in the renal cortex is approximately 100 h, leading to renal accumulation of the drug and toxicity. In clinical trials, the advantages of once-daily dosing compared to two- to three-times daily administration has not been consistently shown, in part because often very potent betalactam combination therapy partners were used and treatment durations often were too short to fully assess differences in toxicity. Nevertheless, once-daily dosing of aminoglycosides is now recommended for most indications including treatment of patients with fever and neutropenia if betalactam monotherapy is unreliable.

There has been controversy about the relative risks of nephrotoxicity for gentamicin versus tobramycin (and netilmicin), respectively. In various animal models, gentamicin was more nephrotoxic than tobramycin if given at identical doses, and netilmicin at the same dose, in turn, was less nephrotoxic than tobramycin. Clinical studies in humans also provided some evidence for the greater potential of gentamicin to cause nephrotoxicity [38, 102]. Accordingly, gentamicin often is limited to combination therapy of enterococcal or streptococcal endocarditis where only low doses are required for synergistic action with penicillin. In patients with Gram-negative infection or suspected Gram-negative infection such as patients with fever and neutropenia (or urinary tract and abdominal sepsis and nosocomial pneumonia), higher doses are useful that make tobramycin, netilmicin, or amikacin drugs of choice.

Table 14.5 shows salient features of aminoglycoside therapy today. It should be noted that resistance rates may vary substantially between hospitals and regions depending among other things on what is the proportion of cephalosporin-resistant *Enterobacteriaceae* and carbapenem-resistant *P. aeruginosa* (which are often coresistant in particular against gentamcin and tobramycin) and on which aminoglycoside is being used most commonly.

Therapeutic drug monitoring (TDM) is still recommended. The measurement of peak levels, however, is rarely needed, and trough levels are usually not required before day 5 of treatment in patients with normal creatinine clearance. So-called high-intensity TDM programs may not be cost-effective [11, 100], and simple linear dose adjustment according to aminoglycoside serum

Table 14.5 Salient features of commonly used aminoglycosides

Drug	Typical MIC (µg/mL) in wild-type cells			Break*k*-points for resistance (µg/mL)	Resistance rates			Daily dose (per body weight) in subjects with normal renal function	Post-infusion plasma drug levels (µg/mL)		
	E. coli	*K. pneumoniae*	*P. aeruginosa*		*E. coli*	*K. pneumoniae*	*P. aeruginosa*		Mean peak levels	Target levels at 8–12 h	Target trough levels (24 h)
Gentamicin	0.25–1	0.25–1	1–4	>4	5 %	11 %	15 %	1×4 mg/kg	10–20	<5	<1
Tobramycin	0.5–2	0.5–1	0.5–1	>4	4 %	8 %	6 %	1×5–6 mg/kg	15–25	<5	<1
Amikacin	2–4	1–2	2–8	>16	<2 %	<2 %	<2 %	1×15–20 mg/kg	30–60	<15	<5

The distribution of MICs and the breakpoints for resistance are according to EUCAST. Resistance rates may vary locally. Dosage per bodyweight need a correction in morbidly obese patients. Infusion time, 1h concentrations is usually sufficient [13, 78]. Drug accumulation may be more sensitively detected by measuring 8–12 h post-infusion levels than just 24 h trough levels. Patients with fever and neutropenia often (like many patients with severe sepsis) have a relatively large volume of distribution in the acute phase which helps to avoid toxic levels if large doses are administered [9]. Audiometry for screening ototoxicity is routinely recommended in patients receiving >14 days of therapy.

14.3 Agents Against Gram-Positive Bacteria

14.3.1 Glycopeptides

Vancomycin and teicoplanin are narrow-spectrum glycopeptides in clinical use since decades [84]. Both compounds are active in vitro against most clinically relevant Gram-positive bacteria including Gram-positive anaerobes with a few exceptions. Members of the genera *Leuconostoc* and *Pediococcus*, certain members of the *Lactobacillus* family (except *L. acidophilus*), *Erysipelothrix*, and certain *Enterococcus* species (*E. casseliflavus/flavescens, E. gallinarum*) are intrinsically resistant.

Glycopeptides have been the standard drugs in cases of infection due to methicillin-resistant staphylococci, ampicillin-resistant enterococci, and high-level penicillin-resistant pneumococci. For bactericidal activity multiples of the MIC are required, and a proportion of MRSA and many enterococci show a so-called "tolerance" phenomenon, i.e., the difference between minimal inhibitory and cidal concentrations is 32-fold or higher [101]. Typical vancomycin MIC values for staphylococci and enterococci are 0.5–2 μg/mL [35]. The activity against pneumococci is slightly better (MIC, 0.25–0.5 μg/mL). Teicoplanin shows a similar MIC distribution in staphylococci. Teicoplanin, however, is slightly more active in enterococci (MIC, 0.25–1 μg/mL) and much more active in pneumococci (MIC, 0.032–0.125 mg/mL) [35].

A major problem has been acquired vancomycin resistance, notably in enterococci (VRE) and in *S. aureus* (VISA or hetero-VISA). Acquired vancomycin resistance in enterococci has become frequent in *E. faecium* and remains rare in *E. faecalis*. Most VRE show the "VanA"-type resistance, meaning that both vancomycin and teicoplanin (but not oritavancin) are inactive with MIC values often being extremely high (>100 μg/mL). "VanB"-type resistance is less frequent. VanB-VRE show lower MICs of vancomycin and are usually susceptible to teicoplanin. VISA show an intermediate susceptibility to vancomycin (hence the name VISA) according to previous breakpoints. MICs of vancomycin typically are 8–16 μg/mL (CLSI breakpoints for resistance were formerly >32 μg/mL). Often VISA are heteroresistant. Only a subpopulation of the cells grow in the presence of otherwise inhibitory concentrations of vancomycin. Heteroresistance can also be observed in vancomycin-susceptible cells and leads to the emergence of VISA. VISA tend to develop thick cell walls. They show an increased cell-wall turnover (likely trapping vancomycin)

Table 14.6 Recommended doses and dose adjustments for glycopeptides and daptomycin

Drug	Creatinine clearance (mL/min)				Intermittent hemodialysis	Continuous RRT
	>80	80–50	50–10	<10		
Vancomycin[a]	1,000 every 12 h	500 every 8 h	500 every 24 h	500 every 72 h	500 every 72 h	1,000 every 24 h
Teicoplanin[b]	400–800 every 24 h	400 every 24 h	400 every 24 h	400 every 72	400 every 72 h	400 every 24 h
Daptomycin	500–700 every 24 h	500 every 24 h	500 every 24 h	500 every 48 h	500 every 48 h	500 every 24 h

Doses (in mg) are per day for an adult patient with a bodyweight of ~70 kg according to renal function. Therapeutic drug monitoring may be required to optimize efficacy and/or reduce toxicity

[a]Some clinicians give a loading dose of 15–20 mg/kg bodyweight

[b]A loading dose of 1,200 mg (in divided doses) on the first day is recommended. High doses may be required in staphylococcal infection

and increased positive cell-wall charge responsible for a repulsion mechanism towards vancomycin, teicoplanin, and daptomycin [17].

Vancomycin is administered as 1–2 h intravenous infusion at a dose of 1 g every 12 h in subjects with normal renal function. Peak plasma concentrations are 20–40 μg/mL. The drug's half-life is approximately 6 h [84]. It has been suggested that trough levels in severe infections should be ~20 μg/mL, but often trough levels after conventional dosing are in the range of 10–15 μg/mL. In one study in stem-cell transplant patients, trough levels after standard dosing were <10 μg/mL in >50 % of the subjects [48]. Therapeutic drug monitoring is therefore recommended to optimize dosing in severe infection and to minimize toxicity and allow dose adaptation in case of drug accumulation. Many investigators use target trough levels of 15–20 μg/mL rather than higher levels to adjust doses. Vancomycin is primarily excreted by the renal route. Doses need to be adjusted according to creatinine clearance. Table 14.6 shows recommended dose adjustments for glycopeptides (and daptomycin).

Teicoplanin has a very long half-life (4–7 days). It is highly protein-bound. Loading doses of 6–10 mg/kg bodyweight every 8–12 h for three doses are required. Maintenance doses are (6-) 10 mg/kg every 24 h. Teicoplanin has a role in the treatment of enterococcal infection but has appeared less reliable for the treatment of severe staphylococcal infections.

Both vancomycin and teicoplanin can be given by mouth (capsules or oral solution) to treat *Clostridium difficile* infection (CDI). Vancomycin at a dose 125 mg every 6 h is a recommended therapy in moderate to severe CDI or in patients failing metronidazole. In severe cases the dose can be increased up to 500 mg every 6–8 h. Direct intracolonic administration is also possible as a retention enema using 500–1,000 mL of saline with 500 mg vancomycin every 6–12 h.

14.3.2 Daptomycin

Daptomycin is a relatively new addition to the armamentarium to treat Gram-positive bacterial infection due to multidrug-resistant organisms. It is a lipopeptide antibiotic discovered in the 1980s, but further developed to market not until 2003 (USA) and 2006 (Europe). Its mode of action is different from that of the glycopeptides since it binds via a calcium-dependent process to the bacterial cell membrane and disrupts the membrane potential rather than inhibiting cell-wall synthesis [84]. The antimicrobial activity is good against staphylococci with MICs of 0.25–1 μg/mL, and in vitro, the drug is usually bactericidal at these concentrations. Enterococci are less susceptible with MICs typically ranging from 0.25 to 8 μg/mL [35]. The EUCAST breakpoint for resistance has been set at >1 μg/mL. The recommended dose for infections other than skin and soft tissue infection is 6 mg/kg every 24 h. With this dose, patients with neutropenia have shown peak plasma concentrations of 20–75 μg/mL, but most of the drug is protein-bound. The mean half-life of daptomycin was 11 h and has shown considerable interindividual variation [14].

Many clinicians use higher doses (8–12 mg/kg every 24 h) in severe staphylococcal infection, and experience in cancer patients is accumulating [14, 19, 67, 70, 98, 99]. There has been repeated (anecdotal) evidence of treatment failures with lower doses, and the safety of high-dose daptomycin appears acceptable. Up to 10 % of the patients develop (mostly asymptomatic) creatine phosphokinase elevation depending on the dose and treatment duration. Daptomycin does not have antimicrobial activity in pulmonary tissue.

14.3.3 Linezolid

Linezolid is a member of a new class of narrow-spectrum agents, the oxazolidinones. It is available for both intravenous and oral administration [84]. The drug shows ~100 % oral bioavailability. The spectrum of activity includes most clinically relevant Gram-positive pathogens including most MRSA, VRE and VISA, *Nocardia*, and some anaerobic bacteria (*Peptostreptococcus*, *Clostridium*, *Prevotella*, and *Fusobacterium*), with MIC values between 0.5 and 4 μg/mL [35]. MICs are 2–8 μg/mL for *Legionella*, *Moraxella*, *Pasteurella*, and *Bacteroides*, but other Gram-negative bacteria are resistant as a result of enhanced drug efflux out of the bacterial cell. The drug is bacteriostatic. The (EUCAST) breakpoint for resistance is >4 μg/mL. Doses of 600 mg every 12 h produce peak plasma concentrations of 15–20 μg/mL and trough concentrations of 3–6 μg/mL. Under steady-state conditions, approximately 30 % of the dose appears in the urine as unchanged drug. Virtually no unchanged linezolid appears in the feces [32, 104]. Tissue penetration is excellent, and the concentration in cerebrospinal fluid is similar to the plasma concentration [32, 104, 105]. In MRSA lung infection linezolid has been found superior to vancomycin.

Linezolid has been compared with vancomycin for empirical therapy in patients with fever and neutropenia. This double-blind trial in 605 cancer patients with proven (24 %) or suspected Gram-positive infections showed equivalent efficacy between vancomycin and linezolid in achieving clinical (87 % vs. 86 %) and microbiological (58 % vs. 50 %) success, with no differences in survival [56]. There were fewer drug-related adverse events with linezolid (17 % vs. 24 %; $p=0.04$). Other observational studies confirm the efficacy of linezolid for the treatment of Gram-positive infection in neutropenia, particularly VRE bacteremia. Here, responses and cure rates were encouraging [84].

Adverse effects of linezolid included hematotoxicity (anemia, thrombocytopenia and/or neutropenia) and neurotoxicity (peripheral and optic neuropathies) [52, 60, 85]. Both appear to be dose-related and are observed much more frequently in patients treated for >2 weeks [10]. In indications that need long-term treatment (such as MDR tuberculosis), the linezolid dose is usually reduced by 30–50 % to prevent toxicity. Other uncommon but serious adverse effects associated with linezolid include lactic acidosis and serotonin syndrome [52, 85].

14.4 Tetracyclines

Tetracyclines are broad-spectrum agents with activity against intracellular bacteria. Due to emerging resistance they can no longer be used for common indications but may now be valuable options in the treatment of infections due to resistant organisms. Tetracycline resistance rates in MRSA, for example, has now become quite low in many regions, and minocycline or doxycycline have been used successfully in MRSA infection. Both compounds also have some useful activity against *A. baumannii* and *C. difficile*. Like with linezolid patients treated with doxycycline are less likely to develop CDI compared with patients receiving other antibiotics. Most pneumococci, *Haemophilus*, and *Moraxella* species are susceptible [35].

Tigecycline is a new tetracycline. It is derived from minocycline but shows enhanced activity against enterococci (including VRE), *Listeria*, anaerobes, and many Gram-negative organisms with the exception of *P. aeruginosa, Proteus, Providencia, Morganella,* and (extracellular) *Legionella* [35, 74]. *A. baumannii* typically shows MICs in the range of 0.125–2 μg/mL which is not very different from the range of MICs seen with doxycycline or minocycline (0.125–1 μg/mL) [35].

The drug is available for intravenous application. The currently recommended doses of 50 mg every 12 h for adults produce low plasma levels (~1 μg/mL) which are very near to previously defined breakpoints for resistance in Gram-negative bacteria (>2 μg/mL) and are likely to be associated with more failures and increased mortality, compared to other antibiotic therapies, especially in ventilator-associated pneumonia. Higher dosages are poorly tolerated due to nausea and other gastrointestinal disturbances. The breakpoint definitions are likely to be revised and adapted to those already recommended for several Gram-positive organisms (>0.5 μg/mL).

Interestingly, tigecycline was evaluated in combination therapy with a variety of drugs in cancer and transplant patients [15, 21]. In a prospective multicenter trial of empirical therapy for patients with fever and neutropenia, successful outcomes were reported in 126 of 164 (74 %) treated with piperacillin-tazobactam plus tigecycline compared with 90 of 190 (47 %) patients treated with piperacillin-tazobactam monotherapy ($p<0.01$), but there was no difference in mortality. Improved success rates were observed in bacteremia and in clinically documented infections [15]. These results, however, have not been reproduced so far and need to be interpreted with caution since the trial was open-label and details have not yet been published.

Tigecycline should be considered as an adjunct in the combination therapy of infections due to multidrug-resistant *Enterobacteriaceae* and possibly *A. baumannii*. In addition, it is a valuable option for patients with very severe CDI and with VRE infection.

14.5 Fluoroquinolones

Fluoroquinolones were marketed in the 1980s and have rapidly been evaluated as potential alternatives to trimethoprim-sulfamethoxazole or oral nonabsorbable drugs given for antibacterial prophylaxis in neutropenia [46, 55, 73, 108]. Most fluoroquinolones primarily target *Enterobacteriaceae* and *P. aeruginosa*. They have useful activity against other Gram-negative organisms such as gonococci, meningococci, *Legionella*, *Helicobacter*, *Yersinia*, *Francisella*, *Bacillus*, and others [2].

Norfloxacin was the first fluoroquinolone studied as chemoprophylaxis in leukemia patients. It is not active systemically due to very rapid renal elimination but has some effect on the intestinal microflora relevant for the prevention of Gram-negative infection. Ofloxacin – later replaced by levofloxacin – and ciprofloxacin were later developments, and these drugs are still being used for treatment of systemic infection. Newer fluoroquinolones still on the market include moxifloxacin and gatifloxacin which both show enhanced activity against streptococci and anaerobes, but also have some interesting activity against tuberculosis. Ciprofloxacin has the best activity against *P. aeruginosa* [2].

Due to the development of resistance among many *Enterobacteriaceae*, in particular *E. coli*, the fluoroquinolones are now less commonly used in cancer patients. Rates of resistance in cancer centers may be >50 % among *E. coli*. Such high rates of resistance may be associated both with inefficacy of the drugs for chemoprophylaxis as well as with failures in therapeutic indications such as fever and neutropenia [12, 93, 111]. However, low-risk patients (not given fluoroquinolone prophylaxis) may still benefit from fluoroquinolone therapy in the situation of fever and neutropenia. A recently published international trial that compared moxifloxacin with the combination of ciprofloxacin plus amoxicillin/clavulanic acid reported few failures: only 1 fluoroquinolone-resistant out of 19 (rate, 5 %) Gram-negative bloodstream isolates (without *P. aeruginosa*) causing primary infection among 333 patients [64]. This rate was comparable with that reported in a similar trial performed in the late 1990s [63].

An advantage of the fluoroquinolones is their good or excellent oral bioavailability. For ciprofloxacin, it is approximately 70 % with no substantial loss by first pass metabolism. Ciprofloxacin maximum serum concentrations are 2.5 (500 mg dose) or 4 μg/mL (750 mg dose). A 750 mg oral dose given every 12 h has been shown to produce an AUC at steady-state equivalent to that produced by an intravenous infusion of 400 mg given over 60 min every 8 h [20]. Such "high" doses are required for the treatment of systemic infections (outside the urinary tract) [53]. Approximately 40–50 % of an orally administered dose of ciprofloxacin is excreted in the urine as unchanged drug. Approximately 20–35 % of an oral dose is recovered from the feces within 5 days after dosing through biliary clearance and transintestinal elimination.

The oral bioavailabilities of levofloxacin (>95 %) and moxifloxacin (>90 %) are higher than that of ciprofloxacin. Both moxifloxacin (~11 h) and levofloxacin (~7 h) have longer half-lives than ciprofloxacin (~4 h) and are usually given once daily. The elimination through urine is >90 % of the total dose for levofloxacin but <30 % for moxifloxacin, respectively. All fluoroquinolones have been associated with phototoxicity, ruptures of tendons (including shoulder, hand and Achilles tendon), various adverse central nervous system events, serious reactions such as cardiac arrest or seizures after coadministration with theophylline, cholestatic jaundice and hepatitis, hypersensitivity reactions, and pseudomembranous colitis. The concurrent administration with magnesium/aluminum antacids, sucralfate, products containing calcium, iron, or zinc or dairy products (like milk or yogurt) or calcium-fortified juices impairs fluoroquinolone absorption and should be avoided.

14.6 Co-trimoxazole

Both sulfamethoxazole and trimethoprim are folate synthesis inhibitors. The spectrum of activity includes many Gram-negative bacteria (*Acinetobacter*, *Haemophilus*, *Moraxella*, *Enterobacteriaceae*, *Burkholderia*, *S. maltophilia*, *Vibrio cholerae*, *Brucella*), *Listeria monocytogenes*, many *Nocardia* species, *Tropheryma whipplei*, pneumococci, and staphylococci. The combination has also variable activity against various protozoa including *Plasmodium*, *Isospora belli*, and *Cyclospora* and some activity against *Pneumocystis jiroveci* and some other rare fungi [28, 35, 50]. In early studies, many culture media contained thymidine in a concentration sufficient to antagonize the folate synthesis inhibitory effects of sulfa drugs. Many streptococci and staphylococci therefore appeared resistant in vitro, and it was speculated that the in vivo activity of the drug and drug combination (co-trimoxazole) in (staphylococcal) abscesses might be severely impaired and circumvented due to thymidine uptake by *S. aureus*. *S. aureus* thermonuclease can release thymidine from polymerized DNA originating from inflammatory cells and injured tissues in the abscess.

The fixed combination preparation contains a 1:5 ratio of trimethoprim to sulfamethoxazole which in vivo changes to about 1:20 at steady state. Staphylococci exhibit wild-type MICs of ~1–2 μg/mL (tested at this trimethoprim:sulfamethoxazole 1:20 ratio), and the in vitro activity against most Gram-negative species is similar.

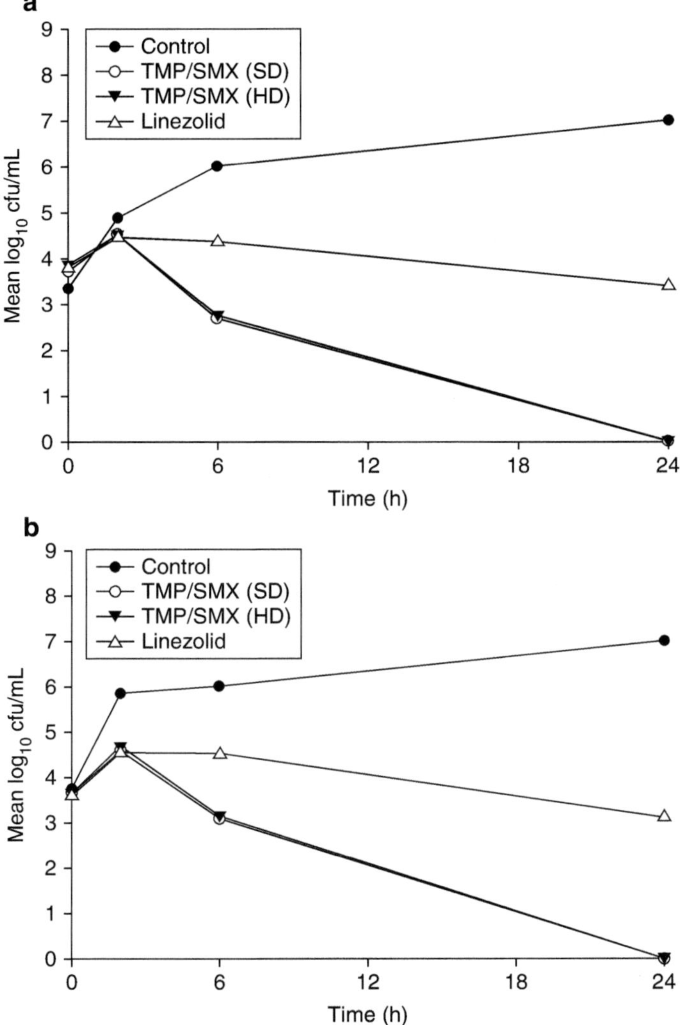

Fig. 14.3 The in vitro bactericidal activity of co-trimoxazole standard dose and high dose against *S. aureus* (two test strains (**a**) methicillin-susceptible *S. aureus* reference strain ATCC 29213, (**b**) MRSA strain MSU 33) compared with the static activity of linezolid (Data are from Stein et al. [105], with permission)

Of note is the bactericidal activity against *S. aureus* (Fig. 14.3) [105]. The (EUCAST) breakpoint for susceptibility (in most bacterial species including staphylococci) is ≤40 (2/38) μg/mL. *Stenotrophomonas maltophilia* is considered susceptible at a breakpoint of ≤80 (4/76) μg/mL, while enterococci and *Listeria* are considered susceptible only at a breakpoint of ≤1 μg/mL. According to the MIC distribution, almost all *Listeria* are highly susceptible and most enterococci have only intermediate susceptibility.

Both drugs are readily absorbed after oral administration and are distributed into body tissues and fluids, including sputum, aqueous humor, middle ear fluid, bronchial secretions, prostatic fluid, vaginal fluid, bile, and even cerebrospinal fluid [105]. Peak serum concentrations after a so-called double strength tablet (160/800 mg) are ~2–3 μg/mL for trimethoprim and 40–70 μg/mL for sulfamethoxazole, respectively. Urine concentrations of both sulfamethoxazole and trimethoprim are considerably higher than the concentrations in the blood. The average percentage of the dose recovered in urine from 0 to 72 h after a single oral dose is ~80–90 % for the sulfa part and 60–70 % for free trimethoprim. The half-life of trimethoprim is slightly shorter (~8 h) than that of sulfamethoxazole (~10 h). In renal insufficiency, the sulfamethoxazole component of the combination accumulates more rapidly than trimethoprim.

Infections outside the urinary tract due to less susceptible organisms may require higher daily dosages than the typically recommended 160/800 mg every 12 h. A higher dosage of 12/60 mg per kg bodyweight (divided into two or three doses per day, corresponding to two double strength tablets every 8–12 h in an adult) yields peak serum concentrations of ~8/200 μg/mL which are adequate for treatment of infections due to *Nocardia* and *S. maltophilia*.

Even higher dosages (20/100 mg per kg bodyweight divided into three or four doses per day) have been recommended for treatment of *P. jiroveci* pneumonia, but such high doses may relatively rapidly lead to accumulation of sulfamethoxazole and an elevated risk of associated hematotoxicity. In patients with renal dysfunction receiving high-dose therapy, it is wise to monitor trough blood levels in order to avoid too low levels of trimethoprim and too high and toxic levels of sulfamethoxazole [66].

Adverse events include allergic skin reactions (3–4 %) that can be severe (including erythema multiforme, Lyell's syndrome, and Stevens-Johnson syndrome) and inhibition by trimethoprim of renal creatinine secretion, leading to high serum creatinine levels, hyperkalemia, and cytopenias [1].

The drugs were introduced into the market in the 1960s and 1970s. Today, *E. coli* is often resistant to the drug (~20–40 %). Uses in cancer patients are primarily for *P. jiroveci* pneumonia prophylaxis or therapy and therapy of rare infections, for example, due to *Nocardia* or *S. maltophilia*. In addition, cotrimoxazole may be a very valuable oral drug for the treatment of *S. aureus* infection.

14.7 Colistin and Polymyxin B

Colistin (polymyxin E) and polymyxin B are increasingly needed and used as the last-resort treatment options against infections caused by MDR Gram-negative bacteria [4, 33, 37, 51, 75]. The two substances are large polypeptide antibiotics that are not absorbed from the intestinal tract. Previously, they have only rarely been used as intravenous drugs since more efficient and less toxic compounds were available. The recent reevaluation of these old polypeptides for the treatment of infection due to MDR Gram-negative bacteria has yielded some new insights with practical implications in particular for dosing.

Colistin is available as colistin methanesulfonate (CMS) that, after parenteral administration, undergoes conversion in vivo to form colistin, which is responsible for antibacterial activity [47, 75, 90, 110]. Thus, CMS is considered as an inactive prodrug. CMS has been assigned a potency of 12,500 IU/mg (one million units corresponding to 80 mg). Some recommendations regarding dosing refer to CMS units rather than weight, while some (older) recommendations refer to colistin base activity (given in units) rather than to CMS, and it is highly recommended to carefully pay attention to these details in order to avoid possible confusion and inadequate dosing [110]. With conventional dosing (typically one to two million units of CMS [80–160 mg] every 8 h), it will take 2–3 days before the steady-state concentration of colistin is obtained, and peak plasma concentrations often are in the range of only 1–2 μg/mL. This conventional dosing usually does not allow to reach an AUC/MIC of ≥60 that was predicted to produce in vivo bactericidal activity and found to yield acceptable clinical responses. A revised CMS dosing schedule is to give a loading dose of nine million units (720 mg), and subsequent twice-daily fractioned maintenance doses of up to ten million units (800 mg), titrated on renal function [26, 47, 90]. Infections due to microorganisms with an MIC >1 μg/mL remain difficult to be treated even with these higher doses, and monotherapy with colistin cannot be recommended in such cases.

Colistin can also be administered by inhalation [92]. Doses typically are one million units of CMS (80 mg) every 8–12 h. Intrathecal administration with doses of 10 mg of CMS per day has been reported as successfully eradicating MDR Gram-negative bacteria in cerebrospinal shunt infection.

Polymyxins are only active against Gram-negative bacteria. The EUCAST breakpoint for resistance is >2 μg/mL for *Enterobacteriaceae* and *Acinetobacter* and >4 μg/mL for *Pseudomonas*, respectively. The distribution of MICs for members of these groups of organisms is shown in Fig. 14.4. Natural resistance to polymyxins is seen in *Neisseria*, *Moraxella*, *Helicobacter*, *Proteus mirabilis*, *Serratia marcescens*, *Morganella morganii*, *Chromobacterium*, *Pandoraea* and *Burkholderia* associated with cystic fibrosis, and *Brucella*. Acquired resistance has been observed in MDR Gram-negative bacteria, notably in *Klebsiella* and *Pseudomonas*. Heteroresistance against polymyxins associated with regrowth observed at 24 h after an early concentration-dependent killing was demonstrated in *Acinetobacter* and *Klebsiella*.

Nephrotoxicity and neurotoxicity are the most common adverse effects of polymyxins. Total cumulative CMS dose is associated with kidney damage. The incidence is probably not much higher than that associated with aminoglycosides. Close monitoring of renal function is mandatory. The incidence of neurotoxicity is lower. Dizziness, weakness, visual disturbance, and neuromuscular blockade have been reported in rare cases.

For the treatment of infection due to MDR Gram-negative organisms, colistin should be combined with a second drug that is active or at least partially active, if possible, with meropenem, doxycycline or tigecycline, or fosfomycin [4]. If coadministered with an active aminoglycoside, enhanced nephrotoxicity is of concern.

Colistin has also been used in oral regimens for "selective decontamination of the digestive tract" (SDD) in an attempt to reduce intestinal tract colonization with

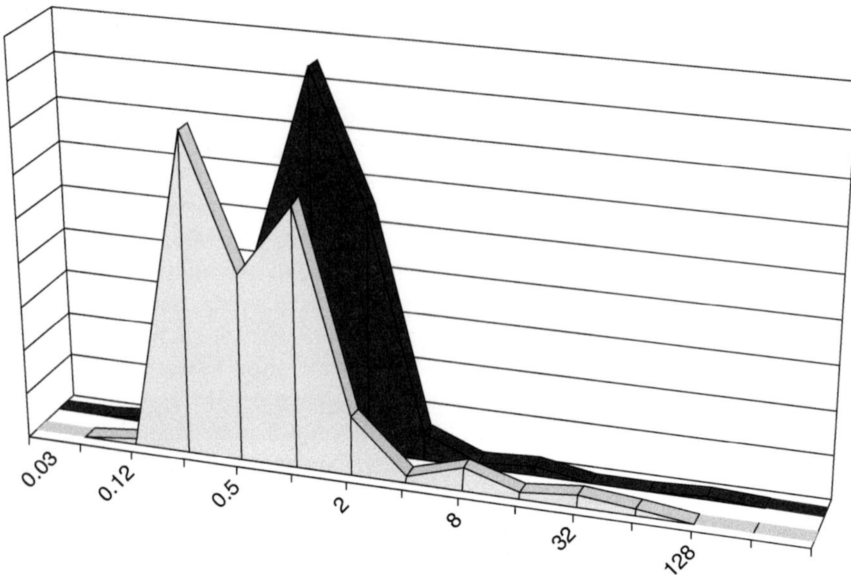

Fig. 14.4 The in vitro activity of colistin (μg/mL) with the distribution of MICs for *Acinetobacter baumannii* (*gray area*) and *Pseudomonas aeruginosa* (*black area*), respectively (Data are from EUCAST [35]). The EUCAST breakpoint for resistance is >2 μg/mL for *Acinetobacter* and >4 μg/mL for *Pseudomonas*, respectively. Recent PK-PF data indicate that infections due to microorganisms with an MIC >1 μg/mL remain difficult to be treated even with these higher doses of colistin, and monotherapy with colistin cannot be recommended in such cases

Gram-negative bacteria and associated infection in both leukemia patients and in patients admitted to intensive care. Whether intestinal decolonization with this or similar regimens is possible in the situation of MDR Gram-negative bacteria is unknown.

References

1. Ackerman BH, Patton ML, Guilday RE, et al. Trimethoprim-induced hyperkalemia in burn patients treated with intravenous or oral trimethoprim sulfamethoxazole for methicillin-resistant Staphylococcus aureus and other infections: nature or nurture? J Burn Care Res. 2013;34:127–32.
2. Appelbaum PC, Hunter PA. The fluoroquinolone antibacterials: past, present and future perspectives. Int J Antimicrob Agents. 2000;16:5–15.
3. Ariano RE, Nyhlén A, Donnelly JP, et al. Pharmacokinetics and pharmacodynamics of meropenem in febrile neutropenic patients with bacteremia. Ann Pharmacother. 2005;39:32–8.
4. Averbuch D, Orasch C, Cordonnier C, et al. European guidelines for empirical antibacterial therapy for febrile neutropenic patients in the era of growing resistance: summary of the 2011 4th European Conference on Infections in Leukemia. Haematologica. 2013;98:1826–35.
5. Baglie S, Rosalen PL, Franco LM, et al. Comparative bioavailability of 875 mg amoxicillin tablets in healthy human volunteers. Int J Clin Pharmacol Ther. 2005;43:350–4.

6. Berry V, Thorburn CE, Knott SJ, et al. Bacteriological efficacies of three macrolides compared with those of amoxicillin-clavulanate against Streptococcus pneumoniae and Haemophilus influenzae. Antimicrob Agents Chemother. 1998;42:3193–9.
7. Berthoin K, Le Duff CS, Marchand-Brynaert J, et al. Stability of meropenem and doripenem solutions for administration by continuous infusion. J Antimicrob Chemother. 2010;65:1073–5.
8. Blaser J, König C. Once-daily dosing of aminoglycosides. Eur J Clin Microbiol Infect Dis. 1995;14:1029–38.
9. Bhavnani SM, Hammel JP, Cirincione BB, Wikler MA, Ambrose PG. Use of pharmacokinetic-pharmacodynamic target attainment analyses to support phase 2 and 3 dosing strategies for doripenem. Antimicrob Agents Chemother. 2005;49(9):3944–7.
10. Boak LM, Rayner CR, Grayson ML, et al. Clinical population pharmacokinetics and toxicodynamics of linezolid. Antimicrob Agents Chemother. 2014;58:2334–43.
11. Bookstaver PB, Johnson JW, McCoy TP, et al. Modification of diet in renal disease and modified Cockcroft-Gault formulas in predicting aminoglycoside elimination. Ann Pharmacother. 2008;42:1758–65.
12. Bow EJ. Point: fluoroquinolone-based antibacterial chemoprophylaxis in neutropenic cancer patients works for defined outcomes in defined populations, but must be used wisely. J Natl Compr Canc Netw. 2004;2(5):433–44.
13. Boyer A, Gruson D, Bouchet S, et al. Aminoglycosides in septic shock: an overview, with specific consideration given to their nephrotoxic risk. Drug Saf. 2013;36:217–30.
14. Bubalo JS, Munar MY, Cherala G, et al. Daptomycin pharmacokinetics in adult oncology patients with neutropenic fever. Antimicrob Agents Chemother. 2009;53:428–34.
15. Bucaneve G, Miccozzi A, for the GIMEMA Infection Program. Prospective, randomised, multicentre controlled trial on empiric antibiotic therapy in febrile neutropenic cancer patients: piperacillin and tazobactam plus tigecycline versus piperacillin or tazobactam monotherapy. 51st ICAAC, Am Soc Microbiol. 2011, Abstract L1-1503a.
16. Burgess DS, Summers KK, Hardin TC. Pharmacokinetics and pharmacodynamics of aztreonam administered by continuous intravenous infusion. Clin Ther. 1999;21:1882–9.
17. Cafiso V, Bertuccio T, Spina D, et al. Modulating activity of vancomycin and daptomycin on the expression of autolysis cell-wall turnover and membrane charge genes in hVISA and VISA strains. PLoS One. 2012;7:e29573.
18. Casapao AM, Davis SL, Barr VO, et al. A large retrospective evaluation of the effectiveness and safety of ceftaroline fosamil therapy. Antimicrob Agents Chemother. 2014;58:2541–6.
19. Casapao AM, Kullar R, Davis SL, et al. Multicenter study of high-dose daptomycin for treatment of enterococcal infections. Antimicrob Agents Chemother. 2013;57:4190–6.
20. Catchpole C, Andrews JM, Woodcock J, et al. The comparative pharmacokinetics and tissue penetration of single-dose ciprofloxacin 400 mg i.v. and 750 mg po. J Antimicrob Chemother. 1994;33:103–10.
21. Chemaly RF, Hanmod SS, Jiang Y, et al. Tigecycline use in cancer patients with serious infections: a report on 110 cases from a single institution. Med (Baltimore). 2009;88:211–20.
22. Chytra I, Stepan M, Benes J, et al. Clinical and microbiological efficacy of continuous versus intermittent application of meropenem in critically ill patients: a randomized open-label controlled trial. Crit Care. 2012;16:R113.
23. Cometta A, Calandra T, Gaya H, et al. Monotherapy with meropenem versus combination therapy with ceftazidime plus amikacin as empiric therapy for fever in granulocytopenic patients with cancer. Antimicrob Agents Chemother. 1996;40:1108–15.
24. Crandon JL, Nicolau DP. Human simulated studies of aztreonam and aztreonam-avibactam to evaluate activity against challenging gram-negative organisms, including metallo-β-lactamase producers. Antimicrob Agents Chemother. 2013;57:3299–306.
25. Daikos GL, Markogiannakis A. Carbapenemase-producing Klebsiella pneumoniae: (when) might we still consider treating with carbapenems? Clin Microbiol Infect. 2011;17:1135–41.
26. Dalfino L, Puntillo F, Mosca A, et al. High-dose, extended-interval colistin administration in critically ill patients: is this the right dosing strategy? A preliminary study. Clin Infect Dis. 2012;54:1720–6.

27. Dandekar PK, Maglio D, Sutherland CA, et al. Pharmacokinetics of meropenem 0.5 and 2 g every 8 hours as a 3-hour infusion. Pharmacotherapy. 2003;23:988–91.
28. de Aguiar CR, Mourão CI, Rocha MF, et al. Antifolates inhibit Cryptococcus biofilms and enhance susceptibility of planktonic cells to amphotericin B. Eur J Clin Microbiol Infect Dis. 2013;32:557–64.
29. de Pauw BE, Deresinski SC, Feld R, et al. Ceftazidime compared with piperacillin and tobramycin for the empiric treatment of fever in neutropenic patients with cancer. A multicenter randomized trial. The Intercontinental Antimicrobial Study Group. Ann Intern Med. 1994;120:834–44.
30. del Favero A, Menichetti F, Martino P, et al. A multicenter, double-blind, placebo-controlled trial comparing piperacillin-tazobactam with and without amikacin as empiric therapy for febrile neutropenia. Clin Infect Dis. 2001;33:1295–301.
31. Docobo-Pérez F, López-Cerero L, López-Rojas R, et al. Inoculum effect on the efficacies of amoxicillin-clavulanate, piperacillin-tazobactam, and imipenem against extended-spectrum β-lactamase (ESBL)-producing and non-ESBL-producing Escherichia coli in an experimental murine sepsis model. Antimicrob Agents Chemother. 2013;57:2109–13.
32. Dryden MS. Linezolid pharmacokinetics and pharmacodynamics in clinical treatment. J Antimicrob Chemother. 2011;66 Suppl 4:7–15.
33. Durakovic N, Radojcic V, Boban A, et al. Efficacy and safety of colistin in the treatment of infections caused by multidrug-resistant Pseudomonas aeruginosa in patients with hematologic malignancy: a matched pair analysis. Intern Med. 2011;50:1009–13.
34. Egerer G, Goldschmidt H, Salwender H, et al. Efficacy of continuous infusion of ceftazidime for patients with neutropenic fever after high-dose chemotherapy and peripheral blood stem cell transplantation. Int J Antimicrob Agents. 2000;15:119–23.
35. EUCAST Antimicrobial wild type distributions of microorganisms. 2014. http://mic.eucast.org/Eucast2/. Accessed 1 Feb 2014.
36. Fainstein V, Bodey GP, Elting L, et al. A randomized study of ceftazidime compared to ceftazidime and tobramycin for the treatment of infections in cancer patients. J Antimicrob Chemother. 1983;12(Suppl A):101–10.
37. Falagas ME, Rafailidis PI, Ioannidou E, et al. Colistin therapy for microbiologically documented multidrug-resistant gram-negative bacterial infections: a retrospective cohort study of 258 patients. Int J Antimicrob Agents. 2010;35:194–9.
38. Feig PU, Mitchell PP, Abrutyn E, et al. Aminoglycoside nephrotoxicity: a double blind prospective randomized study of gentamicin and tobramycin. J Antimicrob Chemother. 1982;10:217–26.
39. Feld R, dePauw B, Berman S, et al. Meropenem versus ceftazidime in the treatment of cancer patients with febrile neutropenia: a randomized, double-blind trial. J Clin Oncol. 2000;18:3690–8.
40. Fleischhack G, Hartmann C, Simon A, et al. Meropenem versus ceftazidime as empirical monotherapy in febrile neutropenia of paediatric patients with cancer. J Antimicrob Chemother. 2001;47:841–53.
41. Fraschini F, Scaglione F, Falchi M, et al. Pharmacokinetics and tissue distribution of amoxicillin plus clavulanic acid after oral administration in man. J Chemother. 1990;2:171–7.
42. Freifeld AG, Bow EJ, Sepkowitz KA, et al. Clinical practice guideline for the use of antimicrobial agents in neutropenic patients with cancer: 2010 update by the Infectious Diseases Society of America. Clin Infect Dis. 2011;52:e56–93.
43. Freifeld AG, Walsh T, Marshall D, et al. Monotherapy for fever and neutropenia in cancer patients: a randomized comparison of ceftazidime versus imipenem. J Clin Oncol. 1995;13:165–76.
44. Fugate JE, Kalimullah EA, Hocker SE, et al. Cefepime neurotoxicity in the intensive care unit: a cause of severe, underappreciated encephalopathy. Crit Care. 2013;17:R264.
45. Fujisawa Y, Oyake T, Mine T, et al. Doripenem versus meropenem for empirical antimicrobial therapy in high risk febrile neutropenic patients with hematological malignancies: a randomized, controlled trial. ASH 2013 Annual Meeting Abstracts. Blood. 2013;122:4716.

46. Gafter-Gvili A, Fraser A, Paul M, et al. Antibiotic prophylaxis for bacterial infections in afebrile neutropenic patients following chemotherapy. Cochrane Database Syst Rev. 2012;(1):CD004386.
47. Garonzik SM, Li J, Thamlikitkul V, et al. Population pharmacokinetics of colistin methanesulfonate and formed colistin in critically ill patients from a multicenter study provide dosing suggestions for various categories of patients. Antimicrob Agents Chemother. 2011; 55:3284–94.
48. Ghehi MT, Rezaee S, Hayatshahi A, et al. Vancomycin pharmacokinetic parameters in patients undergoing hematopoietic stem cell transplantation (HSCT). Int J Hematol Oncol Stem Cell Res. 2013;7:1–9.
49. Gibson J, Date L, Joshua DE, et al. A randomised trial of empirical antibiotic therapy in febrile neutropenic patients with hematological disorders: ceftazidime versus azlocillin plus amikacin. Aust N Z J Med. 1989;19:417–25.
50. Goldberg E, Bishara J. Contemporary unconventional clinical use of co-trimoxazole. Clin Microbiol Infect. 2012;18:8–17.
51. Hachem RY, Chemaly RF, Ahmar CA, et al. Colistin is effective in treatment of infections caused by multidrug-resistant Pseudomonas aeruginosa in cancer patients. Antimicrob Agents Chemother. 2007;51:1905–11.
52. Hachem RY, Hicks K, Huen A, et al. Myelosuppression and serotonin syndrome associated with concurrent use of linezolid and selective serotonin reuptake inhibitors in bone marrow transplant recipients. Clin Infect Dis. 2003;37:e8–11.
53. Haeseker M, Stolk L, Nieman F, et al. The ciprofloxacin target AUC: MIC ratio is not reached in hospitalized patients with the recommended dosing regimens. Br J Clin Pharmacol. 2013;75:180–5.
54. Hatala R, Dinh TT, Cook DJ. Single daily dosing of aminoglycosides in immunocompromised adults: a systematic review. Clin Infect Dis. 1997;24:810–5.
55. Imran H, Tleyjeh IM, Arndt CA, et al. Fluoroquinolone prophylaxis in patients with neutropenia: a meta-analysis of randomized placebo-controlled trials. Eur J Clin Microbiol Infect Dis. 2008;27:53–6.
56. Jaksic B, Martinelli G, Perez-Oteyza J, et al. Efficacy and safety of linezolid compared with vancomycin in a randomized, double-blind study of febrile neutropenic patients with cancer. Clin Infect Dis. 2006;42:597–607.
57. Jaruratanasirikul S, Limapichat T, Jullangkoon M, et al. Pharmacodynamics of meropenem in critically ill patients with febrile neutropenia and bacteraemia. Int J Antimicrob Agents. 2011;38:231–6.
58. Jaruratanasirikul S, Sriwiriyajan S, Punyo J. Comparison of the pharmacodynamics of meropenem in patients with ventilator-associated pneumonia following administration by 3-hour infusion or bolus injection. Antimicrob Agents Chemother. 2005;49:1337–9.
59. Jean SS, Lee WS, Bai KJ, et al. Relationship between the distribution of cefepime minimum inhibitory concentrations and detection of extended-spectrum β-lactamase production among clinically important Enterobacteriaceae isolates obtained from patients in intensive care units in Taiwan: results from the Surveillance of Multicenter Antimicrobial Resistance in Taiwan (SMART) in 2007. J Microbiol Immunol Infect. 2013. pii: S1684–1182(13)00118–7. doi: 10.1016/j.jmii.2013.07.002. [Epub ahead of print].
60. Joshi L, Taylor SR, Large O, et al. A case of optic neuropathy after short-term linezolid use in a patient with acute lymphocytic leukemia. Clin Infect Dis. 2009;48:e73–4.
61. Kahan FM, Kropp H, Sundelof JG, et al. Thienamycin: development of imipenem-cilastatin. J Antimicrob Chemother. 1983;12(Suppl D):1–35.
62. Kalil AC. Is cefepime safe for clinical use? A Bayesian viewpoint. J Antimicrob Chemother. 2011;66:1207–9.
63. Kern WV, Cometta A, de Bock R, et al. Oral versus intravenous empirical antimicrobial therapy for fever in patients with granulocytopenia who are receiving cancer chemotherapy. International Antimicrobial Therapy Cooperative Group of the EORTC. N Engl J Med. 1999;341:312–8.

64. Kern WV, Marchetti O, Drgona L, et al. Oral antibiotics for fever in low-risk neutropenic patients with cancer: a double-blind, randomized, multicenter trial comparing single daily moxifloxacin with twice daily ciprofloxacin plus amoxicillin/clavulanic acid combination therapy – EORTC Infectious Diseases Group Trial X. J Clin Oncol. 2013;31:1149–56.
65. Kim PW, Wu YT, Cooper C, et al. Meta-analysis of a possible signal of increased mortality associated with cefepime use. Clin Infect Dis. 2010;51:381–9.
66. Klinker H, Langmann P, Zilly M, et al. Drug monitoring during the treatment of AIDS-associated Pneumocystis carinii pneumonia with trimethoprim-sulfamethoxazole. J Clin Pharm Ther. 1998;23:149–54.
67. Kullar R, Casapao AM, Davis SL, et al. A multicentre evaluation of the effectiveness and safety of high-dose daptomycin for the treatment of infective endocarditis. J Antimicrob Chemother. 2013;68:2921–6.
68. Kuti JL, Nightingale CH, Knauft RF, et al. Pharmacokinetic properties and stability of continuous-infusion meropenem in adults with cystic fibrosis. Clin Ther. 2004;26:493–501.
69. Kwon KT, Cheong HS, Rhee JY, et al. Panipenem versus cefepime as empirical monotherapy in adult cancer patients with febrile neutropenia: a prospective randomized trial. Jpn J Clin Oncol. 2008;38:49–55.
70. Lai CC, Sheng WH, Wang JT, et al. Safety and efficacy of high-dose daptomycin as salvage therapy for severe gram-positive bacterial sepsis in hospitalized adult patients. BMC Infect Dis. 2013;13:66.
71. Landersdorfer CB, Kirkpatrick CM, Kinzig-Schippers M, et al. Population pharmacokinetics at two dose levels and pharmacodynamic profiling of flucloxacillin. Antimicrob Agents Chemother. 2007;51:3290–7.
72. Lee LS, Kinzig-Schippers M, Nafziger AN, et al. Comparison of 30-min and 3-h infusion regimens for imipenem/cilastatin and for meropenem evaluated by Monte Carlo simulation. Diagn Microbiol Infect Dis. 2010;68:251–8.
73. Leibovici L, Paul M, Cullen M, et al. Antibiotic prophylaxis in neutropenic patients: new evidence, practical decisions. Cancer. 2006;107:1743–51.
74. Livermore DM, Warner M, Mushtaq S, et al. What remains against carbapenem-resistant Enterobacteriaceae? Evaluation of chloramphenicol, ciprofloxacin, colistin, fosfomycin, minocycline, nitrofurantoin, temocillin and tigecycline. Int J Antimicrob Agents. 2011;37:415–9.
75. Luque S, Grau S, Valle M, et al. Differences in pharmacokinetics and pharmacodynamics of colistimethate sodium (CMS) and colistin between three different CMS dosage regimens in a critically ill patient infected by a multidrug-resistant acinetobacter baumannii. Int J Antimicrob Agents. 2013;42:178–81.
76. MacVane SH, Kuti JL, Nicolau DP. Prolonging β-lactam infusion: a review of the rationale and evidence, and guidance for implementation. Int J Antimicrob Agents. 2014;43:105–13.
77. Manji A, Lehrnbecher T, Dupuis LL, et al. A systematic review and meta-analysis of anti-pseudomonal penicillins and carbapenems in pediatric febrile neutropenia. Support Care Cancer. 2012;20:2295–304.
78. Mareville J, Gay J, Cliquennois E, et al. Therapeutic drug monitoring of aminoglycosides in acute myeloid leukaemia patients. Scand J Infect Dis. 2012;44:398–401.
79. Martínez JA, Cobos-Trigueros N, Soriano A, et al. Influence of empiric therapy with a beta-lactam alone or combined with an aminoglycoside on prognosis of bacteremia due to gram-negative microorganisms. Antimicrob Agents Chemother. 2010;54:3590–6.
80. Mavros MN, Polyzos KA, Rafailidis PI, et al. Once versus multiple daily dosing of aminoglycosides for patients with febrile neutropenia: a systematic review and meta-analysis. J Antimicrob Chemother. 2011;66:251–9.
81. McKinnon PS, Paladino JA, Schentag JJ. Evaluation of area under the inhibitory curve (AUIC) and time above the minimum inhibitory concentration (T>MIC) as predictors of outcome for cefepime and ceftazidime in serious bacterial infections. Int J Antimicrob Agents. 2008;31:345–51.
82. Micek ST, Welch EC, Khan J, et al. Empiric combination antibiotic therapy is associated with improved outcome against sepsis due to gram-negative bacteria: a retrospective analysis. Antimicrob Agents Chemother. 2010;54:1742–8.

83. Munckhof WJ, Grayson ML, Turnidge JD. A meta-analysis of studies on the safety and efficacy of aminoglycosides given either once daily or as divided doses. J Antimicrob Chemother. 1996;37:645–63.
84. Nailor MD, Sobel JD. Antibiotics for gram-positive bacterial infections: vancomycin, teicoplanin, quinupristin/dalfopristin, oxazolidinones, daptomycin, dalbavancin, and telavancin. Med Clin North Am. 2011;95:723–42.
85. Narita M, Tsuji BT, Yu VL. Linezolid-associated peripheral and optic neuropathy, lactic acidosis, and serotonin syndrome. Pharmacotherapy. 2007;27:1189–97.
86. Paul M, Dickstein Y, Schlesinger A, et al. Beta-lactam versus beta-lactam-aminoglycoside combination therapy in cancer patients with neutropenia. Cochrane Database Syst Rev. 2013;(6):CD003038.
87. Paul M, Yahav D, Bivas A, et al. Anti-pseudomonal beta-lactams for the initial, empirical, treatment of febrile neutropenia: comparison of beta-lactams. Cochrane Database Syst Rev. 2010;(11):CD005197.
88. Pea F, Viale P, Damiani D, et al. Ceftazidime in acute myeloid leukemia patients with febrile neutropenia: helpfulness of continuous intravenous infusion in maximizing pharmacodynamic exposure. Antimicrob Agents Chemother. 2005;49:3550–3.
89. Pizzo PA, Hathorn JW, Hiemenz J, et al. A randomized trial comparing ceftazidime alone with combination antibiotic therapy in cancer patients with fever and neutropenia. N Engl J Med. 1986;315:552–8.
90. Plachouras D, Karvanen M, Friberg LE, et al. Population pharmacokinetic analysis of colistin methanesulfonate and colistin after intravenous administration in critically ill patients with infections caused by gram-negative bacteria. Antimicrob Agents Chemother. 2009;53:3430–6.
91. Poulikakos P, Falagas ME. Aminoglycoside therapy in infectious diseases. Expert Opin Pharmacother. 2013;14:1585–97.
92. Quon BS, Goss CH, Ramsey BW. Inhaled antibiotics for lower airway infections. Ann Am Thorac Soc. 2014;11:425–34.
93. Rangaraj G, Granwehr BP, Jiang Y, et al. Perils of quinolone exposure in cancer patients: breakthrough bacteremia with multidrug-resistant organisms. Cancer. 2010;116:967–73.
94. Reed MD. Clinical pharmacokinetics of amoxicillin and clavulanate. Pediatr Infect Dis J. 1996;15:949–54.
95. Rigge DC, Jones MF. Shelf lives of aseptically prepared medicines – stability of piperacillin/tazobactam in PVC and non-PVC bags. J Pharm Biomed Anal. 2005;39:339–43.
96. Rodríguez-Baño J, Navarro MD, Retamar P, et al. β-lactam/β-lactam inhibitor combinations for the treatment of bacteremia due to extended-spectrum β-lactamase-producing Escherichia coli: a post hoc analysis of prospective cohorts. Clin Infect Dis. 2012;54:167–74.
97. Rodríguez-Baño J, Oteo J, Ortega A, et al. Epidemiological and clinical complexity of amoxicillin-clavulanate-resistant Escherichia coli. J Clin Microbiol. 2013;51:2414–7.
98. Rolston KV, Besece D, Lamp KC, et al. Daptomycin use in neutropenic patients with documented gram-positive infections. Support Care Cancer. 2014;22:7–14.
99. Rolston KV, McConnell SA, Brown J, et al. Daptomycin use in patients with cancer and neutropenia: data from a retrospective registry. Clin Adv Hematol Oncol. 2010;8:249–56.
100. Ryzner KL. Evaluation of aminoglycoside clearance using the modification of diet in renal disease equation versus the Cockcroft-Gault equation as a marker of glomerular filtration rate. Ann Pharmacother. 2010;44:1030–7.
101. Safdar A, Rolston KV. Vancomycin tolerance, a potential mechanism for refractory gram-positive bacteremia observational study in patients with cancer. Cancer. 2006;106:1815–20.
102. Schentag JJ, Plaut ME, Cerra FB. Comparative nephrotoxicity of gentamicin and tobramycin: pharmacokinetic and clinical studies in 201 patients. Antimicrob Agents Chemother. 1981;19:859–66.
103. Shea KM, Cheatham SC, Smith DW, et al. Comparative pharmacodynamics of intermittent and prolonged infusions of piperacillin/tazobactam using Monte Carlo simulations and steady-state pharmacokinetic data from hospitalized patients. Ann Pharmacother. 2009;43:1747–54.

104. Smith PF, Birmingham MC, Noskin GA, et al. Safety, efficacy and pharmacokinetics of linezolid for treatment of resistant gram-positive infections in cancer patients with neutropenia. Ann Oncol. 2003;14:795–801.
105. Stein GE, Throckmorton JK, Scharmen AE, et al. Tissue penetration and antimicrobial activity of standard- and high-dose trimethoprim/sulfamethoxazole and linezolid in patients with diabetic foot infection. J Antimicrob Chemother. 2013;68:2852–8.
106. Stephens C, López-Nevot M, Ruiz-Cabello F, et al. HLA alleles influence the clinical signature of amoxicillin-clavulanate hepatotoxicity. PLoS One. 2013;8:e68111.
107. Thabet F, Al Maghrabi M, Al Barraq A, et al. Cefepime-induced nonconvulsive status epilepticus: case report and review. Neurocrit Care. 2009;10:347–51.
108. van de Wetering MD, de Witte MA, Kremer LC, et al. Efficacy of oral prophylactic antibiotics in neutropenic afebrile oncology patients: a systematic review of randomised controlled trials. Eur J Cancer. 2005;41:1372–82.
109. Veeraraghavan B. Newer β-lactam and β-lactamase inhibitor combinations available in India: consensus and controversies. Indian J Med Microbiol. 2011;29:315–6.
110. Velkov T, Roberts KD, Nation RL, et al. Pharmacology of polymyxins: new insights into an 'old' class of antibiotics. Future Microbiol. 2013;8:711–24.
111. Vesole DH, Oken MM, Heckler C, et al. Oral antibiotic prophylaxis of early infection in multiple myeloma: a URCC/ECOG randomized phase III study. Leukemia. 2012;26:2517–20.
112. Viaene E, Chanteux H, Servais H, et al. Comparative stability studies of antipseudomonal beta-lactams for potential administration through portable elastomeric pumps (home therapy for cystic fibrosis patients) and motor-operated syringes (intensive care units). Antimicrob Agents Chemother. 2002;46:2327–32.
113. Viscoli C, Cometta A, Kern WV, et al. Piperacillin-tazobactam monotherapy in high-risk febrile and neutropenic cancer patients. Clin Microbiol Infect. 2006;12:212–6.
114. Wolfensberger A, Sax H, Weber R, et al. Change of antibiotic susceptibility testing guidelines from CLSI to EUCAST: influence on cumulative hospital antibiograms. PLoS One. 2013;8:e79130.
115. Yahav D, Paul M, Fraser A, et al. Efficacy and safety of cefepime: a systematic review and meta-analysis. Lancet Infect Dis. 2007;7:338–48.
116. Zhanel GG, Lawson CD, Adam H, et al. Ceftazidime-avibactam: a novel cephalosporin/β--lactamase inhibitor combination. Drugs. 2013;73:159–77.
117. Zhanel GG, Lawson CD, Zelenitsky S, et al. Comparison of the next-generation aminoglycoside plazomicin to gentamicin, tobramycin and amikacin. Expert Rev Anti Infect Ther. 2012;10:459–73.

Antifungal Agents 15

George R. Thompson III and Thomas F. Patterson

Contents

15.1 Introduction

Invasive fungal infections (IFIs) are responsible for significant morbidity and mortality, particularly in the immunocompromised host. Although mortality from invasive candidiasis has decreased in recent years, an overall increase in the number of

G.R. Thompson III (✉)
Department of Medical Microbiology and Immunology, Coccidioidomycosis Serology Laboratory, University of California – Davis,
One Shields Avenue, Tupper Hall, Davis, CA 95616, USA

Division of Infectious Diseases, Department of Internal Medicine,
University of California Davis Medical Center, 4150 V Street, Suite G500,
Sacramento, CA 95817 USA
e-mail: grthompson@ucdavis.edu

T.F. Patterson
Division of Infectious Diseases, Department of Internal Medicine, University of Texas Health Science Center at San Antonio and South Texas Veterans Health Care System,
San Antonio, TX 78229, USA

G. Maschmeyer, K.V.I. Rolston (eds.), *Infections in Hematology*,
DOI 10.1007/978-3-662-44000-1_15

deaths from IFIs has been noted, largely due to invasive aspergillosis [1–4]. The number of patients at risk has also increased as a greater number of patients are exposed to immunosuppressive therapy and more intensive chemotherapy regimens [5]. Fortunately, the number of agents available to treat fungal infections has continued to increase. This greater number of therapeutic choices necessitates a detailed knowledge of each drug class and potential differences in efficacy, spectrum of antifungal activity, bioavailability, pharmacokinetics, and side-effect profiles.

15.2 Polyenes

Amphotericin B (AMB) and nystatin are the only polyenes currently available and nystatin is limited solely to topical therapy. The polyenes bind to ergosterol present within the fungal cell membrane and disrupt cell permeability causing fungal death (Fig. 15.1). There is also evidence that AMB acts as a proinflammatory agent by stimulating the release of immunologic mediators such as cytokines and chemokines; however, this mechanism is likely also responsible for the infusion-related toxicity related to AMB administration.

Clinical outcomes in susceptible isolates are best predicted by the peak serum level to MIC ratio. Serum drug levels are infrequently measured and are typically available only in the research setting [6]. Resistance to AMB is common in *Aspergillus terreus*, *Pseudallescheria boydii* complex, *Scedosporium prolificans*, *Trichosporon* spp., and *Candida lusitaniae* (Table 15.1). Resistance has been reported in other species and changes in ergosterol biosynthesis and/or the synthesis

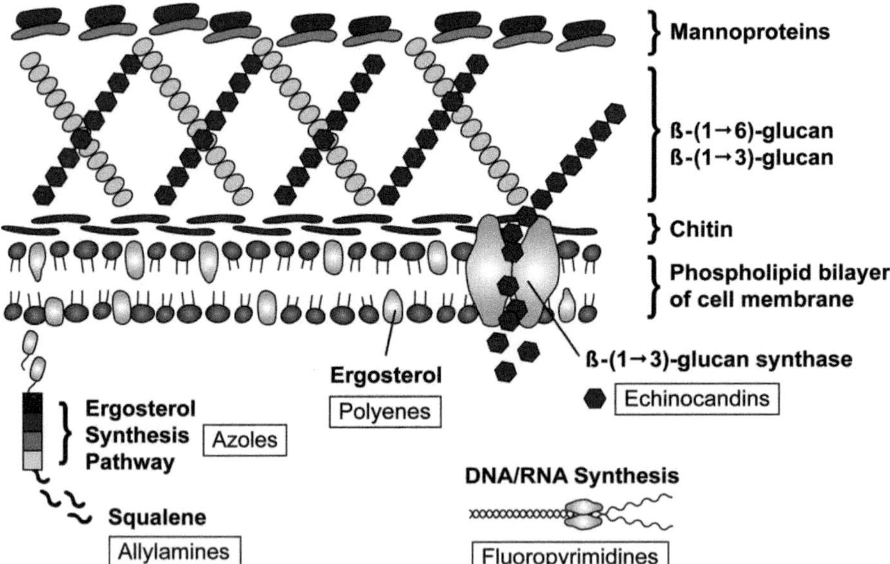

Fig. 15.1 Targets of systemic antifungal agents

Table 15.1 Antifungal spectrum of activity against common molds and yeast

Organism	AMB	FLU	ITR	POS	VOR	ANI	MFG	CAS	5FC
Aspergillus fumigatus	+	–	+	+	+	+	+	+	–
Aspergillus flavus	+/–	–	+	+	+	+	+	+	–
Aspergillus terreus	–	–	+	+	+	+	+	+	–
Aspergillus niger	+	–	+/–	+	+	+	+	+	–
Candida albicans	+	+	+	+	+	+	+	+	+
Candida glabrata	+	+/–	+/–	+	+	+	+	+	+
Candida krusei	+	–	+/–	+	+	+	+	+	+/–
Candida parapsilosis	+	+	+	+	+	+/–	+/–	+/–	+
Cryptococcus spp.	+	+	+	+	+	–	–	–	+
Blastomyces spp.	+	+	+	+	+	+/–	+/–	+/–	–
Histoplasma spp.	+	+/–	+	+	+	+/–	+/–	+/–	–
Coccidioides spp.	+	+	+	+	+	–	–	–	–
Fusarium spp.	+/–	–	–	+	+	–	–	–	–
Phaeohyphomycoses[a]	+	–	+	+	+	+	+	+	–
Scedosporium apiospermum	+/–	–	+/–	+	+	–	–	–	–
Scedosporium prolificans	–	–	–	+/–	+/–	–	–	–	–
Mucorales[b]	+/–	–	–	+	–	–	–	–	–

AMB amphotericin, *FLU* fluconazole, *ITR* itraconazole, *POS* posaconazole, *VOR* voriconazole, *ANI* anidulafungin, *MFG* micafungin, *CAS* caspofungin, *5FC* flucytosine
(+) implies antifungal activity against isolates, (–) implies no or limited activity against isolate, (+/–) implies variable activity against isolates
[a]Infection requires debridement in almost all circumstances
[b]Formerly Zygomycetes

of alternative sterols is the proposed mechanism for reduced AMB activity in these isolates [7].

AMB is available in inhalational, oral, and intravenous formulations. The well-known nephrotoxicity seen with intravenous amphotericin B deoxycholate (AmBd; Fungizone) has prompted the development of lipid formulations with more favorable side-effect profiles so that in patients with hematological malignancies lipid formulations of AMB have largely replaced the use of AmBd. Liposomal amphotericin B (L-AMB; Ambisome), amphotericin B lipid complex (ABLC; Abelcet), and amphotericin B colloidal dispersion (ABCD; Amphotec, Amphocil) are all currently available lipid formulations with a high degree of protein binding (>95 %, primarily to albumin) and comparably long half-lives.

Cerebrospinal fluid levels are low (<5 % of concurrent serum concentration) yet AMB remains the drug of choice for cryptococcal meningitis [8]. Intrathecal AMB has been used in the salvage setting for both coccidioidal and candidal meningitis; however, this practice is seldom used due to poor patient tolerability, the difficulty of administration, and the availability of alternative agents.

Similarly, AMB has low vitreous penetration (0–38 %) and intraocular injections are often required in the treatment of deep-seated ophthalmologic fungal infections including candidal endophthalmitis [9, 10]. The route of elimination of AMB remains unknown and dosing need not be adjusted in patients with a reduced glomerular filtration rate.

The broad antifungal spectrum and experience with the use of amphotericin B accounts for its continued use despite toxicity concerns. Liposomal amphotericin B remains a recommended antifungal during the treatment of neutropenic fever following an open-label, randomized international trial comparing L-AMB to voriconazole [11]. A recent meta-analysis also suggests L-AMB is associated with lower mortality during empiric treatment of neutropenic fever [12].

AMB was previously the preferred first-line agent during the treatment of invasive aspergillosis; however, a comparative trial has now demonstrated a lower mortality rate when voriconazole is administered in this setting [13, 14]. AMB remains the agent of choice for treatment of mucormycosis and a delay in the prescribing of an AMB formulation in this population is associated with a twofold greater risk of death [15].

AMB in combination with flucytosine remains the drug of choice in the treatment of cryptococcal meningitis and in most cases a lipid formulation is preferred due to the decreased incidence of nephrotoxicity. Severe infection caused by one of the endemic mycoses (histoplasmosis, coccidioidomycosis, blastomycosis, and sporotrichosis) should also be treated with an AMB formulation.

Intravenous AmBd is typically given in doses of 0.7–1 mg/kg, while the lipid formulations are given in higher doses (3–5 mg/kg). Recently, in an attempt to define the efficacy of even higher doses of lipid formulations, doses of L-AmB (3 mg/kg vs 10 mg/kg) were given in a randomized trial of invasive mold infections. Success rates were similar in both arms although more nephrotoxicity was seen in those receiving higher L-AmB doses [16]. Despite these findings, in cases of severe or life-threatening disease, escalating doses of lipid AMB formulations may be indicated.

Local delivery of amphotericin B has been attempted through use of aerosolized therapy. Lipid preparations are preferred for inhalation and aerosolized delivery has been found effective in the prevention of pulmonary IFIs in lung transplantation and in bone marrow transplant recipients [17, 18].

Side effects of AmBd infusion include fever, chills, rigors, myalgias, bronchospasm, nausea and vomiting, tachycardia, tachypnea, and hypertension [19]. The use of lipid formulations has decreased the incidence of these untoward effects although ABCD has been associated with the development of dyspnea and hypoxia and L-AMB has been associated with back pain during infusion [9]. The potential nephrotoxicity of amphotericin B is well known and may occur in up to 30 % of patients. Vascular smooth muscle dysfunction with resultant vasoconstriction and ischemia are the presumed mechanism of renal injury following AMB administration [20]. Lipid preparations have lower rates of nephrotoxicity and studies have shown that when AmBd is replaced by a lipid formulation after the development of acute kidney injury, renal function stabilizes or improves in a significant proportion of patients [21]. Despite the higher drug costs of lipid AMB formulations, the reduction in hospital days when toxicity is avoided has proven the lipid formulations more cost-effective than AmBd [21].

15.3 Triazoles

The triazoles exert their effects within ergosterol synthesis by inhibition of cytochrome P450 (CYP)-dependent 14-α-demethylase preventing the conversion of lanosterol to ergosterol (Fig. 15.1). This class has demonstrated both species- and strain-dependent fungistatic or fungicidal activity in vitro and the area under the curve to MIC ratio (AUC/MIC) is the best predictor of drug efficacy.

Azoles differ in their affinity for the 14-α-demethylase enzyme and these differences are largely responsible for their varying antifungal potency and spectrum of activity. Cross-inhibition of several human CYP-dependent enzymes (3A4, 2C9, and 2C19) is responsible for the majority of the clinical side effects and drug-drug interactions within this class. Itraconazole and posaconazole act as inhibitors of 3A4 and 2C9 with little effect on 2C19 and voriconazole acts as both an inhibitor and a substrate on all three isoenzymes. Although comprehensive lists of triazole drug interactions can be found elsewhere, concurrent administration should be avoided with most HMG-CoA reductase inhibitors, benzodiazepines, phenytoin, carbamazepine, cyclosporine, tacrolimus, sirolimus, methylprednisolone, buspirone, alfentanil; the dihydropyridine calcium channel blockers; the sulfonylureas, rifampin, rifabutin, vincristine, busulfan, docetaxel, trimetrexate; and the protease inhibitors ritonavir, indinavir, and saquinavir [22–28].

The triazoles have also been associated with QTc prolongation and coadministration with other agents known to have similar effects should be avoided. This class is additionally embryotoxic and teratogenic and is secreted into breast milk, so that administration should be avoided during pregnancy or while lactating [29–31].

15.3.1 Fluconazole

Fluconazole (Diflucan) remains one of the most prescribed triazoles due to its favorable bioavailability, tolerability, and side-effect profile. Greater than 80 % of ingested drug is found in the circulation, and excellent urine and tissue penetration (CSF levels 70 % of matched serum levels) are seen. A half-life of 27–34 h allows once daily dosing for most patients; however, in those with a reduced creatinine clearance, the normal dose should be reduced by 50 %.

Fluconazole is active against most *Candida* spp. with the exception of *C. krusei* and *C. glabrata* (Table 15.1). Susceptible *C. glabrata* isolates should be treated with higher doses (12 mg/kg/daily) of fluconazole than other species [10].

Fluconazole remains one of the first-line agents in the treatment of oropharyngeal candidiasis (OPC) [10] and patients with frequent relapse should remain on chronic suppressive fluconazole until immune reconstitution has been documented as chronic therapy is well tolerated when necessary [32].

Fluconazole has also been used for antifungal prophylaxis in high-risk patients. Initiation of 400 mg/day of fluconazole for the first 75 days following bone marrow transplantation (BMT) has been found effective in reducing cases of candidemia [33].

Following induction therapy with AMB and flucytosine, fluconazole is used for suppression of cryptococcosis following CNS disease until immunologic derangements have abated – otherwise life-long therapy is recommended [8]. Recent data has examined the use of high-dose fluconazole monotherapy during induction treatment of cryptococcal meningitis; however, this practice should be used only in resource limited settings and not when AMB is available [34].

Headache, alopecia, and anorexia are the most common side effects (10 %) with transaminase elevation in <10 %.

15.3.2 Itraconazole

Itraconazole is currently available as both capsules and an oral solution suspended in hydroxypropyl-β-cyclodextrin (HPCD). The intravenous preparation is no longer available in all developed countries. Itraconazole capsules are dependent upon an acidic environment for maximal absorption, and the concomitant administration of H_2-receptor antagonists or proton pump inhibitors causes unpredictable drug absorption, and it is recommended that itraconazole capsules be taken with food or an acidic beverage [35, 36].

Itraconazole solution allows for greater oral bioavailability and the AUC and peak concentrations are both increased by 30 % when itraconazole solution is taken in the fasting state [37]. Oral loading (200 mg three times daily for 3 days) allows for more rapid attainment of therapeutic serum levels. Itraconazole is also highly protein bound with less than 1 % available as free drug and has a relatively high volume of distribution.

The recent development of more effective antifungal agents (i.e., voriconazole) has relegated itraconazole to second-line therapy during the treatment of invasive aspergillosis. Itraconazole does, however, remain the drug of choice for those with mild to moderate infection caused by histoplasmosis [38]. Itraconazole is also approved for allergic bronchopulmonary aspergillosis (ABPA) [14].

The recommended dosage of oral itraconazole in adults is 400 mg/day (capsules) and 2.5 mg/kg twice daily (HPCD solution) [14]. Dose adjustment is not indicated with use of the oral formulations of itraconazole when used in patients with renal insufficiency or those receiving hemodialysis. The half-life of itraconazole is prolonged in patients with hepatic dysfunction and dose adjustment, liver function testing, and drug interactions should be carefully assessed in this circumstance [39].

The most frequent side effects include nausea and vomiting (<10 %), hypertriglyceridemia (9 %), hypokalemia (6 %), liver enzyme elevations (5 %), skin rashes/pruritus (2 %), headache and dizziness (<2 %), and pedal edema (1 %) [30]. Gastrointestinal intolerance (46 %) is common with the oral solution at doses greater than 400 mg per day and may require discontinuation in up to 30 % of patients. The myocardial depressant effects of itraconazole are also well known and cases of congestive heart failure have been reported [40]. Past studies examining the effects of itraconazole have observed adverse events leading to discontinuation of treatment in up to 30 % of patients [41–43].

15.3.3 Posaconazole

Posaconazole is a lipophilic second-generation antifungal triazole. Its spectrum of activity includes agents of mucormycoses (formerly zygomycoses) and has improved in vitro activity against *Aspergillus* spp. compared to itraconazole.

Posaconazole is insoluble in water and no intravenous formulation is currently available and it is thus administered as a cherry-flavored suspension. Absorption is maximized when posaconazole is given as 2–4 divided doses administered with food or a liquid nutritional supplement. H_2-receptor antagonists and proton pump inhibitors may decrease posaconazole serum levels and, if possible, coadministration should be avoided.

Posaconazole has demonstrated dose-dependent pharmacokinetics with saturable absorption above 800 mg per day; thus, oral loading is not possible therefore delaying attainment of therapeutic drug levels [44]. This prolonged time required to reach steady-state impacts the use of posaconazole as primary therapy for IFIs. Posaconazole is hepatically metabolized and renal clearance plays a minor role in the clearance of posaconazole which is predominantly eliminated fecally.

Oral posaconazole has proven effective in the prevention of proven or probable invasive aspergillosis in neutropenic patients with acute myelogenous leukemia (AML) and in allogeneic hematopoietic stem cell transplant recipients with GVHD [45, 46]. Following these landmark trials 200 mg three times daily is recommended for prophylaxis, and 800 mg divided in 2 or 4 doses is recommended in the salvage setting. For patients not tolerating food, a liquid nutritional supplement has been recommended to increase absorption [47].

Posaconazole is usually well tolerated and infrequently requires discontinuation due to adverse events. The most frequent side effects are gastrointestinal (14 %), with transaminase elevation and hyperbilirubinemia occurring in 3 % [46].

Posaconazole is not significantly metabolized through the cytochrome P450 system and posaconazole serum levels are unlikely to be increased by concomitant administration of P450 inhibitors. However, posaconazole is known to both increase and decrease other medications metabolized through the cytochrome P450 system and the clinician should be aware of potential drug-drug interactions.

15.3.4 Voriconazole

Voriconazole is a low-molecular weight water-soluble second-generation triazole with a broad spectrum of activity against molds with the exception of the mucormycetes (Table 15.1).

Available in both oral and intravenous formulations, the intravenous form is dependent upon sulfobutyl ether β–cyclodextrin (SBECD) for solubility [48]. When 3–6 mg/kg of daily voriconazole is administered, steady-state levels are reached in 5–6 days, although if oral or intravenous loading is prescribed, steady-state levels can be reached within 24 h [49]. Fatty foods have been found to reduce bioavailability by 80 % [50].

Although voriconazole in children has demonstrated linear pharmacokinetics, adults exhibit nonlinear metabolism, likely secondary to saturable metabolic processes [49]. Interpatient serum concentration variability has been attributed to polymorphisms within CYP2C19, the major metabolic pathway for voriconazole [48]. Up to 20 % of non-Indian Asians have low CYP2C19 activity thereby increasing voriconazole serum levels up to four times higher than those found in white or black populations [51].

For intravenous administration 6 mg/kg twice daily on day 1 followed by 4 mg/kg IV twice daily for the duration of therapy is recommended. The oral dosages in adults are also weight based. For those weighing greater than 40 kg, 400 mg twice daily on day 1 followed by 200 mg twice daily until completion of therapy is suggested, although weight-based dosing has been recommended for oral therapy in patients with severe infection [14, 48]. Pediatric patients are "loaded" with an intravenous dose of 7 mg/kg twice daily followed by oral dosing of 200 mg twice daily [52]. In patients with liver dysfunction, standard loading doses should be given, but the maintenance dose reduced by 50 %, although dosing in severe liver disease remains uncertain. Although no dosage adjustment is required if oral drug is given to patients with impaired renal function, the presence of a cyclodextrin within the IV formulation has caused concerns about vehicle accumulation and IV administration is best avoided in patients with a CrCl <50 mL [48].

Voriconazole is typically reasonably well tolerated and the side-effect profile is similar to other triazoles. However, voriconazole is notable for the side effect of abnormal vision (up to 23 %) that is transient, infusion related, and without sequelae. This unique effect typically occurs 30 min after infusion and abates 30 min after onset.

Other well-known effects of voriconazole therapy include skin rash and transaminase elevation [31]. Elevated voriconazole serum levels have been attributed to the majority of side effects encountered in clinical practice, and higher levels (>5.5 mg/L) have been associated with encephalopathy and/or hallucinations [53].

Voriconazole has become the drug of choice for most cases of invasive aspergillosis [13]. In a study evaluating the use of voriconazole for empirical antifungal therapy in febrile neutropenic patients, there were significantly fewer breakthrough infections in the voriconazole-treated group as compared with liposomal amphotericin B, although predetermined non-inferiority criteria were not met [11]. Voriconazole has also been evaluated for use during infection caused by *Fusarium* and *Scedosporium* spp., and although a retrospective study, a favorable response was seen in 63 % of voriconazole-treated patients with these difficult infections.

15.3.5 Therapeutic Drug Monitoring (TDM)

Commercial assays are available for monitoring the serum concentrations of all currently available triazoles; however, at this time existing guidelines recommend only itraconazole TDM [14]. The newer triazoles, posaconazole and voriconazole, have received attention due to unpredictable absorption (posaconazole) and interpatient serum level variability (voriconazole). Posaconazole and voriconazole serum drug levels have been shown to predict efficacy and TDM should be considered when drug interactions or poor absorption is a concern. The frequency with which to monitor these newer triazoles remains to be determined.

15.4 Echinocandins

Echinocandins (caspofungin, micafungin, anidulafungin) inhibit the synthesis of (1→3)-β-D-glucan by inhibiting the activity of glucan synthase leading to impaired cell wall integrity and cell lysis (Fig. 15.1). Their clinical use is limited primarily to *Candida* and *Aspergillus* spp. as they lack activity against *Mucorales*, *Cryptococcus* spp., and other important mycoses (Table 15.1). Although resistance rates remain low, mean inhibitory concentrations (MICs) are elevated (>1 μg/mL) in a majority of *C. parapsilosis* and *C. guilliermondii* isolates, and other species may develop resistance on therapy [54].

Echinocandin efficacy is predicted by the peak-to-MIC ratio, yet therapeutic drug monitoring of echinocandins is seldom required and not routinely recommended. Echinocandins have poor oral absorption and current agents are available only in the intravenous formulation. Echinocandins are highly protein bound (anidulafungin 84 %, caspofungin 97 %, and micafungin 99 %) and have a half-life of 26, 30, and 15 h, respectively. Their vitreal and CSF penetration is negligible and alternative antifungals should be used for IFIs at these sites. No discernible clinical differences have been found between the currently available echinocandins.

Caspofungin was the first available agent of this class and is metabolized by both hepatic hydrolysis and N-acetylation. Inactive metabolites are subsequently eliminated in the urine albeit in small quantities. Severe hepatic dysfunction mandates caspofungin dose reduction [9]. Caspofungin has several drug interactions with agents metabolized through the cytochrome P450 system and serum levels are reduced in the presence of rifampin and caspofungin may increase levels of sirolimus, nifedipine, and cyclosporine [9]. Micafungin is metabolized by non-oxidative metabolism within the liver and anidulafungin undergoes nonenzymatic degradation within the kidney. Both agents are eliminated in stool. These agents therefore do not require dosage adjustment with hepatic impairment [9].

The side-effect profile of the echinocandins is very favorable with minimal toxicity and these agents are typically well tolerated. An infusion-related reaction has been described during overly rapid administration with tachycardia, hypotension, and/or thrombophlebitis noted by some patients. Clinically relevant drug interactions are uncommon. For example, although interaction with cyclosporin is described for caspofungin, the clinical impact of that interaction is minimal.

The increased proportions of triazole-resistant *Candida* spp. such as C. *krusei* and *C. glabrata* in invasive candidiasis reported from several institutions worldwide and the fungicidal activity of the echinocandins against yeasts have prompted some authorities to recommend these agents as first-line therapy for invasive candidiasis.

Additionally, their proven efficacy, infrequency of side effects, and favorable drug interaction profiles make them attractive options over other available antifungals [19, 55–57].

The echinocandins have been found at least equally efficacious and better tolerated than other systemic antifungals in the treatment of invasive candidiasis, predominantly candidemia. In one trial, caspofungin (70 mg loading dose followed by 50 mg daily) was compared to amphotericin B deoxycholate (0.6–1 mg/kg) in the treatment of invasive candidiasis. Although *C. albicans* was more common in the AMB arm, modified intention to treat (MITT) revealed similar survival in each group, with a trend towards increased survival and a statistically significant decrease in drug side effects in those receiving caspofungin [19].

Micafungin (100 mg IV daily) has been compared to liposomal amphotericin B (L-AmB) 3 mg/kg IV daily in an international, double-blind trial. This study assigned patients to 14 days of intravenous treatment and outcomes were equivalent in each group, yet fewer treatment-related adverse events – including those that were serious or led to treatment discontinuation – were seen in those who received micafungin [55].

Micafungin and caspofungin have been directly compared in a recent study assigning patients to one of three different treatment groups: micafungin 100 mg/day IV daily, micafungin 150 mg IV daily, or caspofungin 70 mg IV loading dose followed by 50 mg IV daily. No differences in response to therapy, treatment or microbiologic failure, or all cause mortality were found in the intention to treat analysis [57]. Although this trial found that higher echinocandin doses do not necessarily equate to higher response rates, no increase in toxicity was seen with these higher doses. Therefore, in unusual circumstances or in morbid obesity, dose escalation is thought to be safe.

Anidulafungin has been directly compared with fluconazole for the treatment of invasive candidiasis. Treatment was successful in 75.6 % of patients treated with anidulafungin, compared with only 60.2 % of those treated with fluconazole which was statistically superior in terms of outcome, but not for overall survival [56]. The echinocandins have also been found efficacious in the second-line treatment of invasive aspergillosis. The known toxicity of AMB and its different formulations and the potential for voriconazole-associated drug-drug interactions or toxicity has increased interest in the echinocandins for use during treatment of IA, and prospective trials are ongoing [58].

15.5 Flucytosine

Flucytosine (5FC) is deaminated to 5-fluorouracil by fungal cytosine deaminase. 5-fluorouracil is then converted to 5-fluorodeoxyuridylic acid which interferes with DNA synthesis (Fig. 15.1) [59]. This agent may be either fungistatic or fungicidal depending upon both fungal species and strain.

Activity has been observed against most fungal pathogens; however, *Aspergillus* spp., *Mucorales*, dermatophytes, and the endemic mycoses are all resistant to 5FC (Table 15.1). Resistance commonly develops when 5FC is used as monotherapy and it should not be used as such except during the treatment of localized candidal infections when alternative agents are unavailable or contraindicated.

5FC has excellent oral bioavailability and 80–90 % of oral drug is absorbed. Peak serum levels occur 1–2 h after ingestion and although possessing a relatively low volume of distribution, bone, peritoneal, and synovial fluid 5FC levels have been demonstrated and urinary levels are several-fold higher than concurrent serum levels. More than 95 % of 5FC is eliminated unchanged in the urine.

Side effects of therapy include rash, diarrhea, hepatic transaminase elevation, and bone marrow suppression. Marrow suppressive effects are common when serum levels exceed 100–125 μg/mL and in the presence of prolonged therapy (>7 days) or with alterations in renal function, serum drug monitoring is recommended [60]. Other side effects such as abdominal pain or diarrhea are often indirect markers of elevated 5FC levels and therapy is typically stopped in these circumstances. 5FC is teratogenic and should not be administered during pregnancy.

5FC is primarily used only in the treatment of cryptococcosis (combined with AMB). Despite overlapping toxicity concerns, the synergistic effects of dual therapy in cryptococcosis allow for more rapid cerebrospinal fluid clearance [34].

Conclusion

The incidence of infection with invasive mycoses continues to rise with the increasing immunosuppressed patient population. The recently expanded antifungal armamentarium offers the potential for more effective and less toxic therapy and these agents offer distinct pharmacologic profiles and indications for use necessitating a working knowledge of each agent.

References

1. Chamilos G, Luna M, Lewis RE, et al. Invasive fungal infections in patients with hematologic malignancies in a tertiary care cancer center: an autopsy study over a 15-year period (1989–2003). Haematologica. 2006;91(7):986–9.
2. Pappas PG, Alexander BD, Andes DR, et al. Invasive fungal infections among organ transplant recipients: results of the Transplant-Associated Infection Surveillance Network (TRANSNET). Clin Infect Dis. 2010;50(8):1101–11.
3. Kontoyiannis DP, Marr KA, Park BJ, et al. Prospective surveillance for invasive fungal infections in hematopoietic stem cell transplant recipients, 2001–2006: overview of the Transplant-Associated Infection Surveillance Network (TRANSNET) Database. Clin Infect Dis. 2010;50(8):1091–100.
4. Pagano L, Caira M, Candoni A, et al. Invasive aspergillosis in patients with acute myeloid leukemia: a SEIFEM-2008 registry study. Haematologica. 2010;95(4):644–50.
5. Leventakos K, Lewis RE, Kontoyiannis DP. Fungal infections in leukemia patients: how do we prevent and treat them? Clin Infect Dis. 2010;50(3):405–15.
6. Andes D. In vivo pharmacodynamics of antifungal drugs in treatment of candidiasis. Antimicrob Agents Chemother. 2003;47(4):1179–86.
7. Rex JH, Pfaller MA. Has antifungal susceptibility testing come of age? Clin Infect Dis. 2002;35(8):982–9.
8. Saag MS, Graybill RJ, Larsen RA, et al. Practice guidelines for the management of cryptococcal disease. Infectious Diseases Society of America. Clin Infect Dis. 2000;30(4):710–8.

9. Dodds Ashley ES, Lewis R, Lewis JS, Martin C, Andes D. Pharmacology of systemic antifungal agents. Clin Infect Dis. 2006;43(s1):S28–39.
10. Pappas PG, Rex JH, Sobel JD, et al. Guidelines for treatment of candidiasis. Clin Infect Dis. 2004;38(2):161–89.
11. Walsh TJ, Pappas P, Winston DJ, et al. Voriconazole compared with liposomal amphotericin B for empirical antifungal therapy in patients with neutropenia and persistent fever. N Engl J Med. 2002;346(4):225–34.
12. Goldberg E, Gafter-Gvili A, Robenshtok E, Leibovici L, Paul M. Empirical antifungal therapy for patients with neutropenia and persistent fever: systematic review and meta-analysis. Eur J Cancer. 2008;44(15):2192–203.
13. Herbrecht R, Denning DW, Patterson TF, et al. Voriconazole versus amphotericin B for primary therapy of invasive aspergillosis. N Engl J Med. 2002;347(6):408–15.
14. Walsh TJ, Anaissie EJ, Denning DW, et al. Treatment of aspergillosis: clinical practice guidelines of the Infectious Diseases Society of America. Clin Infect Dis. 2008;46(3):327–60.
15. Chamilos G, Lewis RE, Kontoyiannis DP. Delaying amphotericin B-based frontline therapy significantly increases mortality among patients with hematologic malignancy who have zygomycosis. Clin Infect Dis. 2008;47(4):503–9.
16. Cornely OA, Maertens J, Bresnik M, et al. Liposomal amphotericin B as initial therapy for invasive mold infection: a randomized trial comparing a high-loading dose regimen with standard dosing (AmBiLoad trial). Clin Infect Dis. 2007;44(10):1289–97.
17. Rijnders BJ, Cornelissen JJ, Slobbe L, et al. Aerosolized liposomal amphotericin B for the prevention of invasive pulmonary aspergillosis during prolonged neutropenia: a randomized, placebo-controlled trial. Clin Infect Dis. 2008;46(9):1401–8.
18. Borro JM, Sole A, de la Torre M, et al. Efficiency and safety of inhaled amphotericin B lipid complex (abelcet) in the prophylaxis of invasive fungal infections following lung transplantation. Transplant Proc. 2008;40(9):3090–3.
19. Mora-Duarte J, Betts R, Rotstein C, et al. Comparison of caspofungin and amphotericin B for invasive candidiasis. N Engl J Med. 2002;347(25):2020–9.
20. Saliba F, Dupont B. Renal impairment and amphotericin B formulations in patients with invasive fungal infections. Med Mycol. 2008;46(2):97–112.
21. Kleinberg M. What is the current and future status of conventional amphotericin B? Int J Antimicrob Agents. 2006;27 Suppl 1:12–6.
22. Kramer MR, Marshall SE, Denning DW, et al. Cyclosporine and itraconazole interaction in heart and lung transplant recipients. Ann Intern Med. 1990;113(4):327–9.
23. Varis T, Kaukonen KM, Kivisto KT, Neuvonen PJ. Plasma concentrations and effects of oral methylprednisolone are considerably increased by itraconazole. Clin Pharmacol Ther. 1998;64(4):363–8.
24. Tucker RM, Denning DW, Hanson LH, et al. Interaction of azoles with rifampin, phenytoin, and carbamazepine: in vitro and clinical observations. Clin Infect Dis. 1992;14(1):165–74.
25. Kivisto KT, Lamberg TS, Kantola T, Neuvonen PJ. Plasma buspirone concentrations are greatly increased by erythromycin and itraconazole. Clin Pharmacol Ther. 1997;62(3):348–54.
26. Engels FK, Ten Tije AJ, Baker SD, et al. Effect of cytochrome P450 3A4 inhibition on the pharmacokinetics of docetaxel. Clin Pharmacol Ther. 2004;75(5):448–54.
27. Grub S, Bryson H, Goggin T, Ludin E, Jorga K. The interaction of saquinavir (soft gelatin capsule) with ketoconazole, erythromycin and rifampicin: comparison of the effect in healthy volunteers and in HIV-infected patients. Eur J Clin Pharmacol. 2001;57(2):115–21.
28. Jeng MR, Feusner J. Itraconazole-enhanced vincristine neurotoxicity in a child with acute lymphoblastic leukemia. Pediatr Hematol Oncol. 2001;18(2):137–42.
29. Noxafil (posaconazole) [package insert]. Kenilworth: Schering Corp; 2006.
30. Sporanox (itraconazole) [package insert]. Toronto: Janssen-Ortho; 2001.
31. VFEND (voriconazole) [package insert]. Roering: Pfizer; 2008.
32. Stevens DA, Diaz M, Negroni R, et al. Safety evaluation of chronic fluconazole therapy. Fluconazole Pan-American Study Group. Chemotherapy. 1997;43(5):371–7.
33. Slavin MA, Osborne B, Adams R, et al. Efficacy and safety of fluconazole prophylaxis for fungal infections after marrow transplantation–a prospective, randomized, double-blind study. J Infect Dis. 1995;171(6):1545–52.

34. Perfect JR, Dismukes WE, Dromer F, et al. Clinical practice guidelines for the management of cryptococcal disease: 2010 update by the infectious diseases society of america. Clin Infect Dis. 2010;50(3):291–322.
35. Jaruratanasirikul S, Kleepkaew A. Influence of an acidic beverage (Coca-Cola) on the absorption of itraconazole. Eur J Clin Pharmacol. 1997;52(3):235–7.
36. Lange D, Pavao JH, Wu J, Klausner M. Effect of a cola beverage on the bioavailability of itraconazole in the presence of H2 blockers. J Clin Pharmacol. 1997;37(6):535–40.
37. Van de Velde VJ, Van Peer AP, Heykants JJ, et al. Effect of food on the pharmacokinetics of a new hydroxypropyl-beta-cyclodextrin formulation of itraconazole. Pharmacotherapy. 1996;16(3):424–8.
38. Wheat LJ, Freifeld AG, Kleiman MB, et al. Clinical practice guidelines for the management of patients with histoplasmosis: 2007 update by the Infectious Diseases Society of America. Clin Infect Dis. 2007;45(7):807–25.
39. De Beule K, Van Gestel J. Pharmacology of itraconazole. Drugs. 2001;61 Suppl 1:27–37.
40. Ahmad SR, Singer SJ, Leissa BG. Congestive heart failure associated with itraconazole. Lancet. 2001;357(9270):1766–7.
41. Glasmacher A, Cornely O, Ullmann AJ, et al. An open-label randomized trial comparing itraconazole oral solution with fluconazole oral solution for primary prophylaxis of fungal infections in patients with haematological malignancy and profound neutropenia. J Antimicrob Chemother. 2006;57(2):317–25.
42. Marr KA, Crippa F, Leisenring W, et al. Itraconazole versus fluconazole for prevention of fungal infections in patients receiving allogeneic stem cell transplants. Blood. 2004;103(4):1527–33.
43. Winston DJ, Maziarz RT, Chandrasekar PH, et al. Intravenous and oral itraconazole versus intravenous and oral fluconazole for long-term antifungal prophylaxis in allogeneic hematopoietic stem-cell transplant recipients. A multicenter, randomized trial. Ann Intern Med. 2003;138(9):705–13.
44. Courtney R, Pai S, Laughlin M, Lim J, Batra V. Pharmacokinetics, safety, and tolerability of oral posaconazole administered in single and multiple doses in healthy adults. Antimicrob Agents Chemother. 2003;47(9):2788–95.
45. Cornely OA, Maertens J, Winston DJ, et al. Posaconazole vs. fluconazole or itraconazole prophylaxis in patients with neutropenia. N Engl J Med. 2007;356(4):348–59.
46. Ullmann AJ, Lipton JH, Vesole DH, et al. Posaconazole or fluconazole for prophylaxis in severe graft-versus-host disease. N Engl J Med. 2007;356(4):335–47.
47. Sansone-Parsons A, Krishna G, Calzetta A, et al. Effect of a nutritional supplement on posaconazole pharmacokinetics following oral administration to healthy volunteers. Antimicrob Agents Chemother. 2006;50(5):1881–3.
48. Johnson LB, Kauffman CA. Voriconazole: a new triazole antifungal agent. Clin Infect Dis. 2003;36(5):630–7.
49. Purkins L, Wood N, Ghahramani P, Greenhalgh K, Allen MJ, Kleinermans D. Pharmacokinetics and safety of voriconazole following intravenous- to oral-dose escalation regimens. Antimicrob Agents Chemother. 2002;46(8):2546–53.
50. Lazarus HM, Blumer JL, Yanovich S, Schlamm H, Romero A. Safety and pharmacokinetics of oral voriconazole in patients at risk of fungal infection: a dose escalation study. J Clin Pharmacol. 2002;42(4):395–402.
51. Ikeda Y, Umemura K, Kondo K, Sekiguchi K, Miyoshi S, Nakashima M. Pharmacokinetics of voriconazole and cytochrome P450 2C19 genetic status. Clin Pharmacol Ther. 2004;75(6):587–8.
52. Walsh TJ, Driscoll T, Milligan PA, et al. Pharmacokinetics, safety, and tolerability of voriconazole in immunocompromised children. Antimicrob Agents Chemother. 2010;54(10):4116–23.
53. Zonios DI, Gea-Banacloche J, Childs R, Bennett JE. Hallucinations during voriconazole therapy. Clin Infect Dis. 2008;47(1):e7–10.
54. Pfaller MA, Diekema DJ, Ostrosky-Zeichner L, et al. Correlation of MIC with outcome for Candida species tested against caspofungin, anidulafungin, and micafungin: analysis and proposal for interpretive MIC breakpoints. J Clin Microbiol. 2008;46(8):2620–9.
55. Kuse ER, Chetchotisakd P, da Cunha CA, et al. Micafungin versus liposomal amphotericin B for candidaemia and invasive candidosis: a phase III randomised double-blind trial. Lancet. 2007;369(9572):1519–27.

56. Reboli AC, Rotstein C, Pappas PG, et al. Anidulafungin versus fluconazole for invasive candidiasis. N Engl J Med. 2007;356(24):2472–82.
57. Pappas PG, Rotstein CM, Betts RF, et al. Micafungin versus caspofungin for treatment of candidemia and other forms of invasive candidiasis. Clin Infect Dis. 2007;45(7):883–93.
58. Heinz WJ, Einsele H. Caspofungin for treatment of invasive aspergillus infections. Mycoses. 2008;51 Suppl 1:47–57.
59. Polak A, Scholer HJ. Mode of action of 5-fluorocytosine and mechanisms of resistance. Chemotherapy. 1975;21(3–4):113–30.
60. Stamm AM, Diasio RB, Dismukes WE, et al. Toxicity of amphotericin B plus flucytosine in 194 patients with cryptococcal meningitis. Am J Med. 1987;83(2):236–42.

Part V

Infection Prevention

Antimicrobial Prophylaxis in Hematology

16

Corrado Girmenia and Francesco Menichetti

Contents

C. Girmenia (✉)
Dipartimento di Ematologia, Oncologia, Anatomia Patologica e Medicina Rigenerativa, Azienda Policlinico Umberto I, Rome, Italy
e-mail: girmenia@bce.uniroma1.it

F. Menichetti
Unità Operativa di Malattie Infettive, Azienda Ospedaliero-Universitaria Pisana, Pisa, Italy
e-mail: menichettifrancesco@gmail.com

G. Maschmeyer, K.V.I. Rolston (eds.), *Infections in Hematology*,
DOI 10.1007/978-3-662-44000-1_16

16.1 Introduction

Infectious complications represent an important cause of morbidity and mortality in hematologic patients, especially those receiving intensive chemotherapy or submitted to stem cell transplant (SCT). In recent years, however, the management of these complications has improved greatly, especially in the field of prevention of bacterial, fungal, and viral infections.

The impact of antimicrobial prophylaxis had been much more controversial until recently when new data suggested that chemoprophylaxis might be able not only to reduce the incidence of infectious complications but also to allow the continuation of the underlying hematologic disease treatment with a significant impact on the overall survival also in high-risk patient populations.

16.2 Antibacterial Prophylaxis

16.2.1 Intestinal Decontamination

Risk of bacterial infection is directly related to the severity and duration of neutropenia. Bacterial infections frequently occur when the neutrophil count is below 500/mm^3 and most of the bacteremias are documented when the neutrophils count is below 100/mm^3. The risk of bacterial infections increase proportionally to the duration of neutropenia: virtually all patients with neutropenia duration longer than 2 weeks develop febrile episodes.

The practice of chemoprophylaxis for the prevention of bacterial infections in neutropenic cancer patients is derived from the observation that most of the bacterial pathogens causing infection originated from the patient's endogenous flora of the gastrointestinal tract [1]. Oral and gastrointestinal chemotherapy-induced mucositis represents a main risk for bacterial entry directly into the bloodstream. The administration of nonabsorbable antibiotics aimed at suppressing the intestinal bacterial flora and at preventing the acquisition of exogenous organisms represented the first antibacterial prophylaxis schedule in neutropenic patients. In the first experiences, oral nonabsorbable antibiotics (such as gentamicin, vancomycin, framycetin, colistin, neomycin/polymyxin, in various combinations) were administered with the aim to operate a total intestinal decontamination involving both aerobic and anaerobic microorganisms [2, 3]. However, poor compliance related to gastrointestinal side effects, uncertain data on its efficacy, and the risk of colonization with resistant opportunistic pathogens coming from the hospital flora made this procedure very unpopular in the clinical practice [4]. Afterward, oral nonabsorbable unselective antibiotics were substituted with other antibacterial agents, first of all trimethoprim/sulfamethoxazole, characterized by their activity against bacterial aerobic flora while preserving the anaerobic flora. This practice was defined as selective intestinal decontamination [5, 6].

16.2.2 The Fluoroquinolones

The concept of selective intestinal decontamination with oral absorbable antibiotics, such as trimethoprim/sulfamethoxazole, which operate directly not only in the gastrointestinal tract but also with their systemic action, represented the main reason for the increasing interest in this setting on a new class of oral antibiotics, the fluoroquinolones, which, owing to their antimicrobial activity and pharmacokinetic characteristics, are now the most attractive agents for antibacterial prophylactic use in neutropenic patients. Fluoroquinolones have bactericidal activity and a broad antimicrobial spectrum that includes enterobacteriaceae, *Pseudomonas* spp., and some Gram-positive cocci, but little or no activity on intestinal anaerobic flora (with the exception of moxifloxacin). Most fluoroquinolones are well absorbed by the oral route and, probably due to active intestinal secretion, are excreted in high concentration in the feces. These antibiotics are usually well tolerated with a favorable patient compliance.

Several studies published prior to 2005 showed a reduction in the number of infectious episodes, particularly by Gram-negative pathogens, in neutropenic patients under fluoroquinolone prophylaxis, but failed to demonstrate a reduction in Gram-positive infections and in mortality [7–10]. However, a meta-analysis of placebo-controlled or no treatment-controlled trials of fluoroquinolone prophylaxis demonstrated a relative risk reduction of 48 and 62 % in all-cause mortality and infection-related mortality, respectively, among fluoroquinolone recipients [11]. The patient population who took benefit from prophylaxis had hematologic malignancies or received SCT, with durations of neutropenia typically >7 days, a condition at high risk for bacterial infections.

In view of the need to reevaluate the role of antibacterial prophylaxis in neutropenic cancer patients after 20 years of wide use in clinical practice and to better define the categories of patients that might benefit from chemoprophylaxis, two multicenter, large controlled trials have been conducted in Europe and published in 2005 [12, 13].

The Italian GIMEMA group conducted a double-blind, placebo-controlled trial of 760 hospitalized high-risk adult patients with prolonged neutropenia (<1,000 neutrophils/mm^3 for >7 days) [12]. The trial included patients with acute leukemia, lymphoma, and solid tumors receiving high-dose chemotherapy. Participants were randomized to receive levofloxacin or placebo from the start of chemotherapy until resolution of neutropenia. The study demonstrated a statistically significant reduction in the incidence of fever in patients receiving levofloxacin compared to the placebo group (65 versus 85 %, $p<0.001$) associated with a nonsignificant decrease in mortality in the levofloxacin arm. The second study, the British SIGNIFICANT trial, regarded 1,565 patients receiving cyclical chemotherapy for solid tumors or lymphoma at risk of temporary neutropenia and classified as at low risk [13]. Patients randomly received either levofloxacin or placebo for 7 days during the expected neutropenic period. A significant reduction in febrile episodes was documented in the levofloxacin group during the first cycle of chemotherapy (3.5 versus 7.9 %, $P\leq0.001$) and all cycles of treatment (10.8 versus 15.2 %, $P=0.01$), but no effect on documented infections was observed. These experiences indicate a potentially important role of levofloxacin prophylaxis in high-risk patients with prolonged neutropenia but not in low-risk patient populations.

Based on the above studies, international guidelines on antibacterial prophylaxis have been updated. European and American guidelines have been summarized in Tables 16.1 and 16.2, respectively [14, 20].

16.2.3 The Emerging Problem of Resistance to Fluoroquinolones

The major drawback of the routine use of prophylaxis is the emergence of fluoroquinolone resistance in both Gram-positive and Gram-negative organisms [22–26]. This phenomenon was well described by a retrospective analysis of the database of International Antimicrobial Therapy Group of the European Organization for Research and Treatment of Cancer (IATG-EORTC) from studies

Table 16.1 European Conference on Infection in Leukemia (ECIL) guidelines on antimicrobial prophylaxis in hematology patients [14–17]

Type of prophylaxis and clinical condition	Recommendation and grading[a]
Antibacterial prophylaxis	
Patients with acute leukemia and adult SCT recipients after myeloablative therapy	A fluoroquinolone with systemic activity including *P. aeruginosa* should be used
	Oral levofloxacin: 500 mg od (AI)
	Oral ciprofloxacin: 500 mg bid (AI)
	Oral norfloxacin: 400 mg bid (BI) (Less effective than ciprofloxacin)
	Oral ofloxacin: 200–300 mg bid (BI) (less tested than ciprofloxacin in RCTs and at variable daily doses, lower activity against *P. aeruginosa* spp. and less effective than ciprofloxacin)
Antifungal prophylaxis	
Leukemia patients, induction chemotherapy	Oral Posaconazole (200 mg t.i.d.) (AI)
	Oral or IV Fluconazole (400 mg q.d.) (CI)
	Itraconazole oral solution (2.5 mg/kg b.i.d.) (CI)
	Echinocandins IV: Insufficient data
	Polyenes IV (CI)
	Aerosolized liposomal AmB plus fluconazole (BI)
Allogeneic SCT recipients, initial neutropenic phase	Oral or IV Fluconazole (400 mg q.d.) AI
	Itraconazole (200 mg i.v. followed by oral solution 200 mg b.i.d.) BI
	Posaconazole BII[b]
	Voriconazole (200 mg b.i.d. oral) Provisional BI[b]
	Micafungin (50 mg q.d. iv) CI
	Polyenes i.v.CI
	Aerosolized liposomal AmB plus fluconazole BII

Table 16.1 (continued)

Type of prophylaxis and clinical condition	Recommendation and grading[a]
Allogeneic SCT recipients, GVHD phase	Posaconazole (200 mg t.i.d. oral) AI Oral or IV Fluconazole (400 mg q.d.) CI Itraconazole (200 mg i.v. followed by oral solution 200 mg b.i.d.) BI Voriconazole (200 mg b.i.d. oral) Provisional BI[b] Echinocandins: Insufficient data Polyenes i.v.CI Aerosolized liposomal AmB plus fluconazole Insufficient data
Antiviral prophylaxis	
Herpes simplex virus (HSV)	Antiviral drug prophylaxis is not recommended in HSV-seronegative leukemic patients during chemotherapy or after SCT (DIII). HSV-seropositive patients undergoing allogeneic HSCT for acute leukemia should receive antiviral drug prophylaxis(AI). HSV-seropositive patients treated for acute leukemia by chemotherapy alone should be considered for antiviral drug prophylaxis (BIII) Intravenous (5 mg/kg q12h) or oral acyclovir (from 3 × 200 to 2 × 800 mg/day) (AI) or oral valaciclovir (2 × 500 mg/day) (BIII) should be given prophylactically for 3–5 weeks after start of chemotherapy or after SCT and for longer periods of time in children treated for acute leukemia. Allogeneic SCT recipients, who develop GVHD or receive immunosuppressive treatment, including steroids, usually require prolonged HSV prophylaxis (BII)
Varicella-zoster virus (VZV)	Passive immunization with i.v. VZIG (at a dose of 0.2–1 ml/kg) or i.m. ZIG or IVIG (300–500 mg/kg) should be given within 96 h after exposure to VZV-seronegative leukemic patients on chemotherapy and those receiving steroids and to VZV-seronegative SCT recipients, patients who have chronic GVHD, who are on immunosuppressive treatment, or whose SCT was within 2 years (AII). Where passive immunization is not available, post-exposure prophylaxis with acyclovir (800 mg four times daily; 600 mg/m^2 four times daily for children), valaciclovir (1,000 mg three times daily; 500 mg three times daily for <40 kg body weight), or famciclovir (500 mg three times a day) is recommended, starting during 3–21 days after exposure (AIII). If a second exposure occurs more than 21 days after a dose of passive immunization or after the administration of the antiviral prophylaxis, prophylaxis should be readministered (CIII) Prophylaxis in VZV-seropositive patients is optional (CIII). Determination of VZV IgG serostatus before transplant is recommended for all SCT candidates (AIII). Prophylaxis with oral acyclovir (800 mg twice daily) or valaciclovir (500 mg once or twice daily) is recommended for seropositive allo-SCT recipients for 1 year (AII), or longer in the presence of GVHD and immunosuppressive therapy (BII). Prophylaxis in autologous SCT is controversial

(continued)

Table 16.1 (continued)

Type of prophylaxis and clinical condition	Recommendation and grading[a]
Cytomegalovirus (CMV)	A preemptive antiviral strategy based on the monitoring of CMV (pp65 antigen or quantitative PCR) represents the most widely used approach not only in the allogeneic SCT setting but also in other patient cohorts at risk of CMV infection and disease such as patients with chronic lymphocytic leukemia under alemtuzumab therapy. Antiviral chemoprophylaxis is an alternative to preemptive therapy in subgroups of patients at high risk for CMV disease. Intravenous ganciclovir prophylaxis is an effective strategy for the prevention of CMV disease in subgroups of allo-SCT patients at high risk for CMV disease (BI), but toxicity concerns and the potential for resistance to ganciclovir among CMV hamper its unselected prophylactic use. Also acyclovir or valacyclovir at high doses can be used for CMV prophylaxis in allo-SCT recipients (BI); however, this approach must be combined with serial CMV monitoring and preemptive therapeutic intervention (AI). Immune globulin has no role as prophylaxis against CMV infection (EII). Valganciclovir prophylaxis is effective and reduces the risk of symptomatic CMV infection in patients receiving alemtuzumab (BII)

[a]*Strength of recommendation*: A Good evidence to support a recommendation for use; B Moderate evidence to support a recommendation for use, C Poor evidence to support a recommendation *Quality of evidence*: I Evidence from _1 properly randomized, controlled trial II Evidence from _1 well-designed clinical trial, without randomization; from cohort or case-controlled analytic studies (preferably from 11 center); from multiple time-series; or from dramatic results from uncontrolled experiments; III Evidence from opinions of respected authorities, based on clinical experience, descriptive studies, or reports of expert committees

[b]for ECIL 5, 2013 guidelines see http://www.kobe.fr/ecil/telechargements2013/ECIL5antifungal prophylaxis%2020062014Final.pdf

of empiric antibacterial therapy in neutropenic patients conducted between 1983 and 1993 [26]. During this period the proportion of neutropenic cancer patients who received fluoroquinolone prophylaxis increased from 1.4 to 45 % and an increase in strains of *Escherichia coli* resistant to fluoroquinolones from 0 to 27 % was observed. Based on the above data, guidelines for the management of febrile neutropenia discouraged the widespread use of prophylaxis in neutropenic cancer patients [27].

However, the clinical implications of fluoroquinolone resistance continued to be investigated. A systematic review of the effect of quinolone prophylaxis on antimicrobial resistance in afebrile neutropenic patients which included 7,878 patients in 56 trials has been published in 2007 [28]. Of the 22 trials comparing fluoroquinolones versus placebo or no intervention, only three reported on colonization by resistant organisms by the end of follow-up and eight on the proportion of patients with fluoroquinolone-resistant infections. A nonsignificant increase in colonization with resistant organisms and no difference in the number of infections caused by resistant organism were observed in patients receiving fluoroquinolones. Prophylaxis decreased the overall incidence of infection without affecting the number of resistant infections (51/308 versus 54/154).

Table 16.2 Infectious Diseases Society of America (IDSA) guidelines on antimicrobial prophylaxis in hematology patients [20, 21]

Type of prophylaxis and clinical condition	Recommendation and grading (see Table 16.1 legend)
Antibacterial prophylaxis in high-risk neutropenic patients	Fluoroquinolone prophylaxis should be considered for high-risk patients with expected durations of prolonged and profound neutropenia (ANC <100 cells/mm^3 for >7 days) (BI). Levofloxacin and ciprofloxacin have been evaluated most comprehensively and are considered to be roughly equivalent, although levofloxacin is preferred in situations with increased risk for oral mucositis-related invasive viridans group streptococcal infection. A systematic strategy for monitoring the development of fluoroquinolone resistance among Gram-negative bacilli is recommended (AII). Addition of a Gram-positive active agent to fluoroquinolone prophylaxis is generally not recommended (AI)
Antibacterial prophylaxis in low-risk neutropenic patients	Antibacterial prophylaxis is not routinely recommended for low-risk patients who are anticipated to remain neutropenic for <7 days (AIII)
Prophylaxis against Candida infections in high-risk neutropenic patients	Recommended in patient groups in whom the risk of invasive candidal infections is substantial, such as allogeneic SCT recipients or those undergoing intensive remission induction or salvage induction chemotherapy for acute leukemia (A-I). Fluconazole, itraconazole, voriconazole, posaconazole, micafungin, and caspofungin are all acceptable alternatives
Prophylaxis against Aspergillus infections in high-risk neutropenic patients	Prophylaxis with posaconazole should be considered for selected patients >13 years of age who are undergoing intensive chemotherapy for AML/MDS in whom the risk of invasive aspergillosis without prophylaxis is substantial (BI) Prophylaxis against Aspergillus infection in pre-engraftment allogeneic or autologous transplant recipients has not been shown to be efficacious. However, a mold-active agent is recommended in patients with prior invasive aspergillosis (AIII), anticipated prolonged neutropenic periods of at least 2 weeks (CIII), or a prolonged period of neutropenia immediately prior to HSCT (CIII)
Prophylaxis against Aspergillus infections in allo-SCT recipients with severe GvHD	Antifungal prophylaxis with posaconazole can be recommended in HSCT recipients with GVHD who are at high risk for invasive aspergillosis (AI)
Antifungal prophylaxis in low-risk neutropenic patients	Antifungal prophylaxis is not recommended for patients in whom the anticipated duration of neutropenia is <7 days (AIII)
Antiviral prophylaxis during neutropenia	HSV-seropositive patients undergoing allogeneic HSCT or leukemia induction therapy should receive acyclovir antiviral prophylaxis (AI). Other herpesvirus infections occur in the post-HSCT setting, including infections due to cytomegalovirus and human herpesvirus 6. However, neutropenia is not a predisposition to reactivation of either virus; thus, prevention strategies for these 2 herpes viruses are not discussed

In summary, after more than two decades of use of fluoroquinolones for prophylaxis of infections in neutropenic cancer patients, the problem of resistance and its clinical implication remains controversial. Considering that the impact of fluoroquinolone resistance on the overall outcome of the patients, including survival, has not been clearly established, the increasing levels of resistance in a hematologic unit may be a poor indicator of potential clinical disadvantage or benefit associated with antibacterial prophylaxis. Based on the published data, it does not appear that the risk of resistance offsets the favorable impact of fluoroquinolone prophylaxis on mortality, microbiologically documented infections, number of febrile episodes, and costs. On the other hand, in view of the improved diagnostic strategies and management of febrile neutropenia, which may positively affect the outcome of neutropenic patients and of the increasing phenomenon of fluoroquinolone resistance over time with possible cross-resistance to other antibiotics, it would seem prudent to carefully monitor bacterial resistance and to periodically reevaluate the proficiency of the practice of antibacterial prophylaxis.

16.3 Antifungal Prophylaxis

16.3.1 Rational for Antifungal Prophylaxis

Patients with hematologic malignancies are at high risk of invasive fungal diseases (IFD), predominantly invasive aspergillosis (IA) and candidiasis, during prolonged chemotherapy-induced neutropenia and following allogeneic SCT particularly in case of acute or chronic graft versus host disease (GVHD) requiring immunosuppressive therapy. Considering that an early diagnosis is difficult to obtain, the prophylaxis of such complications is appealing. Prevention strategies are based on environmental precautions and antimicrobial treatment. While there is a general agreement in the role of the air filtration for the control of airborne filamentous fungal infections, the indication of pharmacological prophylaxis is still debated [29–31].

The prophylactic use of antifungals in some categories of hematologic patients has become standard practice of care and may be directed either to primary prevention of invasive fungal infections (primary antifungal prophylaxis or PAP) or to decrease the risk of recurrence of a previous IFD (secondary antifungal prophylaxis or SAP).

However, evidence supporting the efficacy of the prophylactic strategy is subjected to several variables: etiology of IFD (yeast vs. mold infections), underlying disease or conditions (acute leukemia vs. auto-SCT vs. allo-SCT), risk factors or periods (neutropenia vs. GVHD), and obviously different antifungal drugs (azoles, polyenes, nonabsorbable antifungals).

Patient populations likely to benefit from PAP should be identified as well as the impact of this strategy in reducing IFD (yeast vs. molds), overall mortality, fungal-related mortality, use of empiric antifungal therapy, and toxicity. The emergence of resistant fungal pathogens, duration of prophylaxis, and the need for therapeutic drug monitoring (TDM) of blood levels should be also considered [32, 33].

16.3.2 Primary Antifungal Prophylaxis

16.3.2.1 Fluconazole and Itraconazole

Until a few years ago, only fluconazole and itraconazole had been evaluated in randomized, controlled trials for PAP in patients with hematologic disorders [34–42]. In allo-SCT, fluconazole 400 mg once daily reduced the incidence of IFD, overall and attributable mortality, and use of empiric antifungals and was associated with improved long-term survival probably for its potential role in the containment of severe GVHD [34–36]. In autologous SCT, fluconazole showed to reduce attributable mortality, but the impact on reducing overall mortality, IFD, and empiric use of antifungals was less clear [34]. In AML, fluconazole reduced IFD, but no clear impact was documented on overall and attributable mortality and the need for empiric use of antifungals [37, 38].

Itraconazole is an azole with anti-Aspergillus activity and a variable oral absorption. There is a strong link of blood concentrations to drug efficacy and TDM is indicated especially in case of gastrointestinal dysfunction and potentially harmful co-medication. For IFD prophylaxis target trough blood levels should be above 0.5 mg/l [4]. In a meta-analysis, itraconazole showed to be efficacious in reducing IFD, IA, and fungal-related mortality when used in patients with hematologic malignancies [39]. In an open-label trial, itraconazole IV/PO was compared to fluconazole for long-term prophylaxis in allo-SCT. IFD were documented in 9 % of patients treated with itraconazole vs. 25 % of those receiving fluconazole, but overall mortality was similar and gastrointestinal side effects were more frequently documented in the itraconazole group (24 % vs. 9 %) [40]. In another open-label trial, itraconazole was compared to fluconazole in allo-SCT pts. IFD documented while on treatment were 7 % in the itraconazole-treated patients vs. 15 % in those receiving fluconazole, but at the end of follow-up, no difference was noted (13 % vs. 16 %). More patients were discontinued from itraconazole because of toxicity or gastrointestinal intolerance (36 % vs. 16 %) [41]. A further randomized study which compared itraconazole oral solution with fluconazole oral solution as PAP in 494 neutropenic non-transplant patients with hematologic malignancies reported no differences in the efficacy and safety of the two PAP regimens [42]. However, the incidence of IFDs in this study was too low (1.6 % of patients in the itraconazole group and 2 % of patients in the fluconazole group) to detect any significant efficacy difference [42].

Based on these studies, for several years fluconazole and to a less extent itraconazole were the only drugs recommended for primary prophylaxis against *Candida* infection in neutropenic patients and allogeneic SCT recipients [43, 44]. However, a major limitation of a *Candida* oriented prophylaxis is the lack of activity against molds, which now represent the most frequent cause of IFDs in such populations. In the past years, the consciousness of the epidemiological impact of IA and less common molds, including zygomycetes, Fusarium species, and Scedosporium species, has increased worldwide. At the same time, new broad-spectrum and well-tolerated antifungal drugs, in particular second-generation triazoles and echinocandins, became available, and prospective, controlled trials have been conducted to investigate their ability to prevent IFDs in high-risk hematologic patients [18, 19, 45–49].

16.3.2.2 Posaconazole

Posaconazole, a second-generation triazole with broad spectrum of activity, including *Aspergillus* spp. and zygomycetes fungal group, is available in oral formulation only. The pharmacokinetics are characterized by marked interpatient variability mainly due to erratic bioavailability: the absorption of posaconazole is enhanced by co-administration with food, nutritional supplements, and low-pH beverage (cola), while it is reduced with co-administration of omeprazole. TDM is strongly suggested during posaconazole prophylaxis and target trough blood levels should be above 0.5 mg/l [32, 33]. A new tablet oral formulation and an intravenous formulation of posaconazole with less pharmacokinetic problems will soon be available.

Two phase III clinical studies indicated that posaconazole at a dose of 200 mg PO TID was at least non-inferior to a standard-of-care azole antifungal agent for preventing IFDs in acute myeloid leukemia and allo-SCT patients [45, 46]. The first study was a multicenter, randomized, open-label trial that compared posaconazole with fluconazole (400 mg/day) or itraconazole (200 mg/bid) for the prophylaxis of IFDs in 602 patients (aged >13 year) at high risk for neutropenia after receiving standard induction chemotherapy for a new diagnosis or first relapse of acute myelogenous leukemia or myelodysplastic syndrome [45]. Study drugs were administered at the start of each cycle of chemotherapy and were continued for a maximum of 12 weeks or until recovery from neutropenia and complete remission or occurrence of an IFD or adverse reaction to study drug. The primary efficacy end point was the incidence of proven or probable IFDs from randomization to the end of the oral treatment phase. Significantly fewer patients in the posaconazole arm compared with the fluconazole/itraconazole arm developed an IFD during the oral treatment phase (2 % vs 8 %, respectively; $p=0.001$). While there was only a minor difference in the frequency of infections caused by *Candida* spp. between groups during the oral treatment phase, significantly fewer patients in the posaconazole group had IA (1 % vs. 7 %, $p<0.001$). Survival was significantly longer among recipients of posaconazole than among recipients of fluconazole or itraconazole ($p=0.04$). Serious adverse events possibly or probably related to treatment were reported in 6 % and 2 % of patients in the posaconazole and fluconazole or itraconazole group, respectively ($P=0.01$).

The second study was a randomized, double-blind, multicenter trial in which posaconazole was compared with fluconazole (400 mg/day) for prophylaxis of IFDs in 600 allogeneic SCT recipients (aged >13 years) with GVHD [46]. Treatment was continued for 112 days or until the occurrence of a proven or probable IFD. The primary efficacy end point was the incidence of proven or probable IFDs during the period from randomization to day 112. The mean duration of posaconazole and fluconazole therapy was 80 days and 77 days, respectively. At the end of the fixed 112-day treatment period, the overall rates of IFD did not differ significantly between the two drugs (5.3 % in posaconazole group vs 9.0 % in fluconazole group; $p=0.07$). Although the incidence of infections caused by *Candida* spp. was similar in both groups (<1 % of patients in either arm), posaconazole was superior to fluconazole in preventing proven or probable IA (2.3 % vs. 7.0 %; $p=0.006$). During exposure period, in the posaconazole group, as compared with the fluconazole group, there were fewer breakthrough IFDs (2.4 % vs. 7.6 %, $p=0.004$), particularly

IA (1.0 % vs. 5.9 %, $p=0.001$). Overall mortality was similar in the two groups, but the number of deaths from IFDs was lower in the posaconazole group (1 %, vs. 4 %; $p=0.046$). The incidence of treatment-related adverse events was similar in the two groups (36 % in the posaconazole group and 38 % in the fluconazole group), and the rates of treatment-related serious adverse events were 13 % and 10 %, respectively.

16.3.2.3 Voriconazole

Voriconazole, a second-generation triazole with anti-Aspergillus activity, is characterized by a highly variable pharmacokinetic profile (intra- and inter-subjects) either with IV or oral formulation mostly due to differences in the ability to metabolize the drug via the CYP2C19 P450 enzyme. Polymorphisms in the gene encoding this enzyme are common and result in variable rates of voriconazole metabolism. Additional factors that impact voriconazole metabolism are represented by liver disease, age, and co-medications interacting with CYP2C19 and CYP3A. As demonstrated in several studies, a large number of patients receiving voriconazole for therapy or prophylaxis may reach subtherapeutic or too high blood levels; therefore, also for this triazole TDM is strongly suggested in order to obtain plasma through levels ranging from 1 to 6 mg/L [32, 33, 50].

Two controlled studies of PAP with voriconazole have been conducted in allo-SCT patients [18, 19]. In the first study of primary prophylaxis, voriconazole was compared to fluconazole (295 patients vs 305 patients) in a randomized, double blind trial [18]. This study was characterized by a predefined, structured fungal screening program in order to obtain early diagnosis and therapy of fungal infections and to minimize morbidity and mortality. Patients undergoing myeloablative allo-SCT were randomized before transplant to receive study drugs for 100 days or for 180 days in higher risk patients. The primary end point was freedom from IFD or death (fungal-free survival, FFS) at 180 days. Despite trends to fewer IFDs (7.3 % vs. 11.2 %, $p=0.12$), Aspergillus infections (9 vs. 17, $p=0.09$), and less frequent empiric antifungal therapy (24.1 % vs. 30.2 %, p=0.11) with voriconazole, FFS rates at 180 days were similar (75 % with fluconazole vs. 78 % with voriconazole, $p=0.49$). Relapse-free and overall survival and the incidence of severe adverse events were also similar. This study demonstrates comparable efficacy of fluconazole or voriconazole prophylaxis in allo-SCT patients; however, a careful interpretation of the results is required. The study population considered in this trial was at lower risk of IFD as compared to a real-life allo-SCT population. Indeed, about 90 % of patients had a standard disease risk status, over half of transplants were matched related, the HLA match was 6/6 in 96 % of cases, half of patients did not develop acute or chronic GVHD, and the incidence of disease relapse/progression was only about 10 %. One would be interested to evaluate voriconazole's performance in a higher risk population. This consideration is even more valid when looking at the results among patients with acute myeloid leukemia, a population at higher risk for IFD and with a poorer fungal-free survival. Interestingly, in this patient population voriconazole reduced IFDs (8.5 % vs 21 %; $p=0.04$) and improved FFS (78 % vs 61 %; $p=0.04$) compared to fluconazole [51].

The second study of primary prophylaxis compared voriconazole (200 mg b.i.d.) versus itraconazole (200 mg b.i.d.) in 489 patients receiving allogeneic HSCT for at least 100 days and up to 180 days from conditioning [19]. The primary objective was assessed on a composite end point, including survival at 180 days after transplant, no proven or probable breakthrough IFD, and no discontinuation of the study drug for more than 14 days during the 100-day prophylactic period. The voriconazole arm met the criteria for superiority in the primary end point when compared with the itraconazole arm (49.1 versus 34.5 %, $p=0.0004$). The median duration of voriconazole prophylaxis was longer (97 days) than that of itraconazole (68 days), likely because of significantly more gastrointestinal adverse events (nausea, vomiting, and diarrhea) in the itraconazole group. However, the main concern with this study was the low rate of proven or probable IFDs (three in the voriconazole arm and six in the itraconazole arm).

16.3.2.4 Echinocandins

In a randomized, double-blind trial, micafungin, 50 mg/day iv, was compared to fluconazole 400 mg/day in 882 SCT patients during the neutropenic phase [47]. Treatment success was 80 % for micafungin-treated group (340/425) vs. 73.5 % for the fluconazole-receiving patients (336/457) ($p=0.03$). Aspergillosis was documented respectively in 1 vs. 7 cases. Empiric antifungal therapy was needed in 15 % vs. 21 % of the patient population. An increase in *C. albicans* colonization in micafungin arm was also documented. Criticisms were based on few pts, not exclusively high-risk and few proven IFD.

Caspofungin, 50 mg i.v. daily, was compared to IV itraconazole 200 mg as prophylactic antifungal therapy in 192 neutropenic patients with hematologic malignancies. No difference was documented between the treatment groups for success of prophylaxis (52 % vs. 51 %), proven or probable IFD (7 vs. 5), use of systemic antifungals for pneumonia or FUO (37 % vs. 34 %), fungal deaths: (4 vs 2) and tolerability [48].

16.3.2.5 Aerosolized Amphotericin B

Aerosolized liposomal amphotericin B, 10 mg twice weekly, was tested in a single center, double-blind, placebo-controlled trial in 271 patients with hematologic malignancies with neutropenia following chemotherapy or SCT. Both groups received fluconazole. Less proven/probable invasive pulmonary aspergillosis were documented in patients receiving aerosolized liposomal amphotericin B [49].

Based on the above studies, international guidelines on PAP have been updated. European and American guidelines have been summarized in Tables 16.1 and 16.2, respectively [15, 20, 21, 52].

16.3.3 Secondary Antifungal Prophylaxis (SAP)

An evidence-based approach to SAP in patients with a previous IFD and requiring further antileukemic treatment remains a challenging issue. An anti-infective strategy in the leukemia and transplant setting is clinically effective when the control of the infections enables the optimal cure of the underlying hematologic disease. Thanks to the use of antifungal drugs in SAP, an IFD, including IA, is no more an absolute contraindication for continuing care with intensive chemotherapy or SCT. However, very little data exist on the factors that could predict IFD reactivation while under SAP, on the choice of the best antifungal drug, and on the need of preventative surgical resection of residual pulmonary lesions. Mainly retrospective studies on secondary antifungal prophylaxis in patients with heterogeneous baseline characteristics and undefined risk of reactivation have been published so far [53, 54]. The largest series until now reported is represented by a retrospective survey of the Infectious Diseases Working Party of the European Group for Blood and Marrow Transplantation (EBMT) on 129 patients with a previous history of probable or proven IA who underwent allogeneic SCT [53]. The cumulative incidence of IA progression after transplant was 22 % at 2 years and duration of neutropenia post-transplant, status of the underlying disease, and length of anti-Aspergillus therapy pre-transplant represented determinant factors for progression or reactivation of IA while under SAP.

The first prospective experience on SAP in hematologic patients has been published in 2010 [55]. Voriconazole (4 mg/kg/12 h intravenously or 200 mg/12 h orally) was evaluated in a prospective, open-label, multicenter trial as SAP in 45 allogeneic SCT recipients with previous proven or probable IFD (IA in 31 cases). The primary end point of the study was the incidence of proven or probable recurrent of new IFD after transplant. The median duration of voriconazole prophylaxis was 94 days. Eleven patients (24 %) died within 12 months of transplantation, but only one due to an IFD. The 1-year cumulative incidence of IFD was 6.7 ± 3.6 %. Two relapses of infection (one candidemia and one fatal scedosporiosis) and one new breakthrough zygomycosis in a patient with a previous IA occurred post-transplantation. None of the 31 patients with a previous IA experienced recurrence of their infection. Voriconazole was discontinued in only two patients because of treatment-related hepatotoxicity. This study demonstrated that SAP may be useful in patients with previously documented and fully resolved IFD facing a new episode of prolonged neutropenia (usually chemotherapy-induced) or severe immunosuppression (usually transplantation). Different is the evidence of the efficacy of a SAP in patients with active infection or with persistent radiological abnormalities [56]. Strictly speaking, the treatment with antifungal drugs of a not yet resolved IFD should not be designated as SAP. In these cases other terms such as maintenance or continuous antifungal therapy may be more appropriate. On the other hand, previous studies on patients undergoing intensive chemotherapy or SCT after an IFD had been occurred included also patients with residual or active IFD. An evidence-based antifungal approach in patients with an IFD not in complete remission who require urgent antileukemic treatment is a challenging issue. In the real life, a large number of patients with hematologic malignancies undergo allogeneic SCT despite unresolved IFD. When the underlying malignancy is at high risk of relapse or progression, an early transplant procedure may be required without time for a prolonged antifungal therapy and for the achievement of the infection complete remission before transplant. Such situation is increasingly encountered in the clinical practice and represents a serious therapeutic problem. In retrospective studies of patients with prior IFD undergoing allogeneic SCT, the infection was in partial remission, stable phase, or progression in about half of the cases, and persistent radiographic abnormalities were associated with increased risks of post-transplant relapse or progression of the infection and of IFD-related death. Prior IFD no longer represents a contraindication to allogeneic SCT. However, while SAP in patients with a resolved infection is able to minimize the risk of relapse after transplant, patients with an active/not resolved IFD at the time of transplant or chemotherapy continues to be at risk of a potentially fatal reactivation. The role of suppressive/continuous antifungal treatment and of preventive surgical resection of residual pulmonary lesions should be properly investigated in order to identify a tailored antifungal prevention strategy.

16.3.4 Open Issues in Antifungal Prophylaxis of Hematologic Patients

Several open issues in the prophylaxis of IFDs in patients with hematologic disorders deserve careful consideration. Recommendations of international guidelines reflect important progresses obtained in the prevention of IFDs, including those caused by filamentous fungi, but they have been unable to generate a consensus for optimal prophylaxis of IFDs in the complex scenario of hematologic disorders, particularly in the transplant setting. This problem has been underlined in a recent consensus process by the Gruppo Italiano Trapianto di Midollo Osseo (GITMO), which was undertaken to describe and evaluate current information and practice regarding risk stratification and PAP during pre-engraftment and post-engraftment phases after allogeneic SCT [57]. The recommendations were based on the evaluation of recent literature including a large, prospective, multicenter epidemiological study in allogeneic SCT recipients conducted among the GITMO transplant centers during the period 2008–2010 [58]. A new risk stratification of allogeneic SCT patients was proposed for the identification of types and phases of transplant at low, standard, and high risk for IFD according to the underlying disease, transplant and post-transplant factors. The risk stratification was the critical determinant of a tailored PAP approach in the different allogeneic SCT settings [57].

Additional well-designed studies in PAP and SAP are needed, not only to evaluate the efficacy of new antifungal drugs but also to define risk stratification criteria and tailored prevention strategies. An updated epidemiological consciousness is required in order to individualize specific measures aimed at the prophylaxis of IFDs in the different clinical settings of hematologic malignancies.

16.4 Prophylaxis of Pneumocystis Pneumonia

Pneumocystis pneumonia (PcP), caused by *Pneumocystis jirovecii* (formerly *Pneumocystis carinii*), is a common cause of pneumonia among immunocompromised individuals. Although the efficacy of PcP prophylaxis in hematologic and

SCT patients has not been assessed in controlled clinical trials, PcP prophylaxis is currently routine in these patients. PcP prophylaxis is recommended in hematologic patients receiving a glucocorticoid dose equivalent to ≥20 mg of prednisone daily for 1 month or longer, allogeneic SCT recipients, patients with acute lymphoblastic leukemia, patients receiving certain immunosuppressive drugs (e.g., alemtuzumab, purine analogs), and selected autologous SCT recipients (including those who have a lymphoprolipherative malignancy, have undergone graft manipulations as CD34 selection, or have recently received purine analogs).

A review of the literature published in 2007 showed that trimethoprim-sulfamethoxazole prophylaxis is highly effective in preventing PcP infection in immunocompromised non-HIV-infected patients lowering its incidence by 91 % and its mortality by 83 % [59]. Trimethoprim-sulfamethoxazole may be given as one double-strength tablet daily or three times per week or as one single-strength tablet daily. Atovaquone, dapsone, monthly aerosolized pentamidine, clindamycin, and primaquine may be used in patients who cannot tolerate trimethoprim-sulfamethoxazole.

16.5 Antiviral Prophylaxis

16.5.1 Rational for Antiviral Prophylaxis

Several viral infections may occur in patients with hematologic diseases or SCT recipients. There are good reasons to try to prevent viral diseases, however, only for herpesviruses and hepatitis B virus (HBV) prophylactic strategies with antiviral agents have been defined. Both herpesviruses and HBV infections during chemotherapy-related neutropenia or after SCT generally constitute reactivations of viruses.

Up to 80 % of adult patients with leukemia are herpes simplex virus (HSV)-seropositive and HSV lesions in these patients occur in more than 60 % of patients resulting from reactivation of latent virus, whereas primary infection is unusual. Following allogeneic transplantation the risk for HSV reactivation is approximately 80 %, for cytomegalovirus (CMV) is 20–30 %, and for varicella-zoster virus (VZV) is 20–50 %, among seropositive recipients without prophylaxis [60–63]. Reactivation of chronic hepatitis B in patients undergoing immunosuppressive or antineoplastic treatment approximately occurs in 20–50 % of HBsAg-positive patients and can result in fulminant hepatitis [64]. Patients with malignant lymphoma, especially those treated with anthracycline-containing chemotherapy, are significantly at higher risk [65]. HBsAg-positive allogeneic SCT recipients are at risk of developing severe and possibly fatal hepatic disease and so anti-HBs negative donors for HbsAg-positive patients should be vaccinated before stem cell collection if possible. On the contrary, transplantation of an HBsAg-negative patient with stem cells from an HbsAg-positive donor is associated with a high risk of transmission, but few patients develop aggressive acute infection or chronic hepatitis B [66–68].

European and American guidelines of antimicrobial prophylaxis of some viral infections have been summarized in Tables 16.1 and 16.2, respectively [16, 17, 20].

16.5.2 Prophylaxis of HSV Reactivation

Primary HSV infection in patients treated for leukemia is unusual, and antiviral chemoprophylaxis is thus not recommended in HSV-seronegative leukemia patients during chemotherapy or after SCT. On the contrary, prophylaxis with an HSV-active agent, such as acyclovir, should be offered to all HSV-seropositive autologous or allogeneic SCT recipients and patients with acute leukemia undergoing induction or reinduction therapy [17, 20]. Therapy with antiviral agents is aimed both at shortening the duration of HSV disease and at preventing the dissemination of HSV to visceral sites, which can lead to life-threatening conditions. Prophylaxis should be given until recovery of the white blood cell count and resolution of mucositis. Duration of prophylaxis can be extended for persons with frequent recurrent HSV infections or those with GVHD or can be continued as VZV prophylaxis for up to 1 year. In addition to acyclovir, the newer antiviral compounds valaciclovir and famciclovir are active against HSV. Both agents have an oral bioavailability three to five times superior to that of oral acyclovir and, although less well studied, are commonly used for prevention of HSV reactivation during induction chemotherapy for acute leukemia and after SCT.

16.5.3 Prophylaxis of VZV Primary Infection or Reactivation

Seronegative leukemia patients and SCT recipients are at high risk of varicella after a face-to-face contact of 5 min or more with a person with varicella or intimate contact (touching or hugging) with a person with *herpes zoster*. Patients residing in the same household or in hospital in the same room or adjacent beds in a large ward where there is a contagious person are also at risk. Passive immunization with i.v. varicella-zoster-specific immunoglobulins (at a dose of 0.2–1 ml/kg) or i.v. normal immunoglobulin (300–500 mg/kg) should be given as soon as possible after exposure (<96 h) to VZV-seronegative patients with leukemia on chemotherapy, receiving steroids, or submitted to SCT with chronic GVHD. In VZV-seropositive patients the risk of a new infection after exposure is low but not insignificant; therefore, some authors suggest to use passive immunization with immunoglobulins also in these cases [69]. The efficacy of antiviral agents for post-exposure prophylaxis in leukemic patients and recipients of SCT is uncertain, but uncontrolled experiences seem to suggest that acyclovir, valaciclovir, or famciclovir prophylaxis may reduce the incidence of varicella and its severity. The use of antimicrobial prophylaxis after exposure may be particularly indicated if immunoglobulin administration in not possible starting during 3–21 days after exposure.

Although most SCT recipients are VZV-seropositive, they are at risk of virus reactivation for a prolonged period after transplant. Therefore, for VZV-seropositive allo-SCT recipients, prophylaxis with oral acyclovir (800 mg twice daily; for children: 20 mg/kg twice daily) or valaciclovir (500 mg once or twice daily) is recommended for 1 year or longer in the presence of GVHD requiring immunosuppressive therapy [16].

16.5.4 Prophylaxis of CMV Reactivation

The different preventive strategies for CMV disease include the use of antiviral agents, such as chemoprophylaxis, preemptive therapy, or treatment of symptomatic CMV infection. The currently available antiviral agents for prevention of CMV infection and disease are acyclovir, valacyclovir, ganciclovir, valganciclovir, foscarnet, and cidofovir.

A preemptive antiviral strategy based on the serial monitoring of CMV (pp65 antigen and/or quantitative PCR) represents the most widely used approach, not only in the allogeneic SCT setting but also in other patient cohorts at risk of CMV infection and disease such as patients with chronic lymphocytic leukemia under alemtuzumab therapy. The frequency of CMV reactivation in other subgroups of patients such as autologous SCT recipients and acute leukemia patients is high, but the risk of evolution to overt CMV disease is very low; therefore, routine surveillance in these patients is unnecessary and prophylaxis not recommended [16]. However, subgroups of patients including those receiving CD34-selected grafts and prior treatment with fludarabine or other purine analogs are at high risk for acquiring CMV disease; therefore, they should be monitored similar to allogeneic SCT recipients [70].

Antiviral chemoprophylaxis is an alternative to preemptive therapy in subgroups of patients at high risk for CMV disease. Intravenous ganciclovir prophylaxis is an effective strategy for the prevention of CMV disease in subgroups of allo-SCT patients at high risk for CMV disease, but toxicity concerns and the potential for resistance to ganciclovir among CMV hamper its unselected prophylactic use. Also acyclovir or valacyclovir at high doses can be used; however, this approach must be combined with serial CMV monitoring and pre-emptive therapeutic intervention.

16.5.5 Prophylaxis of HHV-6 and HHV-8 Reactivation

Given the low risk of HHV-6 and HHV-8 diseases and the toxicity of the available antiviral drugs, chemoprophylaxis of such viral infections is not recommended [17].

16.5.6 Prophylaxis of HBV Reactivation

Reactivation of hepatitis B is a well-characterized syndrome associated with the reappearance or rise of HBV DNA in the serum of a patient with previously inactive or resolved HBV infection and is frequently accompanied by reappearance of early or late hepatic disease activity. Reactivation of HBV has been reported not only in HBsAg-positive patients undergoing systemic chemotherapy but also in a proportion of HBsAg-negative patients with anti-HBc antibodies. HBsAg-positive patients with hematologic malignancies undergoing immunochemotherapy are at risk of developing severe hepatic disease. However, the most dramatic examples of HBV reactivation have been described in patients undergoing allogeneic SCT. Guidelines published by the US Centers for Disease Control and Prevention recommend that all patients about to receive chemotherapy for malignant disease be tested for HBsAg before cancer treatment is initiated [71].

Controlled clinical trials and several meta-analyses have shown that prophylaxis with nucleoside analogs decreases the incidence of HBV reactivation and the frequency of clinical hepatitis and death from HBV-associated liver injury in patients undergoing chemotherapy or SCT [72–78]. Initiating therapy once reactivation has occurred appears to be ineffective. Although there are several oral agents approved for the treatment of chronic hepatitis B (lamivudine, adefovir, entecavir, tenofovir, telbivudine), the published experience in prevention and treatment of HBV reactivation following chemotherapy is almost entirely limited to lamivudine (100 mg daily). Such therapy should start before starting chemotherapy or transplant and should continue for at least 6 months after stopping chemotherapy or later in situations in which long-term immune suppression is required [79, 80]. A major concern with prolonged use of lamivudine is the possibility of viral breakthrough following the emergence of resistance mutations [81, 82]. Alternative antiviral agents such adefovir, entecavir, or tenofovir are likely to be associated with lower resistance rates. However, adefovir is showing primary treatment failure in 10 % or more of patients and 30 % resistance by the end of 4 years, whereas entecavir and tenofovir are more attractive candidates given their high potency and extremely low resistance rates. Both agents are significantly more expensive than lamivudine.

References

1. Schimpff SC, Young V, Greene E, et al. Origin of infection in acute nonlymphocytic leukemia: significance of hospital acquisition of potential pathogens. Ann Intern Med. 1972;77:707–15.
2. Donnelly JP. Chemoprophylaxis for the prevention of bacterial and fungal infections. Cancer Treat Res. 1995;79:45–82.
3. Hawthorn JW. Critical appraisal of antimicrobials for prevention of infections in immunocompromised hosts. Hematol Oncol Clin N Am. 1993;7:1051–99.
4. Guiot HF, van den Broek J, van der Meer JW, van Furth R. Selective antimicrobial modulation of the intestinal flora of patients with acute nonlymphocytic leukemia: a double blind, placebo-controlled study. J Infect Dis. 1983;147:615–23.
5. Gualtieri RJ, Donowitz GR, Kaiser DL, et al. Double-blind randomized study of prophylactic trimethoprim/sulfamethoxazole in granulocytopenic patients with hematologic malignancies. Am J Med. 1983;74:934–40.
6. Kramer BS, Carr DJ, Rand KH, et al. Prophylaxis of fever and infection in adult cancer patients. A placebo-controlled trial of oral trimethoprim – sulfamethoxazole plus erythromycin. Cancer. 1984;53:329–35.
7. Karp JE, Merz WG, Hendricksen C, et al. Oral norfloxacin for prevention of gram-negative bacterial infections in patients with acute leukemia and granulocytopenia. A randomised double-blind, placebo-controlled trial. Ann Intern Med. 1987;106:1–7.
8. Winston DJ, Ho WG, Champlin RE, et al. Norfloxacin for prevention of bacterial infections in granulocytopenic patients. Am J Med. 1987;82:40–6.
9. Talbot GH, Cassileth PA, Paradiso L, et al. Oral enoxacin for infection prevention in adults with acute nonlymphocytic leukaemia. The Enoxacin Prophylaxis Study Group. Antimicrob Agents Chemother. 1993;37:474–82.

10. Lew MA, Kehoe K, Ritz J, et al. Prophylaxis of bacterial infections with ciprofloxacin in patients undergoing bone marrow transplantation. Transplantation. 1991;51:630–6.
11. Gafter-Gvili A, Fraser A, Paul M, et al. Meta-analysis: antibiotic prophylaxis reduces mortality in neutropenic patients. Ann Intern Med. 2005;142:979–95.
12. Bucaneve G, Micozzi A, Menichetti F, et al. Levofloxacin to prevent bacterial infection in patients with cancer and neutropenia. N Engl J Med. 2005;353:977–87.
13. Cullen M, Steven N, Billingham L, et al. Antibacterial prophylaxis after chemotherapy for solid tumors and lymphomas. N Engl J Med. 2005;353:988–98.
14. Bucaneve G, Castagnola E, Viscoli C, Menichetti F, Leibovici L. Quinolone prophylaxis for bacterial infections in afebrile high risk neutropenic patients. Eur J Cancer. 2007;5 Suppl 2:5–12.
15. Maertens J, Marchetti O, Herbrecht R, et al. European guidelines for antifungal management in leukemia and hematopoietic stem cell transplant recipients: summary of the ECIL 3-2009 Update. Bone Marrow Transplant. 2011;46:709–18.
16. Styczynski J, Reusser P, Einsele H, Second European Conference on Infections in Leukemia, et al. Management of HSV, VZV and EBV infections in patients with hematological malignancies and after SCT: guidelines from the Second European Conference on Infections in Leukemia. Bone Marrow Transplant. 2009;43:757–70.
17. Ljungman P, de la Camara R, Cordonnier C, European Conference on Infections in Leukemia, et al. Management of CMV, HHV-6, HHV-7 and Kaposi-sarcoma herpesvirus (HHV-8) infections in patients with hematological malignancies and after SCT. Bone Marrow Transplant. 2008;42:227–40.
18. Wingard JR, Carter SL, Walsh TJ, et al. Randomized double-blind trial of fluconazole versus voriconazole for prevention of invasive fungal infection after allogeneic hematopoietic cell transplantation. Blood. 2010;116:5111–8.
19. Marks DI, Pagliuca A, Kibbler CC, et al. Voriconazole versus itraconazole for antifungal prophylaxis following allogeneic haematopoietic stem-cell transplantation. Br J Haematol. 2011;155:318–27.
20. Freifeld AG, Bow EJ, Sepkowitz KA, et al. Clinical practice guideline for the use of antimicrobial agents in neutropenic patients with cancer: 2010 update by the Infectious Diseases Society of America. Clin Infect Dis. 2011;52:e56–93.
21. Walsh TJ, Anaissie EJ, Denning DW, et al. Treatment of aspergillosis: clinical practice guidelines of the Infectious Diseases Society of America. Clin Infect Dis. 2008;46:327–60.
22. Kotilainen P, Nikoskelainen J, Houvien P. Emergence of ciprofloxacin resistant coagulase negative staphylococcal skin flora in immunocompromised patients receiving ciprofloxacin. J Infect Dis. 1990;161:41–4.
23. Trucksis M, Hooper DC, Wolfson JS. Emerging resistance to fluoroquinolones in staphylococci: an alert. Ann Intern Med. 1991;114:424–6.
24. Kern WV, Andriof E, Oethinger M, et al. Emergence of fluoroquinolone-resistant *Escherichia coli* at a cancer center. Antimicrob Agents Chemother. 1994;38:681–7.
25. Caratalla J, Fernandez-Sevilla A, Dominguez MA, et al. Emergence of fluoroquinolone-resistant flora of cancer patients receiving norfloxacin prophylaxis. Antimicrob Agents Chemother. 1996;40:503.
26. Cometta A, Calandra T, Bille J, et al. *Escherichia coli* resistant to fluoroquinolone prophylaxis in patients with cancer and neutropenia. N Engl J Med. 1994;330:1240–1.
27. Hughes WT, Armstrong D, Bodey GP, et al. 2002 Guidelines for the use of antimicrobial agents in neutropenic patients with cancer. Clin Infect Dis. 2002;34:730–51.
28. Gafter-Gvili A, Paul M, Fraser A, et al. Effect of quinolone prophylaxis in afebrile neutropenic patients on microbial resistance: systematic review and meta-analysis. J Antimicrob Chemother. 2007;59:5–22.
29. Bow EJ, Laverdière M, Lussier N, Rotstein C, Cheang MS, Ioannou S. Antifungal prophylaxis for severely neutropenic chemotherapy recipients: a meta analysis of randomized-controlled clinical trials. Cancer. 2002;94:3230–46.
30. Robenshtok E, Gafter-Gvili A, Goldberg E, et al. Antifungal prophylaxis in cancer patients after chemotherapy or hematopoietic stem-cell transplantation: systematic review and meta-analysis. J Clin Oncol. 2007;25:5471–89.

31. Girmenia C. Prophylaxis of invasive fungal diseases in patients with hematologic disorders. Haematologica. 2010;95:1630–2.
32. Andes D, Pascual A, Marchetti O. Antifungal therapeutic drug monitoring: established and emerging indications. Antimicrob Agents Chemother. 2009;53:24–34.
33. Girmenia C. New generation azole antifungals in clinical investigation. Expert Opin Investig Drugs. 2009;18:1279–95.
34. Slavin MA, Osborne B, Adams R, et al. Efficacy and safety of fluconazole prophylaxis for fungal infections after marrow transplantation: a prospective, randomized, double-blind study. J Infect Dis. 1995;171:1545–52.
35. Goodman JL, Winston DJ, Greenfield RA, et al. A controlled trial of fluconazole to prevent fungal infections in patients undergoing bone marrow transplantation. N Engl J Med. 1992;326:845–51.
36. Marr K, Seidel K, Slavin M, et al. Prolonged fluconazole prophylaxis is associated with persistent protection against candidiasis-related death in allogeneic marrow transplant recipients: long-term follow-up of a randomized, placebo-controlled trial. Blood. 2000;96:2055–61.
37. Schaffner A, Schaffner M. Effect of prophylactic fluconazole on the frequency of fungal infections, amphotericin B use, and health care costs in patients undergoing intensive chemotherapy for hematologic neoplasias. J Infect Dis. 1995;172:1035–41.
38. Rotstein C, Bow EJ, Laverdiere M, Ioannou S, Carr D, Moghaddam N. Randomized placebo-controlled trial of fluconazole prophylaxis for neutropenic cancer patients: benefit based on purpose and intensity of cytotoxic therapy. The Canadian Fluconazole Prophylaxis Study Group. Clin Infect Dis. 1999;28:331–40.
39. Glasmacher A, Prentice A, Gorschlüter M, et al. Itraconazole prevents invasive fungal infections in neutropenic patients treated for hematologic malignancies: evidence from a meta-analysis of 3,597 patients. J Clin Oncol. 2003;21:4615–26.
40. Winston DJ, Maziarz RT, Chandrasekar PH, et al. Intravenous and oral itraconazole versus intravenous and oral fluconazole for long-term antifungal prophylaxis in allogeneic hematopoietic stem-cell transplant recipients. A multicenter, randomized trial. Ann Intern Med. 2003;138:705–13.
41. Marr KA, Crippa F, Leisenring W, et al. Itraconazole versus fluconazole for prevention of fungal infections in patients receiving allogeneic stem cell transplants. Blood. 2004;103:1527–33.
42. Glasmacher A, Cornely O, Ullmann AJ, et al. An open-label randomized trial comparing itraconazole oral solution with fluconazole oral solution for primary prophylaxis of fungal infections in patients with haematological malignancy and profound neutropenia. J Antimicrob Chemother. 2006;57:317–25.
43. Stevens DA, Kan VL, Judson MA, et al. Practice guidelines for diseases caused by Aspergillus. Infectious Diseases Society of America. Clin Infect Dis. 2000;30:696–709.
44. Rex JH, Walsh TJ, Sobel JD, et al. Practice guidelines for the treatment of candidiasis. Infectious Diseases Society of America. Clin Infect Dis. 2000;30:662–78.
45. Cornely OA, Maertens J, Winston DJ, et al. Posaconazole vs. fluconazole or itraconazole prophylaxis in patients with neutropenia. N Engl J Med. 2007;356:348–59.
46. Ullmann AJ, Lipton JH, Vesole DH, et al. Posaconazole or fluconazole for prophylaxis in severe graft-versus-host disease. N Engl J Med. 2007;356:335–47.
47. van Burik JA, Ratanatharathorn V, Stepan DE, et al. Micafungin versus fluconazole for prophylaxis against invasive fungal infections during neutropenia in patients undergoing hematopoietic stem cell transplantation. Clin Infect Dis. 2004;39:1407–16.
48. Mattiuzzi GN, Alvarado G, Giles FJ, et al. Open-label, randomized comparison of itraconazole versus caspofungin for prophylaxis in patients with hematologic malignancies. Antimicrob Agents Chemother. 2006;50:143–7.
49. Rijnders BJ, Cornelissen JJ, Slobbe L, et al. Aerosolized liposomal amphotericin B for the prevention of invasive pulmonary aspergillosis during prolonged neutropenia: a randomized, placebo-controlled trial. Clin Infect Dis. 2008;46:1401–8.
50. Trifilio SM, Yarnold PR, Scheetz MH, Pi J, Pennick G, Mehta J. Serial plasma voriconazole concentrations after allogeneic hematopoietic stem cell transplantation. Antimicrob Agents Chemother. 2009;53:1793–6.

51. Girmenia C, Aversa F, Micozzi A. Voriconazole prophylaxis and the risk of invasive fungal infection after allogeneic hematopoietic cell transplantation. Blood. 4 February 2011, e-letter for Wingard et al. Blood. 2010;116:5111–8.
52. Pappas PG, Kauffman CA, Andes D, et al. Clinical practice guidelines for the management of candidiasis: 2009 update by the Infectious Diseases Society of America. Clin Infect Dis. 2009;48:503–35.
53. Martino R, Parody R, Fukuda T, et al. Impact of the intensity of the pretransplantation conditioning regimen in patients with prior invasive aspergillosis undergoing allogeneic hematopoietic stem cell transplantation: a retrospective survey of the Infectious Diseases Working Party of the European Group for Blood and Marrow Transplantation. Blood. 2006;108:2928–36.
54. Sipsas NV, Kontoyiannis DP. Clinical issues regarding relapsing aspergillosis and the efficacy of secondary antifungal prophylaxis in patients with hematological malignancies. Clin Infect Dis. 2006;42:1584–91.
55. Cordonnier C, Rovira M, Maertens J, et al. Voriconazole for Secondary Prophylaxis of Invasive Fungal Infections in patients with allogeneic stem cell transplants (VOSIFI) study group; Infectious Diseases Working Party, European Group for Blood and Marrow Transplantation. Voriconazole for secondary prophylaxis of invasive fungal infections in allogeneic stem cell transplant recipients: results of the VOSIFI study. Haematologica. 2010;95:1762–8.
56. Girmenia C. Voriconazole as secondary antifungal prophylaxis in stem cell transplant recipients (reply). Haematologica. 2011;96:e11.
57. Girmenia C, Barosi G, Piciocchi A, et al. Primary prophylaxis of invasive fungal diseases in allogeneic stem cell transplantation: revised recommendations from a consensus process by Gruppo Italiano Trapianto Midollo Osseo (GITMO). Biol Blood Marrow Transplant. 2014;20:1080–8.
58. Girmenia C, Raiola AM, Piciocchi A, et al. Incidence and Outcome of Invasive Fungal Diseases after Allogeneic Stem Cell Transplantation: A Prospective Study of the Gruppo Italiano Trapianto Midollo Osseo(GITMO). Biol Blood Marrow Transplant. 2014;20:872–80.
59. Green H, Paul M, Vidal L, Leibovici L. Prophylaxis of Pneumocystis pneumonia in immunocompromised non-HIV-infected patients: systematic review and meta-analysis of randomized controlled trials. Mayo Clin Proc. 2007;82(9):1052–9.
60. Gratwohl A, Brand R, Frassoni F, et al. Cause of death after allogeneic haematopoietic stem cell transplantation (HSCT) in early leukaemias: an EBMT analysis of lethal infectious complications and changes over calendar time. Bone Marrow Transplant. 2005;36:757–69.
61. Kernan NA, Bartsch G, Ash RC, et al. Analysis of 462 transplantations from unrelated donors facilitated by the National Marrow Donor Program. N Engl J Med. 1993;328:593–602.
62. Maltezou HC, Kafetzis DA, Abisaid D, et al. Viral infections in children undergoing hematopoietic stem cell transplant. Pediatr Infect Dis J. 2000;19:307–12.
63. Sandherr M, Einsele H, Hebart H, et al. Antiviral prophylaxis in patients with haematological malignancies and solid tumours: guidelines of the Infectious Diseases Working Party (AGIHO) of the German Society for Hematology and Oncology (DGHO). Ann Oncol. 2006;17:1051–9.
64. Rossi G, Pelizzari A, Motta M, et al. Primary prophylaxis with lamivudine of hepatitis B virus reactivation in chronic HbsAg carriers with lymphoid malignancies treated with chemotherapy. Br J Haematol. 2001;115:58–62.
65. Yeo W, Chan P, Ho WM, et al. Lamivudine for the prevention of Hepatitis B Virus reactivation in Hepatitis B s-Antigen seropositive cancer patients undergoing cytotoxic chemotherapy. J Clin Oncol. 2004;22:927–34.
66. Locasciulli A, Testa M, Valsecchi MG, et al. The role of hepatitis C and B virus infections as risk factors for severe liver complications following allogeneic BMT: a prospective study by the Infectious Disease Working Party of the European Blood and Marrow Transplantation Group. Transplantation. 1999;68:1486–91.
67. Chiba T, Yokosuka O, Goto S, et al. Successful clearance of hepatitis B virus after allogeneic stem cell transplantation: beneficial combination of adoptive immunity transfer and lamivudine. Eur J Haematol. 2003;71:220–3.

68. Locasciulli A, Alberti A, Bandini G, et al. Allogeneic bone marrow transplantation from HbsAg+ donors: a multicenter study from the Gruppo Italiano Trapianto di Midollo Osseo (GITMO). Blood. 1995;86:3236–40.
69. Weinstock DM, Boeckh M, Boulad F, et al. Postexposure prophylaxis against varicella-zoster virus infection among recipients of hematopoietic stem cell transplant: unresolved issues. Infect Control Hosp Epidemiol. 2004;25:603–8.
70. Holmberg LA, Boeckh M, Hooper H, et al. Increased incidence of cytomegalovirus disease after autologous CD34-selected peripheral blood stem cell transplantation (see comments). Blood. 1999;94:4029–35.
71. Weinbaum CM, Williams I, Mast EE, et al. Recommendations for identification and public health management of persons with chronic hepatitis B virus infection. MMWR Recomm Rep. 2008;57:1–20.
72. Lau GK, Yiu HH, Fong DY, et al. Early is superior to deferred preemptive lamivudine therapy for hepatitis B patients undergoing chemotherapy. Gastroenterology. 2003;125:1742–9.
73. Hsu C, Hsiung CA, Su I-J, et al. A revisit of prophylactic lamivudine for chemotherapy-associated hepatitis B reactivation in non-Hodgkin's lymphoma: a randomized trial. Hepatology. 2008;47:844–53.
74. Kohrt HE, Ouyang DL, Keeffe EB. Systematic review: lamivudine prophylaxis for chemotherapy induced reactivation of chronic hepatitis B virus infection. Aliment Pharmacol Ther. 2006;24:1003–9. 82.
75. Katz LH, Fraser A, Gafter-Gvili A, Leibovici L, Tur-Kaspa R. Lamivudine prevents reactivation of hepatitis B and reduces mortality in immunosuppressed patients: systematic review and meta-analysis. J Viral Hepat. 2008;15:89–102.
76. Lau GK, He ML, Fong DY, et al. Preemptive use of lamivudine reduces hepatitis B exacerbation after allogeneic hematopoietic stem cell transplantation. Hepatology. 2002;36:702–9.
77. Hui CK, Lie A, Au W-Y, et al. Effectiveness of prophylactic anti-HBV therapy in allogeneic hematopoietic stem cell transplantation with HBsAg positive donors. Am J Transplant. 2005;5:1437–45.
78. Tsutsumi Y, Tanaka J, Kawamura T, et al. Possible efficacy of lamivudine treatment to prevent hepatitis B virus reactivation due to rituximab therapy in a patient with non-Hodgkin's lymphoma. Ann Hematol. 2004;83:58–60.
79. Kusumoto S, Tanaka Y, Mizokami M, Ueda R. Reactivation of hepatitis B virus following systemic chemotherapy for malignant lymphoma. Int J Hematol. 2009;90:13–23.
80. Lubel JS, Angus PW. Hepatitis B reactivation in patients receiving cytotoxic chemotherapy: diagnosis and management. J Gastroenterol Hepatol. 2010;25:864–71.
81. Lok AS, Lai CL, Leung N, et al. Long-term safety of lamivudine treatment in patients with chronic hepatitis B. Gastroenterology. 2003;125:1714–22.
82. Kim JS, Hahn JS, Park SY, et al. Long-term outcome after prophylactic lamivudine treatment on hepatitis B virus reactivation in non-Hodgkin's lymphoma. Yonsei Med J. 2007;48:78–89.

Infection Control and Hospital Epidemiology in Hematology Units

17

Maja Weisser and Andreas Widmer

Contents

M. Weisser (✉) • A. Widmer
Division of Infectious Diseases and Hospital Epidemiology, University Hospital Basel, Basel, Switzerland
e-mail: maja.weisser@usb.ch; Andreas.widmer@usb.ch

G. Maschmeyer, K.V.I. Rolston (eds.), *Infections in Hematology*,
DOI 10.1007/978-3-662-44000-1_17

17.1 Introduction

Hospital hygiene or infection control aims at preventing exposure of immunocompromised hosts with infectious agents that may lead to infections with deleterious outcomes. It should be considered at the planning stage of a unit, since many infection control issues must already be implemented in the architecture of the unit such as directed air flow, water supply, and limited traffic of visitors and healthcare workers (HCWs) not working in the unit. The risk of an infection depends on the level of immunosuppression by the underlying disease and/or side effects of chemotherapy and the level of exposure to infectious agents. Treatment procedures in hematology have undergone vast changes in the last 20 years with more specific chemotherapies becoming available (e.g., imatinib) and with different transplantation modalities (e.g., reduced intensity conditioning, cord blood stem cell transplantation) [3], all associated with distinct risks for infectious complications. Particularly in the first two decades after introduction of hematopoietic stem cell transplantation (HCT) into clinical practice, infectious complications were the main cause of transplant-related mortality (TRM) [31]. Besides the immune system itself, natural barriers important for infection control can be damaged, e.g., by chemotherapy-associated mucositis of the gastrointestinal tract or by placement of vascular catheters. After successful HCT with recovery of leukocytes, graft-versus-host disease (GVHD) combined with the necessary immunosuppressive treatment remains one of the most important risk factors. Many institutions have developed their own local infection control guidelines, based on the recently published multidisciplinary guidelines issued by the American Society for Blood and Marrow Transplantation, endorsed by the Infectious Diseases Society of America (IDSA) [71].

As a simplification, the following classifications have been used to assess risk [6]:

(a) Neutropenia

Duration	<1 week: moderate risk
	>1 week: high risk
Absolute neutrophil count (ANC)	<1,000/μL: moderate risk
	<100/μL: high risk
However, the term neutropenia is frequently used in clinical practice as neutrophils <500/μL	

(b) Hematological stem cell transplantation (cellular immunodeficiency)

Donor-derived infections	
Phase I: preengraftment (day 0–30)	After HCT
Phase II: postengraftment (day 31–100)	After HCT
Phase III: late phase (>day 100)	After HCT

(c) Specific immunosuppressive treatments (e.g., monoclonal antibodies, ATG)

Neutropenia <1 week rarely poses a serious risk for infectious complications if no concomitant immunosuppression is present. Special precautions are not warranted, and therefore, this situation will not be further addressed. The focus of most studies on infection control in hematology is the patient after hematological stem cell transplantation, the main focus of this chapter. Not much data exist on hospital infection control measures for neutropenic patients after induction/consolidation chemotherapies or due to the underlying disease. Published guidelines for neutropenia >1 week are usually the same as for the preengraftment period after HCT [71].

Precautions in severely immunocompromised hosts are based on several animal studies and observational clinical trials. GVHD is not observed, if mice are kept in a sterile cage and environment immediately after birth [65]. However, patients are not sterile, and most infections originate from microorganisms colonizing the body rather than from exposure to an exogenous source. Viruses and many bacteria colonizing the body are controlled by the immune system. Cytomegalovirus (CMV), polyoma viruses, and other opportunistic pathogens become clinically relevant with increase of immunosuppression. Therefore, infection control interventions may prevent only up to 50 % of nosocomial infections or at least prevent acquisition of multiresistant pathogens [17, 49]. Before implementing the recommendations of this chapter, the reader should consult regulations and laws of the country and/or their local guidelines. In addition, more specific information can be obtained from the guidelines issued by the European Centre for Disease Prevention and Control (http://www.ecdc.europa.eu/en/publications/guidance/Pages/index.aspx), the Centers for Disease Control and Prevention, Atlanta, USA (CDC) (http://www.cdc.gov/hicpac/pubs.html), or the World Health Organization (WHO) (http://www.who.int).

Prevention has gathered more attention since new antibiotics are unlikely to be developed before 2020, and the IDSA has started the program "10 by '20," meaning 10 new antibiotics by 2020.

17.2 Microorganisms

17.2.1 Bacteria

As outlined above, the endogenous flora of a patient cannot be eliminated, but the flora changes over time during hospitalization. Therefore, infection control aims at preventing exposure to nosocomial multiresistant bacteria rather than controlling any bacteria. The IDSA included among the top five methicillin-resistant *Staphylococcus aureus* (MRSA), vancomycin-resistant enterococci (VRE) or multiresistant *Pseudomonas aeruginosa*, *Acinetobacter baumannii*, and gram-negative bacteria expressing extended broad-spectrum betalactamases (ESBL). In addition, other pathogens expressing plasmid-mediated AmpC betalactamases are of importance [38]. These pathogens – if untreated – have the potential to abrogate a successful hematological treatment by inducing a potentially lethal sepsis. On the other hand, infection with resident bacteria is almost unavoidable when prolonged and severe neutropenia persists over weeks and months. Severe mucositis leads to translocation of bacteria in the gut and ultimately entry into the bloodstream. The commonly required central venous catheter disrupts the skin as a natural barrier and can lead to catheter-related bloodstream infections.

17.2.2 Viruses

Many viruses reside in the body and require treatment only under severe immunosuppression leading to increased replication and symptomatic disease. Endogenous viruses increasing morbidity and mortality in HCT patients are mainly cytomegalovirus (CMV) and other herpesviruses and polyomavirus [4, 36].

The most common viruses transmitted in hospitals are respiratory viruses such as influenza [25], parainfluenza, respiratory syncytial virus (RSV), metapneumovirus, and adenoviruses. Several studies indicate that RSV infection early after HCT has a mortality rate between 30 and 60 % [41]. Less frequent, but highly contagious are *varicella zoster* and measles. Infections with these viruses are preventable by definition and require a source that comes directly or indirectly into contact with the susceptible patient. Visitors, especially children, and HCWs are common vectors for transmission of viruses. These individuals may not feel sick, but carry viruses in the respiratory secretions for prolonged times. Therefore, vaccination of HCWs and family members is a basic infection control procedure and wearing masks and hand hygiene are essential to prevent transmission (see below).

17.2.3 Fungi

The intestinal and respiratory tracts are colonized with bacteria and fungi. Not surprisingly, yeast infections are usually originating from the endogenous gut flora. Prevention of candidiasis with an antifungal prophylaxis has shown to reduce invasive candida infections [40]. Few studies indicate that *Pneumocystis jirovecii* pneumonia (PCP) might be transmitted by the airborne route [46]. Animal studies demonstrated that *P. jirovecii* could be spread through the air, and air samples from areas frequented or occupied by *P. jirovecii*-infected patients were positive for PCP: However, the introduction of routine prophylaxis with TMP/SMX basically eliminated the risk of PCP, independent of the mode of acquisition. Molds and many dimorphic fungi in endemic areas are airborne. High densities of fungal spores occur during construction work in close proximity of the patient [55]. Special air filtration is a mandatory precaution during construction works as are outlined below. More recently, the hospital water supply has also been described as a possible source of molds [1]. Opportunistic molds (e.g., *Aspergillus* and *Fusarium* species) can be cultured from water and on water-related surfaces of hematology units. Studies by Anaissie and colleagues indicated the potential relatedness of environmental and clinical strains among patients with aspergillosis and fusariosis by epidemiological typing [1]. A relative humidity >60 %, especially over 80 %, promotes growth of any molds in any environment. Therefore, air conditioners are frequently set at a humidity of 30–50 %. An extremely humid climate may limit the capacity of the air condition to lower the humidity below 60 %.

17.2.4 Protozoa and Helminths

Transmission of protozoa and helminths in the hospital setting is a rare event. Standard air conditioning prevents exposure to mosquitoes that may transmit malaria in southern countries. Similarly, simple water treatment, required, e.g., by regulatory agencies in Europe as well as in the USA, prevents contamination of the water with helminths. Hospitals in a highly exposed area are referred to special literature in this field.

17.3 Protective Environment (Reverse Isolation) for Hematology Units

The term isolation is most frequently used to describe measures to *protect the hospital* from patients spreading resistant and/or dangerous microorganisms. The term reverse isolation or protective environment (PE) or protective isolation (PI) aims to *protect the patient* from the hospital environment and/or contact with other patients. Many HCWs have difficulties to distinguish PE from, e.g., isolation precautions.

In the first 10–20 years after introduction of allogeneic HCT, sterile nursing in "life islands" with extensive gastrointestinal tract decontamination and sterile food supply had been considered standard of care [14]. In the 1980s, these measures have been abandoned due to lack of appropriate benefit and high costs: these units were replaced by care in single rooms with or without laminar airflow/HEPA air filters. The few randomized trials comparing PE with standard care have conflicting results, but conclude that there is a favorable effect on the infection rate [24, 51, 58] without translating into an improved survival. Few studies support to continue PE in the outpatient setting after HCT [24, 35, 67, 68].

PE must be combined with isolation precautions in patients colonized or infected with multiresistant pathogens or dangerous viruses.

17.3.1 Rooms/Ventilation

Numerous reports in healthcare facilities report airborne transmission of *Aspergillus* spp., Mucorales, *Mycobacterium tuberculosis*, measles (rubeola) virus, and *varicella-zoster* virus [63]. The current recommendations of the CDC to prevent airborne transmission [32] include protective care in single rooms ventilated with ≥12 air exchanges/hour with appropriate fraction of fresh air and central or point-of-use HEPA filters with 99.97 % efficiency for removing particles ≥0.3 μm in diameter, regular replacement of filters, and directed airflow [63, 69]. Twelve air exchanges per hour require a high air volume, which is generated by powerful ventilators. In new construction, noise of ventilators and uncomfortable airflow to the patient should be considered.

Consistent positive air pressure differential between the patient's room and the hallway ≥2.5 Pa (i.e., 0.01 in. by water gauge) [63] and well-sealed rooms prevent the inflow of spore-containing air from outside. Continuous monitoring and self-closing doors prevent drops in positive pressure. Portable HEPA filters in case of shortage of protective environment have been shown to remove airborne fungal spores and mycobacteria [26, 62] and may be useful during constructions. Data to compare central versus portable filters are lacking.

As laminar airflow (LAF) – consisting of HEPA-filtered air moving in a parallel, unidirectional flow – has not improved survival in HCT recipients, it is not generally recommended, but might protect patients from infection during mold outbreaks related to hospital construction [19]. Anterooms to ensure air balance between rooms and hallways are not generally mandatory and are recommended only for certain airborne infections such as tuberculosis, measles, and varicella.

17.3.2 Cleaning

Dust control is a central issue, as dust contains spores causing mold infections. Despite the proven association of surface contamination with nosocomial infections, only little data support the value of routine surface disinfection in general hospital wards [22]. However, lack of appropriate disinfection of the surfaces is a risk factor for VRE and *Clostridium difficile* [37]. In addition, patients colonized or infected with methicillin-resistant *S. aureus* (MRSA) spread their germs all over the room: In fact, more than 50 % of the environment of such patients is contaminated with MRSA [8]. Studies demonstrate that enterococci survive in the environment of hematology units despite vigorous highly active disinfection of the surfaces [21], probably due to rapid recontamination by patients and HCWs.

CDC recommends daily wet-dusting to avoid aerosolization of dust and cleaning of horizontal surfaces with an approved hospital disinfectant [63]. Dust levels can be further reduced by avoiding carpeting and by floor and furniture surfaces with a smooth, nonporous, and washable finish, which has to be compatible with commonly used disinfectants [64]. As vacuum cleaners could aerosolize fungal spores, they should be fitted with HEPA filters. Boyce and colleagues published a new approach with hydrogen vapor to completely disinfect a room using a commercial equipment and reducing contamination and transmission of *C. difficile*[9].

Contamination of floor and surfaces occurs within hours after disinfection of the environment. Therefore, at least once daily disinfection of the environment is recommended in transplant units [63, 77].

Water leaks and moisture of walls lead to mold proliferation. This can easily be detected by a moisture meter. Plants, plant soil, and flower water might contain gram-negative bacteria, especially *Pseudomonas* spp. or molds. Pots can be visibly overgrown with molds. Therefore, most centers do not allow plants and flowers in patient rooms [69]. In addition, HCW handling plants might transmit pathogens from plants to patients, unless meticulous hand hygiene is performed. With the exception of water-retaining bath toys which have been associated with *Pseudomonas aeruginosa* outbreaks [13], toys should not generally be forbidden in pediatric wards but should be washed and disinfected regularly, following guidelines.

17.3.3 Construction

As mold outbreaks have been reported repeatedly during hospital construction/renovation [74], measures to reduce the content of molds in the air should be specially addressed during these high-risk periods and planned in advance [52]. In moderate climates with four seasons, fungal spores are detected in ambient air from spring to late fall. Therefore, constructions should be planned in a low fungal spore season unless LAF with 12 air changes are in place. Dust-proof barriers with airtight seals [63] and a positive pressure difference between patient care and construction or renovation areas prevent dust – and mold spores – from entering patient care areas. Patients/healthcare personnel and medical equipment should not cross construction area; paths for construction workers should be separate. If patients have to cross construction area, they should wear face masks, preferably N95 or FFP2. Air monitoring and infection surveillance should be intensified during construction.

17.3.4 Standard Barrier Precautions

Standard precautions include hand hygiene and wearing of appropriate personal protective equipment (i.e., gloves, surgical masks or eye and face protection, and gowns) during interventions/situations in which emission of blood, body fluids, secretions, or excretions is possible [73]. The WHO has set important guidelines (http://whqlibdoc.who.int/publications/2009/9789241597906_eng.pdf) for hand hygiene that should be followed by all persons entering the patient room before and after each patient contact. Use of alcohol-based hand rubs is superior to hand washing, the latter should be performed in case of soiled hands [11, 76]. Gloves should be worn during all interventions, leading to contact with blood, secretions, and body fluids, but are not recommended as a routine protective precaution, if hand hygiene guidelines are strictly followed. Unfortunately, compliance with hand hygiene rarely exceeds 40 % during daily care. Higher compliance is achieved in clinical studies with reported rates of >60 %, but as soon as observation is suspended, rates drop again. Certain centers use face masks either during winter seasons or even year-round to further reduce the risk of transmission of respiratory viruses. Surgical masks equally prevented transmission of influenza compared to N95 respirator [44]. This approach has not been shown to improve outcome or to reduce nosocomial infection in a randomized controlled clinical trial, but should be considered in severely immunosuppressed patients. On transports in the hospital, CDC recommends patients in the preengraftment period to wear masks. Masks are likely to prevent transmission of viruses and bacteria while in contact with visitors and other patients during transport, especially in elevators. However, a recent randomized study could not show a beneficial effect of well-fitting masks for the risk of invasive aspergillosis in high-risk patients [47]. Patients after HCT but also other immunosuppressed patients should avoid crowded areas and daycare centers for children to prevent exposure to persons with respiratory infections [32].

Airborne, droplet, or contact precautions should be applied only in case of an indication such as *M. tuberculosis* and MRSA colonization [64].

17.3.5 Healthcare Personnel (HCW)

Besides routine hospital hygiene measures as described above, HCW suffering from possibly transmissible infections should abstain from patient contact according to published recommendations [7]. The application of this recommendation is difficult in winter seasons, as many HCWs are coughing. A reasonable approach is to recommend routine wearing of surgical mask when entering patient rooms. Vaccination against transmissible diseases is recommended in most countries and is discussed elsewhere in this textbook. Reported outbreaks with gram-negative bacteria and *Candida* infections lead to the recommendation not to wear artificial fingernails while working in direct patient contact on a transplant unit [33].

17.3.6 Visitors

Visitors must be instructed to follow the general hospital hygiene rules when visiting patients. Hand hygiene should be performed before and after each patient visit. Written policies should be handed out to HCT recipients and candidates, their household contacts, and visitors. Nursing staff should screen visitors for the presence of transmissible diseases. During a symptomatic transmissible infection, after a known recent exposure to a communicable disease (e.g., chickenpox, mumps, measles, pertussis) or after receipt of a live vaccine, visitors should not see immunocompromised patients. The number of visitors should be kept low: in our center, visitors are restricted to three persons at a time.

17.3.7 Preventing Intravascular Catheter-Associated Infections

Bundle approaches to reduce the incidence of catheter-related infections should be strictly implied [54]. Non-tunneled central venous catheters used most frequently due to the need of multiple lumina in HCT patients should be disinfected daily with either chlorhexidine [59] or octenidine hydrochloride [70], which is available only in Europe. Coated catheters may be a reasonable choice for high-risk patients. Importantly, both the intraluminal surface and the extraluminal surface must be coated, e.g., by chlorhexidine [45] or minocycline/rifampin [27]. The exit site should not come into contact with tap water [30].

17.4 Nutrition

There is little data on safety of food in immunocompromised patients and most recommendations are based on uncertainties [28]. Nevertheless, besides general safety in preparation of foods, a low-microbial diet is generally recommended for HCT recipients prior to engraftment in order to reduce exposure to microbes present in food. The recommendations include avoidance of raw or undercooked meat, uncooked eggs, and seafood to prevent infection with *Salmonella enteritidis*, *Vibrio* spp., or *Cryptosporidium parvum* and toxoplasmosis. Recent data indicate that meat may be contaminated by methicillin-resistant *S. aureus* (MRSA) and gram-negative bacteria expressing broad-spectrum betalactamases (ESBL) [34, 42]. Therefore, handling or ingestion of raw meat should be avoided during the acute phase of transplantation. Unroasted raw nuts or nuts in the shell, miso products, raw grain products, non-pasteurized milk products (milk, cheese, yogurt), cheeses containing uncooked vegetables, and cheeses with molds have led to outbreaks in the past and should therefore be avoided. More detailed recommendations have been published recently [71]. Probiotics containing live yeast and bacterial cultures have shown conflicting results regarding prevention of diarrhea, but certainly have been shown to cause serious invasive infections in the severely immunocompromised host and should, therefore, not be recommended [16, 18].

17.5 Monitoring of Water and Air

Routine monitoring of water and air is commonly performed and required by law in some countries. However, there is insufficient evidence to justify routine air sampling. In fact, it is not recommended by the guidelines issued by CDC [63]. The advantage of such a monitoring is the early indication of deviances from baseline values, e.g., during construction. Air sampling for small particles gives a result within seconds, while microbiological sampling for fungal spores takes days and even weeks for full identification of fungi. Therefore, air sampling should be performed with a particulate sampler and with an air sampler for microbiological testing.

Water is frequently contaminated with *Pseudomonas aeruginosa*, depending on the level of chlorine added to the drinking water. Bottled water without gas, especially those from large bottles (eg. 4 L) may be contaminated with *Pseudomonas* spp. as well. However, soft drinks in small bottles are considered to be safe if replaced daily.

17.5.1 Sinks, Shower, and Toilets

Water of hematological units should provide water free of *Legionella* spp., *Pseudomonas* spp. and fungi [2]. Commonly used systems are point-of-use filters at the faucet or a centralized system to ensure germ-free water. The sinks of toilets are almost always contaminated with fecal pathogens. Our own studies clearly demonstrate that aerosolization occurs during flushing (data not shown). Therefore, closing the toilet lid is a reasonable approach to avoid contact with frequently multiresistant *P. aeruginosa*. Shower drains have been shown to cause outbreaks with *P. aeruginosa*. Frequent disinfection of the sinks may reduce the rate of nosocomial *P. aeruginosa* infection [5]. A standard operating procedure should be implemented to decontaminate shower heads before biofilm becomes established, e.g., weekly decontamination with a washer-disinfector cleared by the European agency (EN DIN ISO 15883-1-2006) [23]. Manual reprocessing is also considered safe.

17.6 Surveillance of Clinical Infections

Routine surveillance of epidemiologically important multiresistant pathogens are recommended by CDC [63]. For VRE rapid detection schemes have been established [50]. Contact isolation has been advocated for MRSA and VRE. VRE phenotype VanC does not require isolation, since it is not implicated with outbreaks [72]. Cases of invasive mold infections should routinely be monitored on a stem cell transplant unit. The optimal surveillance definition for nosocomial invasive mold disease is unclear, but has been published for performing clinical studies [66]. Increases in the number of cases or emergence of a new type of mold should trigger evaluation of possible sources in the environment.

17.7 Screening for Multiresistant Pathogens on Admission

Multiresistant pathogens have become a major challenge for the treatment of infectious diseases. Asymptomatic colonization on admission remains frequently unrecognized and becomes evident only after a pathogen becomes invasive, e.g., in septicemia. The colonization status of patients on admission may guide empiric treatment during neutropenic fever. Therefore, screening patients at risk is a reasonable approach for early identification of such pathogens. In addition to protective care, patients should be isolated (e.g., disposable gowns, gloves and face masks for personnel and visitors entering contact isolation, or FFP2/3 masks in case of airborne infections). Charts should be labeled to avoid unnecessary exposure of other patients. Electronic records of colonization status help to avoid unnecessary isolation and improve patient safety (http://www.who.int/patientsafety/en/).

17.7.1 Methicillin-Resistant *Staphylococcus aureus* (MRSA)

MRSA belongs to the most frequently encountered multiresistant pathogens in hospitals. It is associated with increased morbidity and mortality and prolongs hospitalization [20]. Treatment commonly requires intravenous glycopeptide therapy, which is associated with a considerable risk of impaired renal function. Screening of patients at risk has been shown to decrease the prevalence of MRSA colonization [61]. Swabs from nose and throat combine high sensitivity and ease of use to detect carriers of MRSA [48]. New rapid PCR-based techniques are available, but conventional chrome-agar plates are most cost-effective [75]. Once identified, patients can be placed in isolation preventing transmission effectively. In addition, effective decolonization schemes have been published [12].

17.7.2 Vancomycin-Resistant Enterococci (VRE)

The emergence of vancomycin-resistant enterococci (VRE) of phenotype VanA and VanB is a major challenge for hematological patients. Emergence of resistance to vancomycin does almost never occur during active treatment. Resistant strains are usually acquired from the environment. Prevention guidelines have been published more than 15 years ago [60]. According to local epidemiology, screening of patients for VRE in rectal swabs before start of chemotherapy is recommended.

17.7.3 Extended-Spectrum Betalactamases (ESBL), *Klebsiella Pneumonia* Carbapenemases (KPC), Metallobetalactamases (MBL)

Currently, the biggest challenge for the management of multiresistant microorganisms is gram-negative bacteria expressing broad-spectrum betalactamases (ESBL), *Klebsiella pneumonia* carbapenemases, or metallobetalactamases. The resistance genes are encoded on plasmids, which may cross species barriers. Since 2011, screening for ESBL as well as for other multiresistant gram-negative bacteria can be performed using a ChromID agar or equivalent systems [53, 57]. Due to the rapidly evolving epidemiology, screening has not been standardized or universally recommended yet. However, as colonization with multiresistant bacteria precedes invasive infection, screening might have an impact on the choice of empiric antimicrobial treatment for neutropenic fever.

Table 17.1 Suggested contact precautions in patients colonized or infected with multiresistant pathogens

Item	MRSA	VRE	Multiresistant gram-negatives including ESBL[a]	*C. difficile*
Daily cleaning/disinfection	Yes	Yes	Yes	Yes[c]
Single room	Yes	Yes	Yes	Own toilet
Barriers				
Gloves	Yes	Yes	Yes	Yes
Gowns	Yes	Yes	Yes	Yes
Masks	Yes	No	No	No
Screening on admission	Yes	Yes	Preferred[b]	No

[a]The effectiveness of screening depends on the local epidemiology, and this recommendation should be adapted accordingly
[b]The body of evidence is not yet sufficient to recommend routine ESBL screening
[c]Disinfection with a compound active against spores, e.g., oxygen-releasing compounds or high concentration of bleach

17.8 Special Situations

17.8.1 *Legionella* spp.

Legionella spp. has caused outbreaks in transplant units due to contaminated water tanks, showers, tap water faucets, and cooling towers [43, 56]. Sterile water has become standard of care on in transplant units. Water must be monitored and if present, water must be decontaminated according to published recommendations (http://www.legionella.org/).

17.8.2 *Clostridium difficile*

Clostridium difficile has become an increasing healthcare associated problem in most countries with the selection of hypervirulent strains, e.g., type 027 [15]. Contact precautions during acute illness are generally recommended [29, 39]. Hand disinfection with alcohol-based hand rubs is not sporicidal, which makes gloves mandatory. Hand washing may be an option, but is associated with poor compliance. Surprisingly, studies were unable to demonstrate an increase of CDAD infection after switching from hand washing to hand hygiene with an alcohol-based hand rub [10].

No routine test control in the absence of symptoms is recommended. Only with evidence of ongoing transmission of *C. difficile* contact precautions should be prolonged even after diarrhea has resolved (Table 17.1).

References

1. Anaissie EJ, Stratton SL, Dignani MC, Lee CK, Summerbell RC, Rex JH, Monson TP, Walsh TJ. Pathogenic molds (including Aspergillus species) in hospital water distribution systems: a 3-year prospective study and clinical implications for patients with hematologic malignancies. Blood. 2003;101:2542–6.
2. Anaissie EJ, Stratton SL, Dignani MC, Summerbell RC, Rex JH, Monson TP, Spencer T, Kasai M, Francesconi A, Walsh TJ. Pathogenic Aspergillus species recovered from a hospital water system: a 3-year prospective study. Clin Infect Dis. 2002;34:780–9.
3. Appelbaum FR. Hematopoietic-cell transplantation at 50. N Engl J Med. 2007;357:1472–5.
4. Balduzzi A, Lucchini G, Hirsch HH, Basso S, Cioni M, Rovelli A, Zincone A, Grimaldi M, Corti P, Bonanomi S, Biondi A, Locatelli F, Biagi E, Comoli P. Polyomavirus JC-targeted T-cell therapy for progressive multiple leukoencephalopathy in a hematopoietic cell transplantation recipient. Bone Marrow Transplant. 2011;46(7):987–92.
5. Berrouane YF, McNutt LA, Buschelman BJ, Rhomberg PR, Sanford MD, Hollis RJ, Pfaller MA, Herwaldt LA. Outbreak of severe *Pseudomonas aeruginosa* infections caused by a contaminated drain in a whirlpool bathtub. Clin Infect Dis. 2000;31:1331–7.
6. Bodey GP, Buckley M, Sathe YS, Freireich EJ. Quantitative relationships between circulating leukocytes and infection in patients with acute leukemia. Ann Intern Med. 1966;64:328–40.
7. Bolyard EA, Tablan OC, Williams WW, Pearson ML, Shapiro CN, Deitchmann SD. Guideline for infection control in healthcare personnel, 1998. Hospital Infection Control Practices Advisory Committee. Infect Control Hosp Epidemiol. 1998;19:407–63.
8. Boyce JM. Environmental contamination makes an important contribution to hospital infection. J Hosp Infect. 2007;65 Suppl 2:50–4.
9. Boyce JM, Havill NL, Otter JA, McDonald LC, Adams NM, Cooper T, Thompson A, Wiggs L, Killgore G, Tauman A, Noble-Wang J. Impact of hydrogen peroxide vapor room decontamination on *Clostridium difficile* environmental contamination and transmission in a healthcare setting. Infect Control Hosp Epidemiol. 2008;29:723–9.
10. Boyce JM, Ligi C, Kohan C, Dumigan D, Havill NL. Lack of association between the increased incidence of *Clostridium difficile*-associated disease and the increasing use of alcohol-based hand rubs. Infect Control Hosp Epidemiol. 2006;27:479–83.
11. Boyce JM, Pittet D. Guideline for hand hygiene in health-care settings. Recommendations of the Healthcare Infection Control Practices Advisory Committee and the HICPAC/SHEA/APIC/IDSA Hand Hygiene Task Force. Society for Healthcare Epidemiology of America/Association for Professionals in Infection Control/Infectious Diseases Society of America. MMWR Recomm Rep. 2002;51:1–45, quiz CE1-4.
12. Buehlmann M, Frei R, Fenner L, Dangel M, Fluckiger U, Widmer AF. Highly effective regimen for decolonization of methicillin-resistant *Staphylococcus aureus* carriers. Infect Control Hosp Epidemiol. 2008;29:510–6.
13. Buttery JP, Alabaster SJ, Heine RG, Scott SM, Crutchfield RA, Bigham A, Tabrizi SN, Garland SM. Multiresistant *Pseudomonas aeruginosa* outbreak in a pediatric oncology ward related to bath toys. Pediatr Infect Dis J. 1998;17:509–13.
14. Cantoni N, Weisser M, Buser A, Arber C, Stern M, Heim D, Halter J, Christen S, Tsakiris DA, Droll A, Frei R, Widmer AF, Fluckiger U, Passweg J, Tichelli A, Gratwohl A. Infection prevention strategies in a stem cell transplant unit: impact of change of care in isolation practice and routine use of high dose intravenous immunoglobulins on infectious complications and transplant related mortality. Eur J Haematol. 2009;83:130–8.
15. Cartman ST, Heap JT, Kuehne SA, Cockayne A, Minton NP. The emergence of 'hypervirulence' in *Clostridium difficile*. Int J Med Microbiol. 2010;300:387–95.

16. Cesaro S, Chinello P, Rossi L, Zanesco L. *Saccharomyces cerevisiae* fungemia in a neutropenic patient treated with *Saccharomyces boulardii*. Support Care Cancer. 2000;8:504–5.
17. Chaberny IF, Ruseva E, Sohr D, Buchholz S, Ganser A, Mattner F, Gastmeier P. Surveillance with successful reduction of central line-associated bloodstream infections among neutropenic patients with hematologic or oncologic malignancies. Ann Hematol. 2009;88:907–12.
18. Conen A, Zimmerer S, Trampuz A, Frei R, Battegay M, Elzi L. A pain in the neck: probiotics for ulcerative colitis. Ann Intern Med. 2009;151:895–7.
19. Cornet M, Levy V, Fleury L, Lortholary J, Barquins S, Coureul MH, Deliere E, Zittoun R, Brucker G, Bouvet A. Efficacy of prevention by high-efficiency particulate air filtration or laminar airflow against Aspergillus airborne contamination during hospital renovation. Infect Control Hosp Epidemiol. 1999;20:508–13.
20. de Kraker ME, Wolkewitz M, Davey PG, Grundmann H. The clinical impact of antimicrobial resistance in European hospitals: excess mortality and length of hospital stay related to methicillin resistant *Staphylococcus aureus* bloodstream infections. Antimicrob Agents Chemother. 2011;55(4):1598–605.
21. de Regt MJ, van der Wagen LE, Top J, Blok HE, Hopmans TE, Dekker AW, Hene RJ, Siersema PD, Willems RJ, Bonten MJ. High acquisition and environmental contamination rates of CC17 ampicillin-resistant *Enterococcus faecium* in a Dutch hospital. J Antimicrob Chemother. 2008;62:1401–6.
22. Dettenkofer M, Wenzler S, Amthor S, Antes G, Motschall E, Daschner FD. Does disinfection of environmental surfaces influence nosocomial infection rates? A systematic review. Am J Infect Control. 2004;32:84–9.
23. Diab-Elschahawi M, Furnkranz U, Blacky A, Bachhofner N, Koller W. Re-evaluation of current A0 value recommendations for thermal disinfection of reusable human waste containers based on new experimental data. J Hosp Infect. 2010;75:62–5.
24. Dietrich M, Gaus W, Vossen J, van der Waaij D, Wendt F. Protective isolation and antimicrobial decontamination in patients with high susceptibility to infection. A prospective cooperative study of gnotobiotic care in acute leukemia patients. I: clinical results. Infection. 1977;5:107–14.
25. Elting LS, Whimbey E, Lo W, Couch R, Andreeff M, Bodey GP. Epidemiology of influenza A virus infection in patients with acute or chronic leukemia. Support Care Cancer. 1995;3:198–202.
26. Engelhart S, Hanfland J, Glasmacher A, Krizek L, Schmidt-Wolf IG, Exner M. Impact of portable air filtration units on exposure of haematology-oncology patients to airborne *Aspergillus fumigatus* spores under field conditions. J Hosp Infect. 2003;54:300–4.
27. Falagas ME, Rafailidis PI, Kofteridis D, Virtzili S, Chelvatzoglou FC, Papaioannou V, Maraki S, Samonis G, Michalopoulos A. Risk factors of carbapenem-resistant *Klebsiella pneumoniae* infections: a matched case control study. J Antimicrob Chemother. 2007;60:1124–30.
28. Gardner A, Mattiuzzi G, Faderl S, Borthakur G, Garcia-Manero G, Pierce S, Brandt M, Estey E. Randomized comparison of cooked and noncooked diets in patients undergoing remission induction therapy for acute myeloid leukemia. J Clin Oncol. 2008;26:5684–8.
29. Gerding DN, Johnson S, Peterson LR, Mulligan ME, Silva Jr J. *Clostridium difficile*-associated diarrhea and colitis. Infect Control Hosp Epidemiol. 1995;16:459–77.
30. Gillies D, O'Riordan L, Carr D, Frost J, Gunning R, O'Brien I. Gauze and tape and transparent polyurethane dressings for central venous catheters. Cochrane Database Syst Rev. 2003;(4):CD003827.
31. Gratwohl A, Brand R, Frassoni F, Rocha V, Niederwieser D, Reusser P, Einsele H, Cordonnier C. Cause of death after allogeneic haematopoietic stem cell transplantation (HSCT) in early leukaemias: an EBMT analysis of lethal infectious complications and changes over calendar time. Bone Marrow Transplant. 2005;36:757–69.
32. Guidelines for preventing opportunistic infections among hematopoietic stem cell transplant recipients. MMWR Recomm Rep. 2000;49:1–125, CE1-7.
33. Gupta A, Della-Latta P, Todd B, San Gabriel P, Haas J, Wu F, Rubenstein D, Saiman L. Outbreak of extended-spectrum beta-lactamase-producing *Klebsiella pneumoniae* in a neonatal intensive care unit linked to artificial nails. Infect Control Hosp Epidemiol. 2004;25:210–5.

34. Hasman H, Mevius D, Veldman K, Olesen I, Aarestrup FM. beta-Lactamases among extended-spectrum beta-lactamase (ESBL)-resistant Salmonella from poultry, poultry products and human patients in The Netherlands. J Antimicrob Chemother. 2005;56:115–21.
35. Herrmann RP, Trent M, Cooney J, Cannell PK. Infections in patients managed at home during autologous stem cell transplantation for lymphoma and multiple myeloma. Bone Marrow Transplant. 1999;24:1213–7.
36. Hirsch HH, Knowles W, Dickenmann M, Passweg J, Klimkait T, Mihatsch MJ, Steiger J. Prospective study of polyomavirus type BK replication and nephropathy in renal-transplant recipients. N Engl J Med. 2002;347:488–96.
37. Hota B, Blom DW, Lyle EA, Weinstein RA, Hayden MK. Interventional evaluation of environmental contamination by vancomycin-resistant enterococci: failure of personnel, product, or procedure? J Hosp Infect. 2009;71:123–31.
38. Jacoby GA. AmpC beta-lactamases. Clin Microbiol Rev. 2009;22:161–82, table of contents.
39. Johnson S, Gerding DN. *Clostridium difficile* – associated diarrhea. Clin Infect Dis. 1998;26:1027–34; quiz 1035–6.
40. Kanda Y, Yamamoto R, Chizuka A, Hamaki T, Suguro M, Arai C, Matsuyama T, Takezako N, Miwa A, Kern W, Kami M, Akiyama H, Hirai H, Togawa A. Prophylactic action of oral fluconazole against fungal infection in neutropenic patients. A meta-analysis of 16 randomized, controlled trials. Cancer. 2000;89:1611–25.
41. Khanna N, Widmer AF, Decker M, Steffen I, Halter J, Heim D, Weisser M, Gratwohl A, Fluckiger U, Hirsch HH. Respiratory syncytial virus infection in patients with hematological diseases: single-center study and review of the literature. Clin Infect Dis. 2008;46:402–12.
42. Kluytmans JA. Methicillin-resistant *Staphylococcus aureus* in food products: cause for concern or case for complacency? Clin Microbiol Infect. 2010;16:11–5.
43. Kool JL, Fiore AE, Kioski CM, Brown EW, Benson RF, Pruckler JM, Glasby C, Butler JC, Cage GD, Carpenter JC, Mandel RM, England B, Breiman RF. More than 10 years of unrecognized nosocomial transmission of legionnaires' disease among transplant patients. Infect Control Hosp Epidemiol. 1998;19:898–904.
44. Loeb M, Dafoe N, Mahony J, John M, Sarabia A, Glavin V, Webby R, Smieja M, Earn DJ, Chong S, Webb A, Walter SD. Surgical mask vs N95 respirator for preventing influenza among health care workers: a randomized trial. JAMA. 2009;302:1865–71.
45. Maki DG, Stolz SM, Wheeler S, Mermel LA. Prevention of central venous catheter-related bloodstream infection by use of an antiseptic-impregnated catheter. A randomized, controlled trial. Ann Intern Med. 1997;127:257–66.
46. Manoloff ES, Francioli P, Taffe P, Van Melle G, Bille J, Hauser PM. Risk for Pneumocystis carinii transmission among patients with pneumonia: a molecular epidemiology study. Emerg Infect Dis. 2003;9:132–4.
47. Maschmeyer G, Neuburger S, Fritz L, Bohme A, Penack O, Schwerdtfeger R, Buchheidt D, Ludwig WD. A prospective, randomised study on the use of well-fitting masks for prevention of invasive aspergillosis in high-risk patients. Ann Oncol. 2009;20:1560–4.
48. Mertz D, Frei R, Periat N, Zimmerli M, Battegay M, Fluckiger U, Widmer AF. Exclusive *Staphylococcus aureus* throat carriage: at-risk populations. Arch Intern Med. 2009;169:172–8.
49. Moreno A, Cervera C, Gavalda J, Rovira M, de la Camara R, Jarque I, Montejo M, de la Torre-Cisneros J, Miguel Cisneros J, Fortun J, Lopez-Medrano F, Gurgui M, Munoz P, Ramos A, Carratala J. Bloodstream infections among transplant recipients: results of a nationwide surveillance in Spain. Am J Transplant. 2007;7:2579–86.
50. Muto CA, Jernigan JA, Ostrowsky BE, Richet HM, Jarvis WR, Boyce JM, Farr BM. SHEA guideline for preventing nosocomial transmission of multidrug-resistant strains of *Staphylococcus aureus* and enterococcus. Infect Control Hosp Epidemiol. 2003;24:362–86.
51. Nauseef WM, Maki DG. A study of the value of simple protective isolation in patients with granulocytopenia. N Engl J Med. 1981;304:448–53.

52. Nihtinen A, Anttila VJ, Richardson M, Meri T, Volin L, Ruutu T. The utility of intensified environmental surveillance for pathogenic moulds in a stem cell transplantation ward during construction work to monitor the efficacy of HEPA filtration. Bone Marrow Transplant. 2007;40:457–60.
53. Nordmann P, Poirel L, Carrer A, Toleman MA, Walsh TR. How to detect NDM-1 producers. J Clin Microbiol. 2011;49:718–21.
54. O'Grady NP, Alexander M, Dellinger EP, Gerberding JL, Heard SO, Maki DG, Masur H, McCormick RD, Mermel LA, Pearson ML, Raad II, Randolph A, Weinstein RA. Guidelines for the prevention of intravascular catheter-related infections. Centers for disease control and prevention. MMWR Recomm Rep. 2002;51:1–29.
55. Opal SM, Asp AA, Cannady Jr PB, Morse PL, Burton LJ, Hammer 2nd PG. Efficacy of infection control measures during a nosocomial outbreak of disseminated aspergillosis associated with hospital construction. J Infect Dis. 1986;153:634–7.
56. Oren I, Zuckerman T, Avivi I, Finkelstein R, Yigla M, Rowe JM. Nosocomial outbreak of Legionella pneumophila serogroup 3 pneumonia in a new bone marrow transplant unit: evaluation, treatment and control. Bone Marrow Transplant. 2002;30:175–9.
57. Overdevest IT, Willemsen I, Elberts S, Verhulst C, Kluytmans JA. Laboratory detection of extended-spectrum-beta-lactamase-producing Enterobacteriaceae: evaluation of two screening agar plates and two confirmation techniques. J Clin Microbiol. 2011;49:519–22.
58. Petersen F, Thornquist M, Buckner C, Counts G, Nelson N, Meyers J, Clift R, Thomas E. The effects of infection prevention regimens on early infectious complications in marrow transplant patients: a four arm randomized study. Infection. 1988;16:199–208.
59. Pronovost P, Needham D, Berenholtz S, Sinopoli D, Chu H, Cosgrove S, Sexton B, Hyzy R, Welsh R, Roth G, Bander J, Kepros J, Goeschel C. An intervention to decrease catheter-related bloodstream infections in the ICU. N Engl J Med. 2006;355:2725–32.
60. Recommendations for preventing the spread of vancomycin resistance. Recommendations of the Hospital Infection Control Practices Advisory Committee (HICPAC). MMWR Recomm Rep. 1995;44:1–13.
61. Robicsek A, Beaumont JL, Paule SM, Hacek DM, Thomson Jr RB, Kaul KL, King P, Peterson LR. Universal surveillance for methicillin-resistant in 3 affiliated hospitals. Ann Intern Med. 2008;148:409–18.
62. Rutala WA. APIC guideline for selection and use of disinfectants. 1994, 1995, and 1996 APIC Guidelines Committee. Association for Professionals in Infection Control and Epidemiology, Inc. Am J Infect Control. 1996;24:313–42.
63. Sehulster L, Chinn RY. Guidelines for environmental infection control in health-care facilities. Recommendations of CDC and the Healthcare Infection Control Practices Advisory Committee (HICPAC). MMWR Recomm Rep. 2003;52:1–42.
64. Siegel JD, Rhinehart E, Jackson M, Chiarello L. 2007 Guideline for isolation precautions: preventing transmission of infectious agents in health care settings. Am J Infect Control. 2007;35:S65–164.
65. Skopinska E. Some effects of *Escherichia coli* endotoxin on the graft-versus-host reaction in mice. Transplantation. 1972;14:432–7.
66. Stevens DA, Lee JY. Analysis of compassionate use itraconazole therapy for invasive aspergillosis by the NIAID Mycoses Study Group criteria. Arch Intern Med. 1997;157:1857–62.
67. Svahn BM, Bjurman B, Myrback KE, Aschan J, Ringden O. Is it safe to treat allogeneic stem cell transplant recipients at home during the pancytopenic phase? A pilot trial. Bone Marrow Transplant. 2000;26:1057–60.
68. Svahn BM, Remberger M, Myrback KE, Holmberg K, Eriksson B, Hentschke P, Aschan J, Barkholt L, Ringden O. Home care during the pancytopenic phase after allogeneic hematopoietic stem cell transplantation is advantageous compared with hospital care. Blood. 2002;100:4317–24.
69. Tablan OC, Anderson LJ, Besser R, Bridges C, Hajjeh R. Guidelines for preventing health-care–associated pneumonia, 2003: recommendations of CDC and the Healthcare Infection Control Practices Advisory Committee. MMWR Recomm Rep. 2004;53:1–36.

70. Tietz A, Frei R, Dangel M, Bolliger D, Passweg JR, Gratwohl A, Widmer AE. Octenidine hydrochloride for the care of central venous catheter insertion sites in severely immunocompromised patients. Infect Control Hosp Epidemiol. 2005;26:703–7.
71. Tomblyn M, Chiller T, Einsele H, Gress R, Sepkowitz K, Storek J, Wingard JR, Young JA, Boeckh MJ. Guidelines for preventing infectious complications among hematopoietic cell transplantation recipients: a global perspective. Biol Blood Marrow Transplant. 2009;15:1143–238.
72. Tschudin Sutter S, Frei R, Dangel M, Gratwohl A, Bonten M, Widmer AF. Not all patients with vancomycin-resistant enterococci need to be isolated. Clin Infect Dis. 2010;51:678–83.
73. Tschudin-Sutter S, Pargger H, Widmer AF. Hand hygiene in the intensive care unit. Crit Care Med. 2010;38:S299–305.
74. Vonberg RP, Gastmeier P. Nosocomial aspergillosis in outbreak settings. J Hosp Infect. 2006;63:246–54.
75. Wassenberg MW, Kluytmans JA, Box AT, Bosboom RW, Buiting AG, Van Elzakker EP, Melchers WJ, Van Rijen MM, Thijsen SF, Troelstra A, Vandenbroucke-Grauls CM, Visser CE, Voss A, Wolffs PF, Wulf MW, Van Zwet AA, De Wit GA, Bonten MJ. Rapid screening of methicillin-resistant *Staphylococcus aureus* using PCR and chromogenic agar: a prospective study to evaluate costs and effects. Clin Microbiol Infect. 2010;16:1754–61.
76. Widmer AF. Replace hand washing with use of a waterless alcohol hand rub? Clin Infect Dis. 2000;31:136–43.
77. Widmer AF, Frei R. Decontamination, disinfection, sterilization. In: Baron EJ, Murray PR, Pfaller M, Tenover FC, Yolken R, editors. Manual of clinical microbiology. Washington: ASM Press; 2011. p. 138–64.

Myeloid Growth Factors

18

Hartmut Link

Contents

Many cytotoxic substances impair the function of leukocytes and their production from pluripotent and determined hematopoietic stem cells in the bone marrow. Frequent sequelae of cytostatic chemotherapy therefore are anemia, thrombocytopenia, leukocytopenia, and especially neutropenia, which is a significant risk factor for morbidity and mortality associated with infections. Neutropenia is one of the most severe toxicities of chemotherapy, significantly increasing the risk of infection [2, 10, 33]. As the most important dose-limiting toxicity, neutropenia can compromise the success of tumor therapy.

Hematopoietic myeloid growth factors such as G-CSF (granulocyte-colony stimulating factor) or GM-CSF (granulocyte macrophage-colony stimulating factor) stimulate the generation of neutrophils. G-CSF and GM-CSF are increasingly

H. Link
Department Internal Medicine, Hematology and Oncology, Westpfalz-Klinikum, Kaiserslautern, Germany
e-mail: hlink@westpfalz-klinikum.de

G. Maschmeyer, K.V.I. Rolston (eds.), *Infections in Hematology*,
DOI 10.1007/978-3-662-44000-1_18

produced by T cells, macrophages, and monocytes if the neutrophil counts are decreasing to stimulation proliferation and differentiation of determined progenitor cells. They are termed "myeloid" growth factors.

In the 1980s G-CSF was described, biochemically characterized, its gene cloned and developed as recombinant molecule for clinical application [35, 36]. The majority of trials have been performed with G-CSF.

The prophylactic use of recombinant G-CSF (filgrastim, pegfilgrastim, lenograstim) or GM-CSF preparations (molgramostim, sagramostim) after myelosuppressive chemotherapy accelerates the regeneration of granulocytes to protective levels [11, 33, 35].

After autologous bone marrow or stem cell transplantation, G-CSF of GM-CSF accelerates the regeneration of granulopoiesis [13, 22, 31, 33]. Use of G-CSF is associated with faster neutrophil engraftment and shorter length of posttransplant hospital stay without affecting time to platelet engraftment in patients undergoing autologous transplantation. Following allogeneic stem cell transplantation, G-CSF reduces the time to neutrophil recovery, but has no influence on day 30 or day 100 transplant-related mortality. G-CSF did neither affect graft versus host disease nor leukemia-free survival [17].

Duration and severity of neutropenia as well as infection-associated risks can significantly be reduced by prophylaxis with myeloid hematopoietic growth factors. In many cases, a hazardous neutropenia can be prevented completely [1, 19, 33].

18.1 Incidence and Risks of Febrile Neutropenia

Febrile neutropenia (FN) is the most important sign of infection in neutropenic patients. FN is defined as increased oral temperature (≥38 °C) and concomitant decreased granulocyte concentration <500/μ or <1,000/μl, if a decrease of <500/μl within 48 h is anticipated [8, 21].

Fever during neutropenia is caused by an infection in more than 95 % of cases; however, in 50–70 % of patients, no infectious organisms can be detected [16, 21, 23, 29].

In cancer patients, infections are the most frequent therapy-associated causes of death. The risk of febrile neutropenia and of life-threatening infections correlates with the severity and duration of neutropenia [2]. The mortality by neutropenia-associated infections caused by chemotherapy accounts for 2.8 % and is 5.7 % during the early neutropenic phase [15, 18, 19, 23].

A multivariate analysis of 41,779 patients with different cancers and FN showed the following risk factors for a lethal outcome:

Gram-negative sepsis (relative risk: 4.92), invasive aspergillosis 3.48, invasive candidiasis 2.55, pulmonary disease 3.94, cerebrovascular disease 3.26, renal disease 3.16, liver disease 2.89, pneumonia 2.23, gram-positive sepsis 2.29, hypotension 2.12, pulmonary embolism 1.94, heart disease 1.58, leukemia 1.48, lung cancer 1.18, and age ≥65 years 1.12 [18]. An increasing number of concomitant diseases increase mortality [5, 18].

18.2 Relative Dose Intensity of Chemotherapy

Relative dose intensity (RDI) is the proportion of planned dose intensity per planned time interval. With the exception of hematopoietic stem cell transplantation, many therapy protocols achieve the planned relative dose intensity only, if neutropenia and febrile neutropenia are avoided or at least clinically acceptable [33]. This is especially true for dose dense protocols with short intervals between cycles and increased dose intensities, for example, in Hodgkin lymphoma [14], aggressive non-Hodgkin lymphoma [27, 28, 30], and breast cancer [25].

18.3 Reduction of Relative Dose Intensity of Chemotherapy

It is a common strategy reducing dose of chemotherapy in subsequent cycles or prolonging planned intervals, if severe or febrile neutropenia occurred.

Randomized clinical trials showed a relative dose intensity (RDI) of 71.0–95.0 %, with a mean RDI of 86.7 % (median RDI, 88.5 %). Among G-CSF-treated patients, the average RDI ranged from 91.0 to 99.0 %, with a mean RDI of 95.1 % (median RDI, 95.5 %). RDI differences between study arms ranged from 2.8 to 20.0 %, with average differences of 8.4 % ($P=0.001$) [19].

In some tumors, it is shown that reducing the RDI can impair or question the success of chemotherapy. This has been shown in adjuvant chemotherapy with breast cancer [3, 4, 25, 37], in diffuse large cell non-Hodgkin lymphoma [20].

18.4 Risk Factors for Febrile Neutropenia

The most important factors for febrile neutropenia (FN) following chemotherapy are the type of chemotherapy and its dose intensity. Without G-CSF or GM-CSF, the risk of FN is constant for all chemotherapy cycles [6, 9]. However, it is greater following the first cycle only, if growth factors are given for subsequent cycles [12].

If neutropenic complications occur, then the risk of febrile neutropenia remains high for further chemotherapy cycles.

Combination chemotherapy protocols increase the risk of FN compared to monotherapies, as well as drugs toxic to bone marrow or mucous membranes. Significant predictors for severe or febrile neutropenias are high-dose cyclophosphamide or etoposide in the treatment of malignant lymphoma as well as high-dose anthracyclines in early breast cancer [8].

According to various guidelines, the intensity of the chemotherapy protocol correlates directly with the risk of FN. An overview on frequently used protocols is given in Table 18.1, with the risk of FN: high risk ≥20 %, intermediate risk 10–20 %, or low risk <10 %.

Besides the type of chemotherapy, there are patient- and tumor-specific factors influencing the risk of febrile neutropenia (Table 18.2).

Table 18.1 Examples of frequently used chemotherapy protocols with the risk of FN: high risk ≥20 %, intermediate risk 10–20 %, or low risk <10 %

Tumor	FN-Risk (%)	Regimen
Breast cancer	>20	AC docetaxel, doxorubicin/docetaxel, doxorubicin/paclitaxel, TAC
	10–20	AC, EC, docetaxel, FE120C (q4 weeks), CEF
	<10	CMF
Colon cancer	10–20	5-FU/folinic acid
		FOLFIRI (5-FU/folinic acid/irinotecan)
	<10	FOLFOX (5-FU/folinic acid/oxaliplatin)
Hodgkin lymphoma	>20	BEACOPP: bleomycin, etoposide, doxorubicin, cyclophosphamide, vincristine, procarbazine, prednisone
Melanoma	>20	Dacarbazine-based combinations
Non-small cell lung cancer	>20	Docetaxel/carboplatin, etoposide/cisplatin
	10–20	Paclitaxel/cisplatin, docetaxel/cisplatin, vinorelbine/cisplatin
	<10	Paclitaxel/carboplatin, gemcitabine/cisplatin
Non-Hodgkin lymphoma	>20	CHOP (cyclophosphamide/doxorubicin/vincristine/prednisone)
		DHAP (cisplatin, HD-AraC, dexamethasone)
		ESHAP (etoposide, methylprednisolone, cisplatin, cytarabine)
		R-CHOP (rituximab-CHOP)
Ovarian carcinoma	>20	Docetaxel, paclitaxel
	10–20	Topotecan
	<10	Paclitaxel/carboplatin
Small cell lung cancer	>20	ACE, ICE, topotecan
	10–20	Etoposid/carboplatin, topotecan/cisplatin
	<10	Paclitaxel/carboplatin

EORTC guidelines 2006 [1], ASCO guidelines 2006 [33], and NCCN [8]. Refer to guidelines or original publications for incidences of febrile neutropenia, if other protocols are considered
All figures of febrile neutropenia are derived from the original publications and are related to the dosages of the applied chemotherapy protocols
A doxorubicin, *C* cyclophosphamide, *E* etoposide, *F* 5-fluorouracil, *I* ifosfamide, *M* methotrexate, *T* docetaxel

A review of the literature showed that higher age, especially ≥65 years, consistently correlates with a higher risk of febrile neutropenia among the independent patient-specific risk factors [1]. Higher age is an important risk factor as older patients often receive lower or even too low chemotherapy doses in fear of neutropenic complications, although those patients would benefit from an adequate dosed treatment regimen as younger patients [8].

Further independent factors with a high evidence are advanced disease, previous episodes of FN, or missing prophylaxis with G-CSF or antibiotics [1].

Many other patient- or tumor-related factors for FN are known with a lower level of evidence by retrospective analyses such as reduced general condition, impaired nutritional status, or comorbidity.

Patients with malignant diseases of hematopoiesis or lymphopoiesis have an increased risk by the disease itself and the intensity of the treatment than patients with solid tumors.

Table 18.2 Risk factors of febrile neutropenia according National Comprehensive Cancer Network, NCCN 2010) [8] EORTC [1] and ASCO [33]

Chemotherapy-related factors
Type of chemotherapy
Severe neutropenia with previous comparable chemotherapy
>80 % of planned relative dose intensity
Previous neutropenia (<1,000/μl) or lymphocytopenia
Previous extensive chemotherapy
Concomitant or previous radiotherapy with involvement of bone marrow
Therapy with anthracyclines
Mucositis of the whole gastrointestinal tract
Patient risk factors
Age 65 years or older
Female gender
Poor performance status (ECOG ≥2 "Eastern Cooperative Oncology Group")
Poor nutritional status
Impaired immune function
Tumor risk factors
Cytopenias due to tumor bone marrow involvement
Advanced or uncontrolled tumor
Elevated lactate dehydrogenase (LDH) in lymphoma
Leukemia
Lymphoma
Lung carcinoma
Factors with increased risk for infections
Open wounds
Active infection
Comorbidity
Chronic obstructive lung disease
Cardiovascular disorder
Liver disease (elevated bilirubin, alkaline phosphatase)
Diabetes mellitus
Decreased hemoglobin level at diagnosis

If patients older than 70 years are analyzed, then it could be shown that age alone is not a risk factor for severe or febrile neutropenia, but the type of malignancy, a planned dose intensity ≥85 %, therapy with cis-platinum or anthracyclines, previous chemotherapy, increased urea, and increased alkaline phosphatase [32].

18.5 Indication for Prophylaxis of Febrile Neutropenia with Myeloid Growth Factors According to Guidelines

Most evidence regarding the clinical effects of myeloid growth factors is derived from studies with G-CSF.

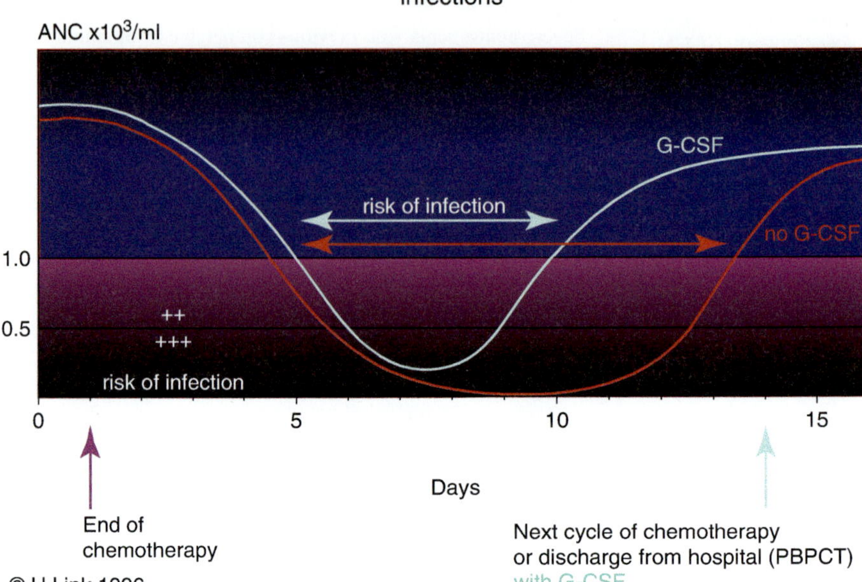

Fig. 18.1 Correlation between incidence of infections including febrile neutropenia and neutrophil recovery

The principle of reducing neutropenia with myeloid growth factors is shown in Fig. 18.1. Neutropenia can be shortened mainly by an accelerated recovery of neutrophils.

The primary prophylaxis with G-CSF halves the incidence of febrile neutropenia (FN) due to chemotherapy with a risk of FN of 40 % [11, 24, 26, 34].

Primary G-CSF prophylaxis to support patients receiving cancer chemotherapy is recommended for all patients judged to be at ≥20 % risk of FN [1, 8, 33].

If using a chemotherapy regimen associated with 10–20 % FN risk, G-CSF prophylaxis should be considered based on treatment intention and individual patient risk factors. The patient's FN risk should be reassessed prior to each cycle of chemotherapy. This is particularly important for chemotherapy regimens with 10–20 % FN risk, as patient-related risk factors may vary throughout chemotherapy cycles, and thus their FN risk could increase throughout the treatment course.

For patients at <10 % FN risk, routine G-CSF prophylaxis is not recommended.

Figure 18.2 shows the algorithm for deciding to use G-CSF after chemotherapy.

18.6 Therapeutic Use of G-CSF or GM-CSF

The aim of therapeutic use of myeloid growth factors is the reduction of morbidity and mortality due to infections including febrile neutropenia.

EORTC and ASCO G-CSF Guideline-Based FN Risk Assessment

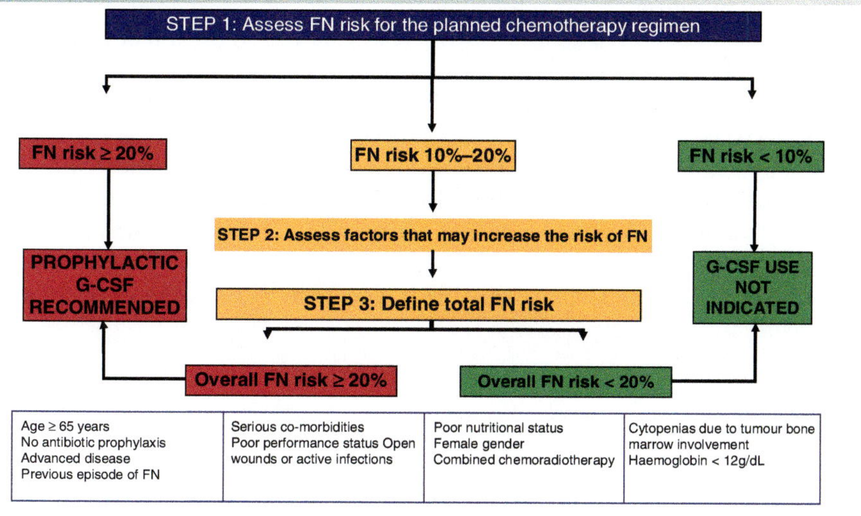

Fig. 18.2 This algorithm is a combined interpretation of the 2006 G-CSF guidelines of European Organisation for Research and Treatment of Cancer (*EORTC*) and American Society of Clinical Oncology (*ASCO*) [1, 33]. All of these organizations recommend that the physician should use their clinical judgment to assess FN risk as greater or less than 20 % according to the estimated risk of expected neutropenic complications, based on the treatment regimen and patient-specific characteristics, including age ≥65 years and experience of FN in a previous chemotherapy cycle

There is less evidence supporting therapeutic use of G- or GM-CSF in addition to antibiotics. However, a meta-analysis showed a shorter hospital stay and shorter time to neutrophil recovery, but no influence on mortality [7].

Myeloid growth factors could be given for patients with risk factors of poor clinical outcome or infection-related complications such as old age (≥65 years), sepsis syndrome, severe neutropenia (absolute neutrophil count <100 μl), or anticipated prolonged (>10 days) neutropenia, pneumonia, invasive fungal infections, or other clinically documented infections, hospitalization, and prior episodes of FN. If risk factors are present, G- or GM-CSF should be considered [8].

Patients under prophylaxis with G-CSF suffering from febrile neutropenia should continue with this treatment.

18.7 Dosing and Administration

Available growth factors are the G-CSFs filgrastim, pegfilgrastim, and lenograstim and the GM-CSFs sargramostim and molgramostim.

18.7.1 G-CSF

G-CSF should be given 24–72 h following the last dose of chemotherapy and continued until the recovery of neutrophils for 3 days above 500 cells/μl or until reaching an ANC of at least 2,000–3,000/μl.

Filgrastim is given subcutaneously (s.c.) at a dose of 5 μg/kg per day and lenograstim at 150 μg/m^2 per day.

The long acting pegylated G-CSF (pegfilgrastim) is given s.c. once 24 h after completion of chemotherapy. Pegfilgrastim 6 mg is given once in each chemotherapy cycle. The 6 mg formulation should not be used in infants, children, or small adolescents weighing <45 kg.

The same day administration of G-CSF within 24 h of chemotherapy is not recommended [8].

18.7.2 GM-CSF

The GM-CSF sargramostim (glycosylated) is indicated for use following chemotherapy in patients with acute myeloid leukemia and for use after autologous or allogeneic bone marrow transplantation. The manufacturer's instructions for administration are limited to those clinical settings. GM-CSF should be initiated on the day of bone marrow infusion and not less than 24 h from the last chemotherapy and 12 h from the most recent radiotherapy. GM-CSF should be continued until an ANC greater than 1,500 cells/μl for 3 consecutive days is obtained. The drug should be discontinued early or the dose be reduced by 50 % if the ANC increases to greater than 20,000 μl. The recommended doses are 250 μg/m2/day for GM-CSF for all clinical settings, given subcutaneously.

The GM-CSF molgramostim (non-glycosylated) is indicated in patients receiving myelosuppressive therapy (cancer chemotherapy) to reduce the severity of neutropenia, thereby reducing the risk of infection and allowing better adherence to the chemotherapeutic regimen, and in patients undergoing autologous or syngeneic bone marrow transplantation to accelerate myeloid recovery.

The recommended dosage regimens are as follows:

Cancer chemotherapy: 5–10 μg/kg per day administered subcutaneously. Treatment should be initiated 24 h after the last dose of chemotherapy and continued for 7–10 days. Dosing may be initiated at 5 μg/kg a day.

Bone marrow transplantation (BMT): 10 μg/kg per day administered by i.v. infusion over 4–6 h, beginning the day after BMT and being continued until the absolute neutrophil count (ANC) is ≥1,000/μl.

The maximum duration of treatment is 30 days.

References

1. Aapro MS, Cameron DA, et al. EORTC guidelines for the use of granulocyte-colony stimulating factor to reduce the incidence of chemotherapy-induced febrile neutropenia in adult patients with lymphomas and solid tumours. Eur J Cancer. 2006;42:2433–53.

2. Bodey GP, Buckley M, Sathe YS, et al. Quantitative relationships between circulating leukocytes and infection in patients with acute leukemia. Ann Intern Med. 1966;64:328–40.
3. Bonadonna G, Valagussa P, Moliterni A, et al. Adjuvant cyclophosphamide, methotrexate, and fluorouracil in node-positive breast cancer: the results of 20 years of follow-up. N Engl J Med. 1995;332:901–6.
4. Budman DR, Berry DA, Cirrincione CT, et al. Dose and dose intensity as determinants of outcome in the adjuvant treatment of breast cancer. The Cancer and Leukemia Group B. J Natl Cancer Inst. 1998;90:1205–11.
5. Caggiano V, Weiss RV, Rickert TS, et al. Incidence, cost, and mortality of neutropenia hospitalization associated with chemotherapy. Cancer. 2005;103:1916–24.
6. Chouaid C, Bassinet L, Fuhrman C, et al. Routine use of granulocyte colony-stimulating factor is not cost-effective and does not increase patient comfort in the treatment of small-cell lung cancer: an analysis using a Markov model. J Clin Oncol. 1998;16:2700–7.
7. Clark OA, Lyman GH, Castro AA, et al. Colony-stimulating factors for chemotherapy-induced febrile neutropenia: a meta-analysis of randomized controlled trials. J Clin Oncol. 2005;23:4198–214.
8. Crawford J. NCCN® Practice Guidelines in Oncology – v.1.2010; myeloid growth factors. NCCN, editor. National Comprehensive Cancer Network; 2010.
9. Crawford J, Althaus B, Armitage J, et al. Myeloid growth factors clinical practice guidelines in oncology. J Natl Compr Canc Netw. 2005;3:540–55.
10. Crawford J, Dale DC, Lyman GH. Chemotherapy-induced neutropenia: risks, consequences, and new directions for its management. Cancer. 2004;100:228–37.
11. Crawford J, Ozer H, Stoller R, et al. Reduction by granulocyte colony-stimulating factor of fever and neutropenia induced by chemotherapy in patients with small-cell lung cancer. N Eng J Med. 1991;325(3):164–70.
12. Crawford J, Wolff DA, Culakova E, et al. First cycle risk of severe and febrile neutropenia in cancer patients receiving systemic chemotherapy: results from a prospective nationwide study. ASH Ann Meet Abstr. 2004;104:2210.
13. Dekker A, Bulley S, Beyene J, et al. Meta-analysis of randomized controlled trials of prophylactic granulocyte colony-stimulating factor and granulocyte-macrophage colony-stimulating factor after autologous and allogeneic stem cell transplantation. J Clin Oncol. 2006;24:5207–15.
14. Diehl V, Franklin J, Pfreundschuh M, et al. Standard and increased-dose BEACOPP chemotherapy compared with COPP-ABVD for advanced Hodgkin's disease. N Engl J Med. 2003;348:2386.
15. Elting LS, Rubenstein EB, Rolston KV, et al. Outcomes of bacteremia in patients with cancer and neutropenia: observations from two decades of epidemiological and clinical trials. Clin Infect Dis. 1997;25:247–59.
16. Hughes WT, Armstrong D, Bodey GP, et al. 2002 guidelines for the use of antimicrobial agents in neutropenic patients with cancer. Clin Infect Dis. 2002;34:730–51.
17. Khoury HJ, Loberiza Jr FR, Ringden O, et al. Impact of posttransplantation G-CSF on outcomes of allogeneic hematopoietic stem cell transplantation. Blood. 2006;107:1712–6.
18. Kuderer NM, Dale DC, Crawford J, et al. Mortality, morbidity, and cost associated with febrile neutropenia in adult cancer patients. Cancer. 2006;106:2258–66.
19. Kuderer NM, Dale DC, Crawford J, et al. Impact of primary prophylaxis with granulocyte colony-stimulating factor on febrile neutropenia and mortality in adult cancer patients receiving chemotherapy: a systematic review. J Clin Oncol. 2007;25:3158–67.
20. Kwak LW, Halpern J, Olshen RA, et al. Prognostic significance of actual dose intensity in diffuse large-cell lymphoma: results of a tree-structured survival analysis. J Clin Oncol. 1990;8:963–77.
21. Link H, Bohme A, Cornely OA, et al. Antimicrobial therapy of unexplained fever in neutropenic patients–guidelines of the Infectious Diseases Working Party (AGIHO) of the German Society of Hematology and Oncology (DGHO), Study Group Interventional Therapy of Unexplained Fever, Arbeitsgemeinschaft Supportivmassnahmen in der Onkologie (ASO) of the Deutsche Krebsgesellschaft (DKG-German Cancer Society). Ann Hematol. 2003;82 Suppl 2:S105–17.
22. Link H, Boogaerts MA, Carella AM, et al. A controlled trial of recombinant human granulocyte-macrophage colony stimulating factor after total body irradiation, high dose chemotherapy and

autologous bone marrow transplantation for acute lymphoblastic leukemia or malignant lymphoma. Blood. 1992;80:2188–95.
23. Link H, Maschmeyer G, Meyer P, et al. Interventional antimicrobial therapy in febrile neutropenic patients. Ann Hematol. 1994;69:231–43.
24. Lyman GH, Kuderer NM, Djulbegovic B. Prophylactic granulocyte colony-stimulating factor in patients receiving dose-intensive cancer chemotherapy: a meta-analysis. Am J Med. 2002;112:406–11.
25. Moebus V, Jackisch C, Lueck HJ, et al. Intense dose-dense sequential chemotherapy with epirubicin, paclitaxel, and cyclophosphamide compared with conventionally scheduled chemotherapy in high-risk primary breast cancer: mature results of an AGO phase III study. J Clin Oncol. 2010;28(17):2874–80.
26. Pettengell R, Gurney H, Radford JA, et al. Granulocyte colony-stimulating factor to prevent dose-limiting neutropenia in non-Hodgkin's lymphoma: a randomized controlled trial. Blood. 1992;80:1430–6.
27. Pfreundschuh M, Trumper L, Kloess M, et al. Two-weekly or 3-weekly CHOP chemotherapy with or without etoposide for the treatment of elderly patients with aggressive lymphomas: results of the NHL-B2 trial of the DSHNHL. Blood. 2004;104:634–41.
28. Pfreundschuh M, Trumper L, Kloess M, et al. Two-weekly or 3-weekly CHOP chemotherapy with or without etoposide for the treatment of young patients with good-prognosis (normal LDH) aggressive lymphomas: results of the NHL-B1 trial of the DSHNHL. Blood. 2004;104:626–33.
29. Schiel X, Link H, Maschmeyer G, et al. A prospective, randomized multicenter trial of the empirical addition of antifungal therapy for febrile neutropenic cancer patients: results of the Paul Ehrlich society for chemotherapy (PEG) multicenter trial II. Infection. 2006;34:118–26.
30. Schmitz N, Kloess M, Reiser M, et al. Four versus six courses of a dose-escalated cyclophosphamide, doxorubicin, vincristine, and prednisone (CHOP) regimen plus etoposide (mega-CHOEP) and autologous stem cell transplantation: early dose intensity is crucial in treating younger patients with poor prognosis aggressive lymphoma. Cancer. 2006;106:136–45.
31. Schmitz N, Linch DC, Dreger P, et al. Randomised trial of filgrastim-mobilised peripheral blood progenitor cell transplantation versus autologous bone-marrow transplantation in lymphoma patients. Lancet. 1996;347:353–7.
32. Shayne M, Culakova E, Poniewierski MS, et al. Dose intensity and hematologic toxicity in older cancer patients receiving systemic chemotherapy. Cancer. 2007 [Epub ahead of print].
33. Smith TJ, Khatcheressian J, Lyman GH, et al. 2006 update of recommendations for the Use of white blood cell growth factors: an evidence-based clinical practice guideline. J Clin Oncol. 2006;24:3187–205.
34. Trillet-Lenoir V, Green J, Manegold C, et al. Recombinant granulocyte colony stimulating factor reduces the infectious complications of cytotoxic chemotherapy. Eur J Cancer. 1993;29A:319–24.
35. Welte K, Gabrilove J, Bronchud MH, et al. Filgrastim (r-metHuG-CSF): the first 10 years. Blood. 1996;88:1907–29.
36. Welte K, Platzer E, Lu L, et al. Purification and biochemical characterization of human pluripotent hematopoietic colony-stimulating factor. Proc Natl Acad Sci. 1985;82:1526–30.
37. Wood WC, Budman DR, Korzun AH, et al. Dose and dose intensity of adjuvant chemotherapy for stage II, node-positive breast carcinoma. N Engl J Med. 1994;330:1253–9.

Index

G. Maschmeyer, K.V.I. Rolston (eds.), *Infections in Hematology*,
DOI 10.1007/978-3-662-44000-1